Psychiatric Intensive Care

Second edition

Edited by

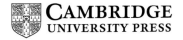

M. Dominic Beer

Oxleas NHS Foundation Trust
University of London

Stephen M. Pereira

Goodmayes Hospital, Essex
University of London

Carol Paton

Oxleas NHS Foundation Trust
Imperial College, London

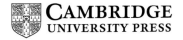

CAMBRIDGE
UNIVERSITY PRESS

CAMBRIDGE UNIVERSITY PRESS
Cambridge, New York, Melbourne, Madrid, Cape Town, Singapore, São Paulo, Delhi

Cambridge University Press
The Edinburgh Building, Cambridge CB2 8RU, UK

Published in the United States of America by Cambridge University Press, New York

www.cambridge.org
Information on this title: www.cambridge.org/9780521709262

First published 2008

Printed in the United Kingdom at the University Press, Cambridge

A catalogue record for this publication is available from the British Library

ISBN 978-0-521-70926-2 paperback

Contents

Contributors

James Anderson
MRCPsych MRCP
Consultant Forensic Psychiatrist
Oxleas NHS Foundation Trust
The Bracton Centre
Dartford
Kent, UK

Zerrin Atakan
FRCPsych
Lead Consultant psychiatrist/Hon Senior Lecturer
National Psychosis Unit
Maudsley and Bethlem Royal Hospitals
Denmark Hill
London, UK

M. Dominic Beer
MD FRCPsych MA (Oxon)
Consultant Psychiatrist in Challenging Behaviour
and Intensive Care Psychiatry (Oxleas NHS
Foundation Trust) and Honorary Senior Lecturer,
Division of Psychological Medicine (Institute of
Psychiatry, University of London)
The Bracton Centre
Dartford
Kent, UK

Christian Betteridge
RMN
Greyfriars Psychiatric Intensive Care Unit
Severn NHS Trust
Wotton Lawn
Gloucester, UK

David Buckle
Approved Social Worker
Montpellier Unit
Severn NHS Trust
Wotton Lawn
Gloucester, UK

Navjyoat Chhina
Specialist Registrar MRCPsych
Kimble PICU
Haleacre Unit
Oxfordshire & Buckinghamshire Mental Health
  Partnership NHS Trust
Amersham Hospital
Amersham
Bucks, UK

Roland Dix
RMN
Consultant Nurse in Psychiatric Intensive Care and
  Secure Rehabilitation
Visiting Research Fellow in the University of the
  West of England
Executive Committee Member NAPICU
Editor in Chief, Journal of Psychiatric Intensive Care
Wotton Lawn
Horton Road
Gloucester, UK

Venugopal Duddu
MRCPsych
Consultant Psychiatrist
Avondale Unit
Royal Preston Hospital
Preston, UK

Stephen Dye
MBBS MRCPsych
Consultant Psychiatrist
Kimble PICU
Haleacre Unit
Oxfordshire & Buckinghamshire Mental Health
  Partnership NHS Trust
Amersham Hospital
Amersham
Bucks, UK

Brenda Flood
MSc Dip NZ OT SROT
Lecturer
Department of Occupational Therapy
Auckland University of Technology
Auckland, New Zealand

Andrew Flynn
MRCPsych
Consultant Psychiatrist
Oxleas NHS Foundation Trust
Bexley Learning Disabilities Team
Stuart House
Sidcup
Kent, UK

Phil Garnham
RMN Dip in Counselling, MA in Counselling and
  Psychotherapy
Head of Nurse Education and Clinical
  Effectiveness
Oxleas NHS Foundation Trust
Dartford
Kent, UK

Harvey Gordon
MRCPsych
Consultant Forensic Psychiatrist, Oxfordshire and
  Buckinghamshire Mental Health
Partnership NHS Trust and
Honorary Senior Lecturer in Forensic Psychiatry,
  University of Oxford
Littlemore Mental Health Centre
Oxford Clinic
Littlemore
Oxon, UK

Caroline L. Holmes
MRCPsych
Consultant Forensic Psychiatrist, The Essex Forensic
  Mental Health Service
Runwell Hospital
Wickford
Essex, UK

Sarah Hooton
BscOT SROT
Formerly Occupational Therapist
Oxleas NHS Foundation Trust
Bracton Centre
Dartford
Kent, UK

Andy Johnston
Hospital Manager RMN
Huntercombe Hospital
Roehampton
London, UK

Faisal Kazi
BSc Hons OT, Senior Occupational
    Therapist
Oxleas NHS Foundation Trust
Bracton Centre
Darford
Kent, UK

Marc Kingsley
BA (Hons) (Applied Psych) MA (Clin Psych) High Dip
Psych (UKCP)
Chartered Clinical Psychologist
North East London Mental Health
    NHS Trust
Goodmayes Hospital
Essex, UK

Maurice Lipsedge
FRCPsych FRCP FFOM (Hons)
Emeritus Consultant Psychiatrist
Guy's Hospital
London, UK

Brian Malcolm McKenzie
MA Clin Psychol (Natal) Dip for Psychotherapy
    (UCL)
Forensic Psychologist
Oxleas NHS Foundation Trust
The Bracton Centre

Dartford
Kent, UK

Gordana Milavić
MD FRCPsych
Clinical Director, Child and Adolescent Mental
    Health Services (CAMHS), The South London
    and Maudsley
NHS Foundation Trust and Lead Clinician,
National and Specialist Services,
CAMHS Directorate
CAMHS
Michael Rutter Centre
Maudsley Hospital
London, UK

Chike I. Okocha
MBBS PhD FRCPsych
Consultant Psychiatrist
Tarn PICU
Oxleas NHS Foundation Trust
Oxleas House
Queen Elizabeth Hospital
Woolwich
London, UK

Mathew J. Page
RN DipHE Dip Msc
Greyfriars Psychiatric Intensive
    Care Unit
Severn NHS Trust
Wotton Lawn
Gloucester, UK

Carol Paton
BSc Dip Clin Pharm
Chief Pharmacist and Honoary Research
    Fellow
Department of Phychological Medicine
Imperial College
University of London
Oxleas NHS Foundation Trust
The Bracton Centre
Kent, UK

Stephen M. Pereira
MD FRCPsych DMSc DPM
Lead Consultant Psychiatrist PICU and
Honorary Senior Lecturer Guy's, King's,
 St Thomas' School of Medicine
Pathways PICU
Goodmayes Hospital
North East London Mental Health NHS Trust
Ilford
Essex, UK

Sabrina Pietromartire
MBBCh FCPsych (SA)
Pathways PICU
Goodmayes Hospital
North East London Mental Health NHS Trust
Ilford
Essex, UK

Andrew W. Procter
FRCPsych
Consultant Psychiatrist, Manchester Royal
 Infirmary
Honorary Senior Clinical Lecturer,
University of Manchester
Manchester, UK

David Ridgers
Ward Manager
Oxford Ward PICU
Manchester Royal Infirmary
Manchester, UK

Helen Simmons
MRCPsych
Consultant Psychiatrist

Trevor Turner
MD FRCPsych
Consultant Psychiatrist and Clinical
 Director (General Adult Psychiatrist),
 East London and The City Mental Health
 NHS Trust
The City and Hackney Centre for Mental
 Health
Homerton University Hospital
London, UK

Kate Woollaston
BSc Psychology
Pathways PICU
Goodmayes Hospital
North East London Mental Health
 NHS Trust
Ilford, UK

Preface to second edition

The first edition of this textbook was published in 2001 and its success surpassed our expectations. The editors have received many positive comments about the usefulness of the text and its relevance to everyday practice. The interest in the care of our most disturbed patients has been highlighted by both sales overseas and by the rapid translation of the text into Czech.

Since the publication of the first edition, the sub-specialities of psychiatric intensive care and low secure care have grown from strength to strength. The Department of Health adopted standards developed by members of National Association of Psychiatric Intensive Care and Low Secure Units (NAPICU) that outline the care that should be delivered in Psychiatric Intensive Care and Low Secure Units (PICUs and LSUs). The publishers of this book have supported NAPICU to develop the first ever journal dedicated to this field: the *Journal of Psychiatric Intensive Care* (http://journals.cambridge.org/jid_JPI). The current chairman of NAPICU, Dr Stephen M. Pereira, played a central role in the development of the National Institute for Health and Clinical Excellence (NICE) guideline on the short-term management of violence; thus influencing the care of acutely disturbed patients beyond the speciality.

NAPICU continues to organise a successful annual national conference and quarterly regional mini-conferences. The majority of UK mental health trusts are now members of NAPICU, and in order to support the infrastructure of a growing organisation, a permanent NAPICU office has been set up in Glasgow. NAPICU continues to produce a quarterly bulletin to keep members up to date with developments in the field. The development of a national clinical governance network, sponsored by the Department of Health, has also been supported and this has overseen clinical quality improvement projects in areas such as responding to emergencies, culture and diversity issues, and user and carer involvement. An award is given to the 'team of the year'. Each year, a travel bursary is awarded to fund a research, clinical audit or good practice project. A national audit of PICUs and LSUs conducted by Dr Pereira's team highlighted environmental issues that led to the Department of Health's investing capital monies to improve buildings.

This edition of the textbook has been expanded to include several new chapters. The interface between PICU/LSU and learning disabilities, child and adolescent psychiatry, general adult psychiatry and substance misuse are covered, as are multidisciplinary team working, the role of social work and user and carer involvement. All other chapters have been updated to include developments such as the publication of NICE guidelines. In the interests of space, the sample unit policies have been removed as most units have now developed their own, usually more comprehensive versions.

We hope that you find the additions to the textbook useful in your practice and look forward to further developments in the speciality of PICU/LSU care. Constructive comments on any aspect of the text are welcome and should be sent to the publisher.

Further details about NAPICU and its activities can be found on the official NAPICU website: www.napicu.org.uk.

The editors would like to thank Sarah Price (Copyeditor), and Jeanette Alfoldi and Chloe Wright from the Cambridge University Press Production team for all their help with the second edition.

M. Dominic Beer
Stephen Pereira
Carol Paton

Preface to first edition

'Why do we need a book about psychiatric intensive care?' 'What *IS* psychiatric intensive care?', 'Is there any difference between intensive care and general psychiatry?' 'Where is the distinction between forensic psychiatry and psychiatric intensive care?, 'What special skills do PICU staff require?' Our first attempt to address some of these questions came at the first national conference on psychiatric intensive care, held at Bexleyheath, England, in 1996. The enthusiasm of the delegates and their thirst for knowledge and networking has led to the publication of this book.

We, as editors, have attempted to cover as many elements of the psychiatric intensive care provision as is possible within one book. We are, however aware of certain deficiencies. Where there is an evidence-base, we have attempted to use it. Where there is not, we have used personal experience and the experience of others to guide us. We believe that psychiatric intensive care is at the heart of psychiatry and its good practice requires a full multidisciplinary team, strong leadership and effective managerial support. We have, therefore, included a wide variety of chapters, all written by professionals who have extensive expertise in this area of care. We have included examples of sample policies, which can be used as a guide, but these obviously need to be adapted and scrutinised for use locally. The editors would welcome any comments and suggestions on this work.

The first section addresses treatment issues. Effective treatment requires input from a wide variety of professionals. We have included contributions on the role of medication, psychological treatments, therapeutic activities, and more controversially, the use of both restraint and seclusion. The development and definition of psychiatric intensive care and the management of the acutely disturbed patient and of the complex needs patient also warrant chapters in their own right.

The second section specifically addresses areas of risk and the interface with forensic services. Contributions from colleagues working in forensic services, we hope, will encourage the breaking down of unnecessary barriers between different services.

The third section addresses management issues such as how to set up and design a new psychiatric intensive care unit and how to manage such a unit effectively once it has been established.

We believe that this book will be of use to all disciplines working in, or interacting with, Psychiatric Intensive Care Units, and also to managers who have the responsibility for commissioning, providing and monitoring this high risk area of care. Although the emphasis is towards practice in the United Kingdom, the general principles should be relevant and applicable in any care setting where the disturbed psychiatric patient is managed.

We would like to thank all the contributors to the book; those who have assisted in the publishing, especially Geoff Nuttall, Nora Naughton, Kathleen Orr and Gavin Smith; our secretarial staff, Mrs Linda Wells, Mrs Lorraine Wright, Miss Michelle Gillham and Mrs Rosemary McCafferty for their considerable hard work; our patients and colleagues who have taught us much; and our families, especially Drs Naomi Beer and Preeti Pereira, for their support and patience through this project.

Dominic Beer
Stephen Pereira
Carol Paton

August, 2000

Foreword

I am delighted to be able to recommend this book to clinicians working at all levels of the multidisciplinary team in psychiatric intensive care, low secure, medium secure and general hospital psychiatry.

Psychiatric intensive care units (PICUs), have now been with us for some 20 years or more and, in that time, have refined and defined their role within the various levels of care offered by individual mental health care trusts. Most patients in the UK have access to intensive care and the importance of this area is emphasised by the continuance and strengthening of the National Association of Psychiatric Intensive Care Units (NAPICU) and the successful founding of the *International Journal of Psychiatric Intensive Care*. The editors of this edition have all been pivotally involved in these developments.

The PICU stands at the interface point between these different levels of care and is often the cornerstone of effective management of the most unwell and difficult to treat within the psychiatrically unwell population. All of those working within this field are consistently faced with complex issues that cut across ordinary boundaries of care. In addition, the biopsychosocial management of PICU patients, from the first break to the chronically treatment resistant, requires the individual practitioner to have access to, and knowledge of, the fullest therapeutic armamentarium.

The first edition of this book published in 2001, represented the 'first definitive and authoritive text in the subject (of PICUs)', and, covered, 'all aspects of the specialty from techniques for rapid tranquillisation through to physical, risk and management issues, as well as interfaces with forensic services'. In the second edition the editors have again gathered and expanded their thoroughly inclusive, clinically experienced and scholarly panel of authors.

For this second edition, the authors and editors have revised, updated and supplemented the text recognising the rapid expansion in the evidence base impacting upon psychiatric intensive care. This includes the routine and rational use of the newer antipsychotics, the implementation of the NICE recommendations, the incorporation of a formal national guideline for PICUs, alterations in guidelines for physical restraint and seclusion, and finally the rapid expansion in forensic psychiatry services within the United Kingdom and the crucial interdependent relationship between these services and PICUs.

The popularity of the first edition of this book, will, I am sure be matched and surpassed by this edition. The authors and editors have produced another landmark publication, which stands at the forefront of the field. The challenges over the coming decade include the advent of new pathophysiologically based diagnoses and treatments for mental illness that will transcend the simple clinical descriptions and 'trial and error' treatments of the past. These developments will be incorporated within ICD-11 and DSM-V within the next 5–8 years. Other,

more local, challenges include further changes in clinical service delivery and the implementation of the European Reform Treaty with its possible impact on human rights legislation.

The second edition of *Psychiatric Intensive Care*, will, in my opinion, prepare the reader to meet the existing and future challenges within this field.

On a final note, the pleasure of writing this foreword is, unfortunately, tinged with a certain sadness. Sadness, that Professor Robert W. Kerwin was unable to write this foreword himself, as he did the foreword for the first edition, due to his untimely death in February of this year. His legacy, however, lives on in the other clinicians and scientists he inspired, myself and several authors of this book included. In addition to projects, like this book, which he avidly supported, Professor Kerwin, though his editorship of the *Maudsley Prescribing Guidelines* and his numerous publications provided the tools for a generation of psychiatrists and mental health professionals to implement rational pharmacological and management strategies for their patients both within and without the PICU.

Rob would have enjoyed studying this book, as I am sure will you.

Michael J. Travis
University of Pittsburgh Medical Center and
Institute of Psychiatry, London

PART I

Therapeutic interventions

Psychiatric intensive care – development and definition

M. Dominic Beer, Stephen M. Pereira and Carol Paton

Historical background

Throughout human history different cultures have had to manage their most behaviourally disturbed and mentally ill members. Turner (1996) has written that historically psychiatry has been judged by its management of the 'furiously mad'. Nearly three thousand years ago the King of Babylon was put to pasture (literally) after he started to behave like a wild animal (Book of Daniel). Two thousand years ago we read in the New Testament of a wild man wandering naked amidst the tombs, having broken the chains that bound him.

Seven hundred and fifty years ago the first 'asylum' for mental patients in England was formed at the Priory of St Mary of Bethlehem in London. 'Bethlem' became the national hospital for the disturbed mentally ill. The patient's parish of origin would pay for a stay of usually up to a year. Abuses however came to light, none better known than the case of William Norris in 1814, which prompted a parliamentary enquiry. The unfortunate man had been kept for seven years in a cell and restrained mechanically so that he could move no more than twelve inches.

Nineteenth century psychiatrists such as John Conolly then embraced 'non-restraint', but many hospitals remained locked. The Mental Treatment Act 1930 introduced the concept of patients being admitted informally and by 1938 such patients constituted 35% of the total (Jones 1993). The Royal Commission on the Law Relating to Mental Illness and Mental Deficiency (1954–57) stressed that patients should be treated informally where possible. The Mental Health Act 1959 confirmed this and laid down strict guidelines for involuntary patients.

In the late 1950s there was another important development in the care of the mentally ill. This was the introduction of chlorpromazine, the first pharmacological treatment for psychotic illness. The potent combination of effective antipsychotic drugs along with the introduction of patients' rights led to the unlocking of many hospital wards. By the early 1960s, only a handful of wards in our own hospital (the former Bexley Hospital, Kent) were still formally locked. Two of these wards housed a stable population of chronically disturbed patients. There was another transient group of acutely disturbed patients who were admitted for brief periods until their behaviour became containable on an open ward. Thus, the Psychiatric Intensive Care Unit (PICU or locked ward) function had evolved as a pragmatic solution to the patient management problems encountered on the open wards.

Secure provision in the 1970s in the UK

By the early 1970s each health region was being encouraged to develop services in district general

Psychiatric Intensive Care, 2nd edn., eds. M. Dominic Beer, Stephen M. Pereira and Carol Paton.
Published by Cambridge University Press. © Cambridge University Press 2008

hospitals. These facilities could not adequately manage difficult patients. The latter joined the mentally abnormal offenders in asylums, prison or special hospitals. The Department of Health and Social Security set up a working party in 1971 to review the existing guidance on security in National Health Service (NHS) psychiatric hospitals and make recommendations on the need for security. Consequently, the Glancy Report (Revised Report of the Working Party on Security in NHS Psychiatric Hospitals) was published (Department of Health and Social Services 1974). The Report noted the almost total lack of secure facilities and recommended 1000 places for England and Wales.

The problem of the mentally abnormal offender was addressed by the Butler Committee which was formed after the case of Graham Young who was convicted of murder whilst on conditional discharge from Broadmoor.

The terms of reference were:
- To consider the criminal law in relation to mental disorder or abnormality and to recommend whether any changes in the powers and procedures were necessary.
- To recommend whether any changes were required in the provision of facilities and treatment for this group of patients.

The Butler Report (Home Office, Department of Health and Social Security 1975), and its interim version of 1974, advocated the development of forensic psychiatric services in the NHS and suggested a figure of 2000 secure beds. This was double the Glancy figure, which was based on the need for security among general psychiatric patients. It was proposed that regional secure units (RSUs) would be crucial in supporting the general psychiatric hospital as well as relieving overcrowding in Special Hospitals and providing a service to courts and prisons.

The RSUs were to be 50- to 150-bedded units closer to major centres of population than the Special Hospitals. A particular point was made regarding difficult long-stay patients – that the RSUs should not be allowed to become blocked with such patients.

If they did then the problem which they were supposed to address would recur; but no clear alternative model of care was proposed for them. The Department of Health and Social Security very quickly made money available for 1000 beds to be provided in RSUs and in Interim Secure Units (ISUs) whilst the former were being built.

These ISUs were usually converted psychiatric wards; most had a double door 'airlock' system to enter the unit and secure external exercise areas, as well as unbreakable glass and alarm systems.

Bluglass (1976) proposed that the admission criteria should include any acutely ill patient whose illness was accompanied by difficult and dangerous behaviour but should exclude wandering demented patients, the severely learning disabled and the difficult acute patients.

Thus, historically, the RSU network has been centrally planned and funded whereas locked beds for acutely ill, non-offender patients (Glancy) have not.

Development of psychiatric intensive care units world-wide

The first publications which described locked PICUs came from the USA. Rachlin (1973) stated that 'an open-door policy cannot provide adequately for the treatment needs of all psychiatric patients'. He described the establishment of a 'locked intensive care unit' serving the Bronx area of New York, 'to treat several types of patients who did not respond on open wards' (p. 829). Half were referred because they were absconders. Crain and Jordan (1979) also reported on a PICU in the Bronx which admitted mainly violent patients, 'who simply cannot be treated with an acceptable level of safety on a regular ward'. It also provided a more humane treatment setting, 'for such individuals whose behaviour ordinarily would provoke angry, punitive responses from the environment' (p. 197).

Other PICUs were described elsewhere in the world. Goldney et al. (1985) described a locked unit for acutely severely ill patients in Adelaide, Australia. Warneke (1986) described a PICU for acutely ill patients in a general medical hospital in Edmonton, Canada. The patients were mainly suicidal and the unit was not locked, nor were the patients legally detained. Musisi *et al.* (1989) described a six-bedded unit in a provincial Toronto psychiatric hospital.

In England the first designated PICU was opened in St James's Hospital, Portsmouth; Mounsey (1979) described the setting up of a twelve-bedded PICU in Salisbury. This was a lockable converted ward for disturbed patients referred from the rest of the psychiatric hospital.

In Scotland, Basson and Woodside (1981, p. 132) described the working of a mixed, 'secure/intensive care/forensic' ward and stated that, 'the pendulum has swung from "open door" hospitals back to a recognition for some security . . .'.

Secure provision in the UK in the 1980s and 1990s

The RSU model was first developed throughout England and Wales and then subsequently in Scotland. Several deficiencies of the RSU model have been noted. Snowden (1990) wrote that

there is a group of patients who are not so dangerous that they require special hospital security but who are chronically ill or poor medication responders and who require a degree of security . . . Some of the more severely ill and disabled patients will not manage in the community and long-term care will not be available . . . The mentally ill who cannot manage in the community may become mentally ill offenders by default, and even if they do not, general psychiatric services could well put pressure on forensic services to take patients that would have been considered appropriate for RSU admission in the past.

In 1991 only 635 medium secure beds existed as compared with 1163 in 1986, according to the Reed Report; this review of Health and Social Services for mentally disordered offenders and others requiring similar services (Department of Health and Home Office 1992) proposed that 1500 beds were needed. It also proposed that, 'access to local intensive care and locked wards should be available more widely' and that, 'secure provision . . . should include provision . . . for those who require long-term treatment and/or care'.

The Reed Report again referred to the lack of service provision.

Many offenders needing in-patient care can be accommodated in ordinary psychiatric provision. But although many offenders can be managed satisfactorily in 'open' wards, there must be also better access to local intensive care and locked wards (Annex J (local services 5.16 Hospital Services, p. 19)).

The Report recognised, 'the need for each Health District to ensure the availability of secure provision . . . [which] should include provision for intensive care'. The Reed Report (Department of Health and Home Office, 1992) referred to ICUs as low secure units.

Smith *et al.* (1990) hypothesised that the role of the RSU was changing. They compared patients admitted to the Butler Clinic RSU in South West England in 1983 and 1989. In the 1983 population there were significantly more patients who had been aggressive towards staff and had histories of absconding. The 1989 population was much more likely to have been referred from the criminal justice system. The authors speculated that the RSU was originally dealing with a 'backlog' of local hospital patients for whom there was no secure provision before the RSU opened.

A survey of RSU patient characteristics in 1994 confirmed that the RSU population had high levels of serious offending (McKenna 1996) and warned that, 'The ability of the RSU to respond quickly, effectively or flexibly to acute difficulties in the services referring potential admissions must in turn be compromised'.

In order to respond quickly, NHS Trusts have now used the low secure wards or PICUs to take up this demand for urgent forensic patients. Dix (1996) pointed out that this group does not necessarily present high levels of behavioural disturbance but requires a degree of security because of their charge or offence. James *et al.* (1996) also referred to a group of patients that had offended but did not require security. The suggestion is that local services should be able to provide low security in order to facilitate diversion of offenders from the criminal justice system, and aid the rehabilitation of patients discharged from Special Hospitals. As Dix (1996) writes, however, 'A significant number of PICUs do not consider themselves as "forensic units" and are reluctant to accept patients who, as a result of legal restrictions, cannot be discharged from the PICU when clinically indicated'. Cripps *et al.* (1995) describe a mixed PICU/forensic unit and discuss some of the advantages and disadvantages of this type of unit. Many would argue that the forensic role conflicts with the more dominant function of local low secure units, namely the modus operandi outlined by Faulk (1995): 'The usual pattern is for the wards to accept the patient briefly, to get them over an acute disturbance, before returning them to the original ward'.

A third role which has been adopted by PICUs is the care of the chronically disturbed patient. Coid (1991a) noted that the private sector was being used increasingly for such patients because of the lack of NHS facilities and he also (Coid 1991b) stated that 'the game of pass the parcel must stop' with reference to 'difficult to place patients'. The Mental Health Act Commission (1995) also reported on the lack of provision for patients who demonstrate longer-term behavioural problems.

The Chief Medical Officer (CMO's update 1996) stated that the number of medium secure beds was planned to be 2350 by the end of 1998 and that there was also a need for a greater diversity of secure beds, particularly those offering longer-term care at medium and low security levels. By 2001 there were some 2000 beds (Sugarman 2002).

Psychiatric Intensive Care Units in the UK in the 1990s

In the UK, PICUs have developed independently of the RSU network, and have provided a range of ser-

vices in line with local circumstances and needs. This development is wholly appropriate. Units may variably describe themselves as PICUs, extra care wards, intensive care, high dependency, special care, challenging behaviour, locked wards or low secure units. None of these terms had a universally agreed definition.

Many PICUs operate in isolation not only from the main hospital wards, but also from other similar units. Zigmond (1995) commented upon his personal experiences of such facilities in his role as a Mental Health Act Commissioner and Second Opinion Appointed Doctor and described them as, 'Physically apart from other inpatient facilities, containing the most seriously disturbed, invariably detained patients who were cared for by staff who rarely rotated around other settings and became brutalised and dehumanised by the constantly high levels of disturbance and violence they faced'.

Psychiatric intensive care, as a specialty in its own right, is only beginning to have an identity. The National Association of Psychiatric Intensive Care and Low Secure Units (NAPICU) was formed as an organisation to provide guidance on PICU issues in the UK to overcome variability of practice and in response to concern of clinicians such as Zigmond (1995).

Aims of NAPICU

- To advance PICU/low secure service
- To discuss and improve mechanisms for the delivery of PICU/low secure care
- To encourage the support of staff working in PICU/low secure services
- To audit the effectiveness of the service provided
- To organise educational opportunities for staff

Unlike the standard services provided by the RSUs, PICUs had developed independently of each other. They sought to provide a service to fulfil local needs. It was therefore impossible to be prescriptive regarding the exact role of any individual PICU, although certain criteria were broadly filled. Patients were generally too disturbed to be nursed on open wards (because of aggression, self-harming behaviour or absconding). There was, therefore, a need for increased nursing and multi-professional input and perimeter security. Admissions and discharges were generally governed by symptoms and behaviour and not by the courts (Dix 1996).

Although there were very few objective data concerning the service that these units provide, three surveys had been published prior to the development of NAPICU. Each of these surveys had a slightly different focus.

Ford and Whiffin (1991) surveyed the 169 Health Authorities in England and asked them, 'about their units providing services to acutely ill clients who require close observation and frequent nursing observation' (p. 48). They identified thirty-nine units in England which admitted in varying proportions those with acute or chronic problems such as aggression or self-harm (in the setting of mental illness) and those with a forensic history.

Mitchell (1992) surveyed psychiatric hospitals in Scotland to determine the numbers and characteristics of their patients. He identified 13 PICUs in Scotland with a total of 219 beds (3% of total inpatient psychiatric beds). Two-thirds of patients were compulsorily detained, half were under 30 years of age; schizophrenia was the most common diagnosis and co-morbid substance abuse/personality disorder was present in 10% of the under 30s.

Beer et al. (1997) identified 110 PICUs in the UK, 45 of which had been operational for less than 3 years. Eleven units were intensive care areas of four to five beds which formed part of acute admission wards; eighteen units were mixed PICU/challenging behaviour or PICU/forensic. The remainder were dedicated PICUs. Bed occupancy rates were high: at the 100% level particularly in the larger dedicated units. There was a wide variation in the level of security provided, ranging from eleven units which were built to medium secure specifications or above through to the twenty-two units which did not have permanently locked doors. Operational policies also differed widely, with many staff feeling that they might as well not have, for example, an admissions policy, because it was frequently overridden in order to accommodate difficult-to-manage patients

who could not be placed elsewhere. Units accepted patients from acute psychiatric wards, prisons, RSUs and special hospitals, and the community, in various combinations. Sixty-three units were willing to admit informal patients and this was irrespective of whether the door was permanently locked or not. The terminology used to describe the patient group who were admitted was confusing. There was no accepted cut-off point between acute and chronic disturbance or between intensive care and challenging behaviour. The point at which a patient was described as 'forensic' is similarly blurred. Medical staffing was also highly variable. Only thirty units had a dedicated consultant psychiatrist with no other inpatient beds. An equal number of units could be accessed by a number of consultants, none of whom had overall responsibility for the daily functioning of the unit. Junior doctors posts were not exclusively filled by experienced Registrars; over half the units accepted rotational Senior House Officers, often with no supervision from a more experienced staff grade doctor or Senior Registrar. Multidisciplinary team working was less developed than in general adult psychiatry and written guidelines or policies covering high-risk areas such as rapid tranquilisation, control and restraint and seclusion were often absent, confirming the informal observations of Zigmond (1995). The implications of these findings have been further developed by Pereira et al. (1999).

The most comprehensive national survey on the Psychiatric Intensive Care and Low Secure Services (Pereira et al. 2006a) identified 170 PICUs and 137 Low Secure Units (LSUs) in UK. This survey resulted in developing a national data set for PICUs and Low Secure Services together with a more comprehensive understanding of the service provision and patient characteristics (Pereira et al. 2006b) within these units. In addition, it also highlighted some of the differences between PICUs and LSUs. The national survey builds upon an earlier London-wide survey conducted on PICUs and LSUs, which described the service structure and functioning of PICUs and LSUs in London (Pereira et al. 2005a) along with the clinical characteristics of patients and the pathways for admission and discharge in the London units (Pereira *et al.* 2005b).

The National Minimum Standards were produced in 2002, recommending specific principles that should be adhered to when planning and managing Psychiatric Intensive Care and Low Secure Services (Pereira and Clinton, 2002). The objective of these standards is to provide users, clinicians, managers and commissioners with a dynamic framework for delivering high-quality services. The standards cover the following core areas of PICU practice, as shown in the following box.

Box 1.1. Mental Health Policy Implementation Guide: National Minimum Standards for General Adult Services in Psychiatric Intensive Care Units (PICU) and Low Secure Environments (Pereira and Clinton 2002)

- Admission criteria
- Core interventions
- Multidisciplinary team (MDT) working
- Physical environment
- Service structure – personnel
- User involvement
- Carer involvement
- Documentation
- Ethnicity, culture and gender
- Supervision
- Liaison with other agencies
- Policies and procedures
- Clinical audit and monitoring
- Staff training
- PICU/Low Secure Support Services

Another important document regarding inpatient care Mental Health Policy Implementation Guide: Adult Acute Care Provision was published by the Department of Health in 2002. This guidance is addressed to all involved in acute mental health care and is useful to all who use, work in, or commission these services. PICU practice is on the spectrum of inpatient care. It covers issues related to the following areas:

Box 1.2. Mental Health Policy Implementation Guide: Adult Acute Inpatient Care Provision (DOH 2002)

- Purpose and aim of adult acute inpatient care
- Integrating inpatient care within a whole systems approach
- Problems with current inpatient provision
- Reshaping the service
- Inpatient care staff
- Specific issues
- Commissioning future inpatient provision
- Developing and sustaining improvement
- This guidance also refers to psychiatric intensive care provision (in section 6.3 of Department of Health 2002)

The innovative MSc Programme in Psychiatric Intensive Care offered by the London South Bank University from 2002 is another milestone in the advancement of psychiatric intensive care. This programme was initiated and developed by Pathways Policy, Research and Development Group in collaboration with South Bank University, following a review of the training needs of PICU staff (Clinton *et al.* 2001). This programme aims to examine a variety of frameworks for the delivery of safe and consistent approaches to psychiatric intensive care and provide practitioners with the necessary confidence to be fit for practice. The course covers in detail the assessment and management of clients in psychiatric intensive care settings together with the therapeutic interventions applied in such settings.

A study was commissioned by the Department of Health to evaluate the costs of addressing physical environment deficits in PICUs and LSUs in England (Pereira *et al.* 2006c). The results showed that approximately 37% of these units did not fulfil the National Minimum Standards for design. This critical study laid the evidence base for the UK Government to release £160 million to address places of safety and for upgrading PICUs and LSUs to meet the National Minimum Standards in England (Pereira and Clinton 2002).

To monitor the development of implementation of the National Minimum Standards, a National PICU Governance Network was created in 2004 as a joint venture of the National Institute of Mental Health in England (NIMHE), North East London Mental Health Trust (NELMHT) and NAPICU (Pereira *et al.* 2006c.) The main aim of this newly created network is to encourage the PICUs to work collaboratively in order to improve service provision, with an objective measurement of the benefits demonstrated. The collaborative nature of this project will enable the different PICUs to share experiences, difficulties and plan improvements drawing upon expertise from both within and outside the network. The Psychiatric Intensive Care Advisory Service (PICAS) was set up as a subsidiary of NAPICU and links with the PICU Governance Network. The main aim of PICAS is to support NHS Trusts/independent providers by providing expert advice and guidance in meeting the National Minimum Standards and to improve the standard and quality of care within the PICU and Low Secure environments across the country.

Definition of psychiatric intensive care

Three features should ideally be present in a PICU. Two of them have parallels with the general medicine ICU; one is unique to psychiatry.

1. 'Psychiatric intensive care is for patients compulsorily detained, usually in secure conditions, who are in an acutely disturbed phase of a serious mental disorder. There is an associated loss of capacity for self-control, with a corresponding increase in risk, which does not enable their safe, therapeutic management and treatment in a general open acute ward' (Pereira and Clinton 2002). PICUs may be permanently locked or just lockable, but they are not absolutely secure settings which can guarantee containment. Admissions from courts or prisons should not be considered if absconding carries serious risk to the public. Behaviours driven by symptoms of mental illness should govern admission, not a court's requirements for security. Such patients should generally be dealt with by the RSUs. There is a need for more facilities than on a general psychiatric ward. There are more facilities on a medical ICU and these are often 'high-tech'. On a PICU resources and facilities will be both environmental and human: more space, a garden, a quiet area, a seclusion suite, snoezelen area, activity and games room are all possible facilities. Just as the patient on a medical ICU is deemed to be in need of special care, so the psychiatric patient often has multiple and complex needs which require extra resources. In human resource terms there will be a need for a multidisciplinary team to address these needs.

2. 'Care and treatment offered must be patient centred, multidisciplinary, intensive, comprehensive, collaborative and have an immediacy of response to critical situations. Length of stay must be appropriate to clinical need and assessment of risk but would ordinarily not exceeed 8 weeks in duration' (Pereira & Clinton 2002). There is the 'intensive' level of care delivered by professionals. This results in both quantitative and qualitative differences from general psychiatric care. The need for increased speed of response is a key element. In terms of nursing, the nurse:patient ratios will be higher than on general wards because of the increased need for monitoring patients exhibiting increased levels of aggression or self-harm, and observing those on large amounts of medication, e.g. for side-effects. Medical staff will also need to be present more often than on general wards because of the need to assess patients rapidly and reach working diagnoses, to formulate and to monitor management plans and to prescribe and review medication. Qualitatively, nursing staff require special training in some areas of expertise such as the management of aggression. Medical staff will need training in the use of medication. The presence of a senior doctor (MRCPsych) on most days will be required to supervise trainees. This parallels the daily consultant ward round on a medical

ICU. Because patients are often locked in and disturbed, they will need more in terms of occupational input and therapeutic activity. Social needs require social workers. Psychological, emotional and behavioural concerns will require a clinical psychologist. Medication issues require the active participation of pharmacists. In addition, all team members need to meet regularly together to discuss all patients.

3. 'Psychiatric intensive care is delivered by qualified staff according to an agreed philosophy of unit operation underpinned by principles of risk assessment and management' (Pereira and Clinton 2002).

Definition of low secure

1. 'Low secure units deliver intensive, comprehensive, multidisciplinary treatment and care by qualified staff for patients who demonstrate disturbed behaviour in the context of a serious mental disorder and who require the provision of security' (Pereira and Clinton 2002).

2. 'This is according to an agreed philosophy of unit operation underpinned by the principles of rehabilitation and risk management. Such units aim to provide a homely secure environment, which has occupational and recreational opportunities and links with community facilities' (Pereira and Clinton 2002).

3. 'Patients will be detained under the Mental Health Act and may be restricted on legal grounds needing rehabilitation, usually for up to 2 years' (Pereira and Clinton 2002).

Conclusion

Psychiatric intensive and low secure care are at the cutting edge of clinical psychiatry. They are developing specialties. Patients in these units are often very unwell and behaviourally disturbed. This book seeks to address the principles and practice of meeting the needs of this group of patients.

Acknowledgement

The authors would like to thank Khadija Chaudhry (Research Psychologist, NELMHT) for providing helpful comments and assistance in writing this chapter.

REFERENCES

Basson JV, Woodside M. 1981 Assessment of a secure/intensive care/forensic ward. Acta Psychiatr Scand 64: 132–141

Beer MD, Paton C, Pereira S. 1997 Hot beds of general psychiatry: a national survey of psychiatric intensive care units. Psychiatr Bull 21: 142–144

Bluglass R. 1976 The design of security units, the type of patient and behaviour patterns. Hosp Eng pp. 5–7

Clinton C, Pereira S, Mullins S. 2001 Training needs of psychiatric intensive care staff. Nursing Standards 15: 33–36

CMO's update 1996 London Department of Health. In: P Snowden. Regional Secure Units and Forensic Services. In: eds. Bluglass R, Bowden P. Principles and Practice of Forensic Psychiatry. London: Churchill Livingstone, 1990, p. 1379

Coid JW. 1991a A survey of patients from five health districts receiving special care in the private sector. Psychiatr Bull 15: 257–262

Coid JW. 1991b Difficult to place patients. The game of pass the parcel must stop. Br Med J 32: 603–604

Crain PM, Jordan EG. 1979 The psychiatric intensive care unit – an in-hospital treatment of violent adult patients. Bull Am Acad Psychiatry Law V11(2): 190–198

Cripps J, Duffield G, James D. 1995 Bridging the gap in secure provision: evaluation of a new local combined locked forensic/intensive care unit. J Forensic Psychiatry 6: 77–91

Department of Health. 2002 Mental Health Policy Implementation Guide: Adult Acute Inpatient Care Provision. London: HMSO

Department of Health and Home Office. 1992 Review of Health and Social Services for Mentally Disordered Offenders and other Requiring Similar Services. (Reed Report). London: DoH/Home Office

Department of Health and Social Services. 1974 Revised Report for the Working Party on Security in NHS Psychiatric Hospitals (Glancy Report). London: DHSS

Dix R. 1996 An investigation into patients presenting a challenge to Gloucestershire's Mental Health Care Services. Gloucester: Gloucestershire Health Authority

Faulk M. 1995 Basic Forensic Psychiatry, 2nd edn. Oxford: Blackwell

Ford I, Whiffin M. 1991 The role of the psychiatric ICU. Nursing Times 87(51): 47–49

Goldney R *et al.* 1985 The psychiatric intensive care unit. Br J Psychiatry 146: 50–54

Home Office, Department of Health and Social Security. 1975 Committee on Mentally Abnormal Offenders (Butler Report). London: HMSO

James AJ, Smith J, Hoogkamer R, Laing J, Donovan M. 1996 Minimum and medium security: the interface: use of Section 17 trial leave. Psychiatr Bull 20: 201–204

Jones K. 1993 Asylums and After. A Revised History of the Mental Health Services: From the Early 18th Century to the 1900s. London: Athlone Press

McKenna J. 1996 In-patient characteristics in a regional secure unit. Psychiatr Bull 20: 264–268

Mental Health Act Commission. 1995 Sixth Biennial Report. London: HMSO

Mitchell GD. 1992 A survey of psychiatric intensive care units in Scotland. Health Bulletin 50(3): 228–232

Mounsey N. 1979 Psychiatric intensive care. Nurs Times 1811–1813

Musisi S, Wasylenski DA, Rapp MS. 1989 A psychiatric intensive care unit in a psychiatric hospital. Can J Psychiatry 34: 200–204

Pereira S, Beer MD, Paton C. 1999 Good practice issues in psychiatric intensive care settings. Findings from a national survey. Psychiatr Bull 23: 397–400

Pereira S, Clinton C. 2002 Mental Health Policy Implementation Guide: National Minimum Standards for General Adult Services in Psychiatric Intensive Care Units (PICU) and Low Secure Environments. London: Department of Health

Pereira SM, Dawson P, Sarsam M. Sept 2006a The National Survey of PICU and Low Secure Services: 2 Unit characteristics. J Psychiatr Intensive Care 2: 13–19

Pereira SM, Dawson P, Sarsam M. Sept 2006b The National Survey of PICU and Low Secure Services: 1 Patient characteristics. J Psychiatr Intensive Care 2: 7–12

Pereira SM, Chaudhry K, Pietromartire S, Dale C, Halliwell J, Dix R. 2006c Design in psychiatric intensive care units: problems and issues. J Psychiatr Intensive Care 2: 70–76

Pereira S, Sarsam M, Bhui K, Paton C. 2005a The London survey of psychiatric intensive care units: service provision and operational characteristics of National Health Service units. J Psychiatr Intensive Care 1: 7–15

Pereira S, Sarsam M, Bhui K, Paton C. 2005b The London survey of psychiatric intensive care units: psychiatric intensive care: patient characteristics and pathways for admission and discharge. J Psychiatr Intensive Care 1: 17–24

Rachlin S. 1973 On the need for a closed ward in an open hospital: the psychiatric intensive-care unit. Hosp Community Psychiat 24: 829–833

Smith J, Parker J, Donovan M. 1990 Is the role of regional secure units changing? Psychiatr Bull 14: 713–714

Snowden P. 1990 Regional secure units and forensic service in England and Wales. In: Bluglass R, Bowden P (eds) Principles and Practice of Forensic Psychiatry. London: Churchill Livingstone, pp. 1375–1386

Sugarman P. 2002 Home Office Statistical Bulletin 22/01: Statistics of MDOs 2000. J Forensic Psychiatry Psychol 13: 385–390.

Turner T. 1996 Commentary on 'Guidelines for the Management of Acutely Disturbed Patients'. Adv Psychiatr Treat 2: 200–201

Warneke L. 1986 A psychiatric intensive care unit in a general hospital setting. Can J Psychiatry 31: 834–837

Zigmond A. 1995 Special care wards: are they special? Psychiatr Bull 19: 310–312

2

Management of acutely disturbed behaviour

M. Dominic Beer, Carol Paton and Stephen M. Pereira

Historically, psychiatry has been judged by its management of the 'furiously mad' (Turner 1996). In the current climate where inquiries into the care of patients are becoming increasingly common, considerable care has to be taken because of the risk of untoward incidents with acutely disturbed patients. On the one hand there is the necessity to protect the patient, their family, carers, the public and staff from the consequences of disturbed behaviour. On the other hand there is the risk that overzealous sedation with inappropriate medication regimens might lead to physical complications for the disturbed patient. Banerjee *et al.* (1995), reviewing eight cases of sudden death in detained patients, concluded that, 'the risk of sudden cardiotoxic collapse in response to neuroleptic medication given during a period of high physiological arousal should be widely publicised'.

There is some evidence to suggest that the level of violence in society is rising (College Research Unit 1998) and that this is reflected in the increasing number of assaults on hospital staff. Psychiatric Intensive Care Unit (PICU) staff are frequently called upon to manage patients who are violent or potentially violent. It is vital that staff work together in an informed and supported environment to minimise the potential risks to themselves and others.

Acute behavioural disturbance requires urgent intervention. It usually manifests with mood, thought or behavioural signs and symptoms and can be transient, episodic or long lasting. It can have either a medical or psychological aetiology and may reflect a person's limited capacity to cope with social, domestic or environmental stressors. The use of illicit substances or alcohol can accompany an episode of acute disturbance, or can be causative. The acute disturbance can involve: threatened or actual violence towards others, destruction of property, emotional upset, psychological distress, active self-harming behaviour, verbal abuse, hallucinatory behaviour, disinhibition, disorientation or confused behaviour and extreme physical overactivity – 'running amok'. More than one patient may be involved and everyday objects such as chairs, table knives or broken cups may be used to threaten or cause damage to others or to property.

Acutely disturbed behaviour can sometimes be anticipated: informing patients of their detention under the Mental Health Act, denial of requests to leave hospital or enforcing medication against a patient's will are all potentially provocative actions. Disturbance can also be unpredictable. A member of staff or another patient may say or do something that is misinterpreted by a paranoid patient who then lashes out. The underlying thought processes may not be obvious to others.

Disturbed behaviour is often transient and associated with the severity of the underlying psychiatric disorder. As the illness responds to treatment, so does the behaviour. Acute disturbance can also become chronic disturbance. Such patients are often

Psychiatric Intensive Care, 2nd edn., eds. M. Dominic Beer, Stephen M. Pereira and Carol Paton.
Published by Cambridge University Press. © Cambridge University Press 2008

described as exhibiting 'challenging behaviour' and may require longer admission and a wide range of pharmacological and psychological treatments. Some patients in this group have associated cognitive deficits (e.g. head injury) or severe problems with impulse control (e.g. borderline personality disorder).

The management of patients with acutely disturbed behaviour is a high-risk activity and it is essential that this risk is recognised and addressed throughout the management hierarchy of the hospital.

The following summarises the relevant issues in PICUs:

• PICU staff should be familiar with the procedures to be followed to facilitate the safe admission of an acutely disturbed patient.
• PICU staff should be trained in risk assessment and in the prediction, prevention and management of aggression.
• The PICU should have a written policy for the management of aggression. This should include advice on psychological and pharmacological interventions and when to involve the police.
• Ward policies on aggression should be communicated to patients as soon as is appropriate after admission.
• Incident forms should be completed after all aggressive incidents. These incident forms should be regularly reviewed and feedback provided to staff.
• Time and resources should be provided for formal debriefing after incidents. Specialist counselling may be required for victims of serious incidents.
• Sufficient appropriately staffed units to manage disturbed behaviour should be available across all levels of security.

Preparing the ward for the arrival of an acutely behaviourally disturbed patient

While many patients admitted to PICUs are already well known to the service, a significant proportion will be being admitted for the first time. A standard admissions procedure will help staff to feel more in control and reduce the variability in approaches that may be seen when less experienced staff or staff unfamiliar with the ward are on duty. Such a procedure could be written in bullet point format and displayed ideally in a prominent position in the nursing office. An example is shown below.

• Ideally, the patient should have been assessed prior to admission by PICU staff and a management plan should be in place.
• All PICU nursing staff should be alerted.
• If the patient is waiting in a police vehicle, he/she should remain there until the PICU is ready to receive him/her.
• If there is no dedicated 'reception suite', ensure that the unit is safe (e.g. lock the servery, TV room, etc.).
• Remove all other patients from the reception area.
• Ensure staff are prepared, e.g. that a control and restraint team is ready if required. Decide which member of staff will be talking to the patient.
• Inform medical staff and discuss any immediate requirement in advance if possible, e.g. a medical examination if the patient is already sedated or a rapid assessment if the patient is still very disturbed and requires sedation.

Nursing observations

Ideally, prior to admission, PICU staff should have assessed the patient and a clear nursing plan should be in place.

For new admissions unknown to staff, the level of nursing observations should be negotiated between the admitting doctor and the most senior nurse on duty.

The levels of observations are:

Level 1 Nominal supervision
Awareness of whereabouts of patient at all times

Level 2 Close attention
15-min checks plus awareness of whereabouts

Level 3 Constant care
Continual presence of nursing staff for observation, but privacy granted for bathing

Level 4   Intensive observations
        Continual presence of nursing staff and constant direct visual observation

On admission, it is wise to be cautious. It is easier to reduce observation levels if the patient is more settled than anticipated than to deal with the consequences of inadequate observation.

The level of nursing supervision should be determined by the multidisciplinary team and reviewed at least once each nursing shift. Nurses trained in the appropriate techniques should carry out close observation. It should be recognised that special observation can exacerbate behavioural disturbance and unobtrusive monitoring can sometimes be used effectively. Episodes of continuous observation lasting less than 72 h have been shown to help two-thirds of patients (Shugar and Rehaluk 1990).

Mental Health Act status

Ideally the PICU should have a policy in place which clearly defines the legal status of patients who may be admitted. This should be subject to local agreement.

Some PICUs may process all Section 136 (police place of safety order) patients and some may accept prison transfers or even patients restricted by the Ministry of Justice. Informal patients may sometimes be admitted although this should be the exception rather than the rule (Department of Health 2002).

Although the Mental Health Act aims to facilitate care and not to be obstructive, it is a fact of life that PICU regimes may compromise basic human rights (Pereira *et al.* 1999) while informal status may compromise the ability of staff to provide optimal care.

In the UK if patients are resisting, aggressive and refusing treatment or threatening to leave the ward and their status is still informal then the appropriate Section-12-approved (approved as having specialist knowledge and experience in psychiatry) doctor (e.g. Consultant, Associate Specialist or Specialist Registrar) should be called to instigate formal detention

under Sections 2 (assessment and treatment) or 3 (treatment) of the Mental Health Act.

If it is immediately necessary, for example to prevent serious injury, intramuscular medication can be given under common law (under the doctrine of necessity). Careful consideration needs to be given to this and clear documentation kept, because professionals may be open to prosecution for assault by an informal patient. Any doctor may use Section 5 (2) to detain a patient for up to 72 h or any registered mental health nurse can use Section 5 (4) to detain a patient for up to 6 h. However, medication cannot be given against the patient's will under Section 5 – but it can under Sections 2, 3 or 4 (as Section 2 but involving only one doctor: valid for up to 72 h). It would be considered good practice to audit the use of these sections in a PICU: they should never be relied upon for routine care.

For the use of control and restraint and for the use of seclusion please see Chapters 8 and 9.

Ensuring a safe environment

- There should be good visibility in all areas of the unit
- Alarms should be within easy reach at all times
- Staff response to alarms should be consistent
- Movable objects should be kept to a minimum; those that exist should be of safe size and construction
- Structured activities should be provided, e.g. gym, garden, games

For further information see Chapter 22 and the National Minimum Standards for General Adult Services in PICU and low secure environments (Department of Health 2002).

Assessment of the acutely disturbed patient

Staff safety

Staff on PICUs should be aware of the basic rules to be followed to reduce the risk to themselves. They should also ensure that other staff who may visit the ward on a sessional basis are aware of these rules.

- When interviewing a patient who has potential for aggressive behaviour always inform colleagues of your intentions and location.
- Try to conduct joint medical and nursing assessments to protect interviewers and to reduce stimulation to the patient.
- Ensure that there are alarms close by at all times. Consideration should be given to providing staff with personal alarms that have the facility to alert others to an emergency and its location.
- Sit at an angle to the patient at a safe distance away and in close proximity to the exit.
- Avoid interviewing with the patient between you and the door.
- Call the police if necessary.

Research performed in PICUs (Walker and Seifert 1994) has shown that a disproportionately high number of violent incidents are perpetrated by a few patients (two patients were responsible for fifteen of the thirty-seven violent incidents). Mortimer (1995) also showed that a few patients caused many incidents. As more staff were trained in control and restraint, the number of incidents fell. It is often very difficult to predict accurately who these patients will be but patients who score heavily from the factors in the lists below should be deemed as those most at risk of disturbed behaviour.

Important factors from the patient's history, which may indicate an increased risk of violence (Royal College of Psychiatrists 1995; College Research Unit 1998), include:

- Previous violence towards others or self
- Young male patients
- Previous forensic history
- Substance misuse
- Antisocial, explosive or impulsive personality traits
- Poor compliance with treatment or services
- Association with a subculture prone to violence
- Evidence of social restlessness or rootlessness
- Presence of precipitants, e.g. loss events
- Access to any named potential victims identified in mental state

The characteristics below have been identified as predicting the 'potential for immediate violence/aggression' (College Research Unit 1998).

Primary characteristics

- Previous history of aggression or violence, overtly aggressive acts, forensic history
- Hostile, threatening verbalisation, boasting of prior abuse
- Suspicious, paranoid ideation
- Delusions of control or hallucinations with violent content
- Poor impulse control
- Non-verbal expression of hostile intent such as increased motor activity, pacing, invading another's personal space, angry facial expression
- Refusal to communicate
- Poor concentration or unclear thought processes
- Possession of a weapon

Secondary characteristics

- Fear, anger, anxiety and pain
- Inappropriate and unrealistic demands
- Exacerbation of psychotic illness particularly the changes in life events, low self-esteem, vulnerability to interpersonal stress
- Inability to verbalise feelings
- Previous substance abuse

Related factors and considerations

- Hypomanic excitement
- Confusional states
- Psychiatric or psychological motivation for problematic behaviour
- Goal structure for aggressive/problematic behaviour

There are also some behavioural clues which have been identified as being predictors of imminent violence (Wykes and Mezey 1994). These are mainly intuitive and include: dishevelled appearance, smell of alcohol, signs of increased physiological arousal, pacing, gesticulating and violent gestures, increased muscle tension such as clenched fists and teeth, flared nostrils, escalating volume of speech, swearing, direct threats, labile affect, and appearing frightened, confused and disorientated.

Precipitants of violent incidents on wards

- Enforcement of ward rules
- Denial of patient's requests
- Confrontational or irritable manner of staff

Staff factors related to incidents

- Staff stability
- Staff training (young untrained more likely to be victims)
- Poor leadership
- Inadequate staff resources

Older, more experienced staff (Hodgkinson *et al.* 1985; James *et al.* 1990; Carmel and Hunter 1991) and those that have been trained in the prevention and management of violence (Carmel and Hunter 1990) are less likely to be physically assaulted. Agency staff (James *et al.* 1990) are more likely to be assaulted, particularly when they are unfamiliar with ward routines (Katz and Kirkland 1990). Several studies support an association between aggression and overcrowding on wards (e.g. Palmstierna *et al.* 1991). Further information can be found in Chapter 12.

Milieu factors

- Access to weapons
- No fresh air
- Lack of privacy
- Environment that is too hot or too cold
- Uncared-for environment
- Lots of hidden corners in building
- Overcrowding
- Unclear staff functions
- Unpredictable routines and structure
- Overstimulation
- Authoritarian conditions

(Katz and Kirkland 1990; Palmstierna *et al.* 1991; College Research Unit 1998.)

Medical causes

Some medical or neurological conditions may present with disturbed behaviour and treatment of the underlying problem is vital. Such problems need to be excluded when accepting an unknown patient into the PICU. The exact screening tests required in any individual patient would depend, of course, on the clinical presentation.

Examples of medical conditions that can present in this way are:
- Head injury with vascular lesions, especially subdural haematoma
- Delirium tremens
- Intoxication with illicit drugs or alcohol
- Overdose with prescribed drugs, e.g. anticholinergics
- Meningitis
- Encephalitis
- Hypoglycaemia
- Diminished cerebral oxygenation of any aetiology, e.g. vascular, metabolic or endocrine
- Hypertensive encephalopathy
- Wernicke's encephalopathy
- Temporal lobe epilepsy
- Neoplastic conditions
- Dementia

On admission, or ideally prior to admission, a comprehensive history should be obtained from as many sources as possible. This may include the patient, family, police, general practitioner, social worker, community psychiatric nurse and previous notes.

Mental State Examination

Mental State Examination should cover the mental state factors known to be associated with violence. These are:
- Evidence of any 'threat/control override' symptoms especially persecutory delusions and delusions of passivity
- Emotions related to violence especially irritability, anger, hostility and suspiciousness
- Erotomania or morbid jealousy symptoms
- Misidentfication phenomena
- Command hallucinations

The severity and nature of the patient's symptoms in the acute situation often limit history taking and detailed examination of the mental state. However, this should be carried out at the first available opportunity.

In the Mental State Examination, special attention should be paid to the level of consciousness, attention and concentration, memory, language abnormalities, mood and affect. Brief and quantifiable tests such as the Mini Mental State Examination can be useful for monitoring the progress of such patients (Folstein *et al.* 1975). Signs of acute organic brain syndrome (delirium) should be suspected until proven otherwise if the following are present:
• Disorientation (especially if worse at night)
• Clouding of consciousness
• Abnormal vital signs
• No previous psychiatric history (especially if over 40 years old)
• Visual hallucinations

Other signs and symptoms would include: an acute onset (hours to days), a reversed sleep–wake cycle, labile mood, shifting delusions, disjointed thoughts, poor attention and impaired memory.

Suicide risk

Some patients are admitted to PICUs because they pose a risk to themselves. The PICU does not offer significant advantages over open acute wards in the management of many suicidal patients. However, in those patients where absconding from the ward in order to self-harm is potentially problematic, then the locked door of the PICU confers additional protection. There are predictors of suicide specific to different diagnostic groups of patients, as follows.

Depression

• Male
• Older
• Single
• Separated
• Socially isolated
• Previous deliberate self-harm/suicide attempt
• Insomnia/hypersomnia
• Self-neglect

• Memory impairment
• Agitation
• Guilt
• Bleakness about the future
• Severe depression

Schizophrenia

• Male
• Younger
• Socially isolated
• Unemployed
• Previous deliberate self-harm/suicide attempt
• Depressive episode
• Severe and relapsing illness
• Insight and fear of deterioration in mental state

Alcohol problems

• Male
• Age 40–60 years
• Depression
• Previous deliberate self-harm/suicide attempt
• Bereavement
• Poor physical health

Management of acutely disturbed behaviour

Attempts should be made to prevent violence by using de-escalation techniques (see Chapter 3). The key points are (adapted from College Research Unit 1998):
• Stay a safe distance from the patient and within easy access to alarms and escape routes
• Stay calm, avoid sudden movements and explain your intentions clearly and confidently
• Engage the patient in conversation and try to reason
• If reasoning fails, consider other interventions depending on circumstances

Turner (1996) states that there is a, 'key need for much better audit and research of acute treatment approaches' in the management of acutely disturbed behaviour. All PICUs should have a written policy for the management of such patients. An example of such a policy is shown in Figure 2.1. The appropriate

MANAGEMENT OF ACUTELY DISTURBED BEHAVIOUR IN ADULTS:
RAPID TRANQUILLISATION (RT)

The aims of RT are threefold:

1. To reduce suffering for the patient: psychological or physical (through self-harm or accidents)
2. To reduce risk of harm to others by managing a safe environment
3. To do no harm (by prescribing safe regimens and monitoring physical health)

Note: *Despite the need for rapid and effective treatment, concomitant use of two or more antipsychotics (antipsychotic polypharmacy) should be avoided on the basis of risk associated with QT prolongation (common to almost all antipsychotics). This is a particularly important consideration in RT where the patient's physical state predisposes to cardiac arrhythmia.*

In an emergency situation	
Step Intervention	
1 De-escalation, time out, placement, etc., as appropriate	

2   Offer **oral** treatment   **Haloperidol** 5 mg or **Olanzapine** 10 mg or **Risperidone** 1–2 mg }
 	
Note that the SPC for haloperidol recommends:
  1. avoiding concomitant antipsychotics
  2. pre-treatment ECG
	With or without lorazepam 1–2 mg If the patient is prescribed regular antipsychotics, lorazepam 1–2 mg alone avoids the risks associated with combining antipsychotics Repeat every 45–60 min Go to step 3 if three doses fail or sooner if the patient is placing themselves or others at significant risk

3 Consider **IM treatment** From this point on: • Have flumazenil to hand in case of lorazepam induced respiratory depression. Consider • The patient's legal status. • Consulting a senior colleague.	**Lorazepam** 2–4 mg or **Haloperidol** 5 mg or **Olanzapine** 5–10 mg Monotherapy with buccal midazolam, 10–20 mg may offer a useful alternative. Note that this preparation is unlicensed Repeat after 30–60 min if insufficient effect **Promethazine** 50 mg IM is an alternative in benzodiazepine-tolerant patients } IM olanzapine should not be combined with an IM benzodiazepine **If haloperidol is used:** • note the warnings above • ensure IM procyclidine is available (5–10 mg) in case of acute dystonia
4 Seek expert advice from the consultant or pharmacist on call	

Figure 2.1. Management of acutely disturbed behaviour in adults. From the Maudsley Prescribing Guidelines, 9th edn. (Taylor *et al.* 2005)

Guidelines for the use of Clopixol Acuphase

Acuphase should only be used after an acutely psychotic patient has required **repeated** injections of short-acting drugs such as haloperidol or olanzapine or sedative drugs such as lorazepam.
Acuphase should only be given when enough time has elapsed to assess the full reponse of previously injected drugs: allow 15 min after IV injections; 60 min after IM.

Acuphase should **never** be administered:
- In an attempt to 'hasten' the antipsychotic effect of other antipsychotic therapy
- For rapid tranquillisation
- At the same time as other parenteral antipsychotics
- Primarily as a 'test dose' for Clopixol injection
- To a patient who is struggling (risk of intravasation & oil emboli)

Acuphase should **never** be used for, or in, the following:
- Patients who accept oral medication
- Patients who are neuroleptic naive
- Patients who have an increased propensity to develop EPSEs
- Patients who are unconscious
- Patients who are pregnant
- Those with hepatitis or renal impairment
- Those with cardiac disease

Onset and duration of action
Sedative effects usually become apparent 2 h after injection and peak after 12 h.
The effects may last up to 72 h.

Dose
Acuphase should be administered in a dose of 50–150 mg, up to a maximum of 400 mg over a 2-week period. This maximum duration ensures that a treatment plan is put in place. It does not indicate that there are known harmful effects from more prolonged administration, although such use should be very exceptional. There is no such thing as a 'course of Acuphase'. The patient should be assessed before each administration.

Injections should be spaced at least 24 hours apart.

Figure 2.2. Guidelines for the use of Clopixol Acuphase (from Taylor *et al.* 2005)

use of Clopixol Acuphase is outlined in Figure 2.2. Monitoring requirements after rapid transquillisation are shown in Figure 2.3.

Detailed discussion of pharmacological management can be found in Chapter 5. Time out, seclusion and control and restraint are discussed in detail in Chapters 8 and 9.

Management after an aggressive incident/debriefing

After all aggressive incidents formal debriefing should be offered, focusing on practical and emo-tional issues at the time; although there is some controversy about the effectiveness of debriefing (Rick *et al.* 1998), victims need sympathy, support and reassurance. For professionals who are assaulted it is advisable for them to return to work as soon as possible to prevent 'the incubation of fear'. Usually the team working at the time of the incident is sufficient to deal with the debriefing. However, in the case of very serious incidents it may be useful to have an external person to ensure that sufficient counselling is provided, particularly to anyone who has sustained significant physical or emotional injury. At the time of a serious aggressive incident, immediate safety

(a)

Rapid tranquillisation: monitoring

After any parenteral drug administration monitor as follows:

Temperature
Pulse
Blood pressure
Respiratory rate

Every 5–10 min for 1 h, then half-hourly until patient is ambulatory.

If the patient is asleep or **unconscious**, the use of pulse oximetry to continuously measure oxygen saturation is desirable. A nurse should remain with the patient until they are ambulatory again.

ECG and haematological monitoring are also strongly recommended when parenteral antipsychotics are given, particularly when higher doses are used. Note that the Summary of Product Characteristics (SPC) for haloperidol recommends that all patients should have an ECG before haloperidol is prescribed (www.medicines.org.uk). Hypokalaemia, stress and agitation place the patient at risk of cardiac arrhythmias.

(b)

Remedial measures in rapid tranquillisation

Problem	Remedial measures
Acute dystonia	**Procyclidine** 5–10 mg IM or IV
Reduced respiratory rate (<10/min) or oxygen saturation (<90%)	Give **oxygen**, raise legs Ensure patient is not lying face down Give **flumazenil** (if benzo implicated) **Mechanical ventilation** (if other drug implicated)
Irregular or slow pulse (<50/min)	**Refer** to medical care immediately
Fall in blood pressure (>30 mmHg orthostatic drop or <50 mmHg diastolic)	**Lie patient flat** Tilt bed towards head
Increased temperature	**Withhold antipsychotics** Check CPK urgently

---

Figure 2.3. a, b. Monitoring requirements after rapid tranquillisation (from Taylor *et al.* 2005)

issues must take precedence over any investigation. The latter should attempt, as sensitively as possible, to compile detailed reports of the incident so as to understand its causes, context and consequences.

The investigation of serious incidents should use 'root cause analysis' where the aim is to identify all contributing factors. Many of these will be related to systems rather than individuals. The organisation has a duty to modify as many systems-related problems as possible (Neal *et al.* 2004; National Patient Safety Agency, Root cause analysis toolkit; available online at http://81.144.177.110/health/resources/root_cause_analysis/conditions).

The following may act as an aide-mémoire for those who are either directly involved in an aggressive incident or who may be required to support colleagues (for further reading, see Wykes and Mezey 1994).

Dealing with the aftermath of an incident if you are the victim

- Acknowledge that you may experience some symptoms of stress and be aware that these may be delayed for several hours
- Do not become helpless, be explicit about what you want or do not want in the way of support
- Do not blame yourself; try and learn from the experience
- Try to return to work soon
- Accept the necessary management investigations
- Follow procedures carefully
- Ensure that you get support, both formal and informal

What colleagues and friends can do

- At the time, give the victim unconditional reassurance
- Show that you are willing to talk at any time
- Reassure the victim's family and ensure that the victim is not left alone after work; for example, offer a lift home

- Help the victim to assimilate the experience and keep a sense of proportion, bearing in mind the nearly universal problem of unrealistic guilt
- Do not treat victims as if they have an infectious disease (they do report being ignored)

What teams and ward managers can do

- Consider the need both for support and debriefing
- Allow time to talk as a group
- Consider what worked well/went wrong and how to prevent/deal with similar incidents in the future
- Consider the feelings involved and make sure you have a chance to express them
- Act on any suggestions which come out of the post-incident debriefing, given the tendency of organisations to experience denial after traumatic events

Whether to charge a patient after an incident

This is often a very difficult decision and it may require considerable time and effort on the part of the clinical team to even persuade the local police service to interview the patient. It is essential for the multidisciplinary team to have a view on whether to press charges and there will be issues for the victim if he or she is part of the clinical team. He or she will need the support of colleagues because there may be emotions such as guilt, which need to be worked through. Factors that may influence the team's decision to press charges may include:

- The patient's mental state
- The capacity of the patient to form intent
- The degree of harm inflicted
- The likely effect on the patient
- Perceived need for more secure placement

Advantages of charges being pressed include

- The possible therapeutic effect for the patient who may understand the concept and value of boundaries
- The responsibility for managing difficult behaviour is shared with the Court/Criminal Justice System professionals

- The patient may get a criminal record/hospital order/restriction order, which will alert others to possible danger in the future
- Resources may be more forthcoming for the treatment of such a patient
- Formal documentation of an incident is made
- The patient has the opportunity to defend himself/herself if he/she feels wrongly accused
- It may increase the chance of compensation for the victim

Further discussion of this subject is in Chapter 14, The interface with forensic services.

'Trust-wide' issues regarding management of disturbed behaviour

- The PICU should have policies on the management of aggression
- Staff should be trained in the management of aggression
- Incident forms should be completed for all aggressive incidents
- These incident forms should be regularly analysed and feedback provided to staff
- Time and resources should be available for formal debriefing after incidents
- Time and resources should be provided for specialist counselling of those victims of a serious incident
- The multidisciplinary team should be expected to confront and counsel patients who exhibit repeated episodes of disturbed behaviour
- Ward policies on aggression designed for patients should be communicated to them as soon as appropriate after admission
- Anger management groups should be provided for patients
- Ensure that staff understand and have experience in risk assessment
- Ensure that there is good cooperation between health and social services
- Ensure that there is good record keeping and communication between community and inpatient facilities
- Ensure that there are sufficient units to manage disturbed behaviour, e.g. intensive care units which

are well staffed and arrange training of staff in the assessment and management of the acutely disturbed patient

Leadership is essential. Basic skills in risk assessment and confidence in the management of disturbed behaviour are core skills that should be shared by all staff working in PICUs/LSUs.

Conclusion

This chapter has shown that there are many factors to the effective management of the acutely disturbed patient. It is essential that services are planned, resourced and supported to ensure the safety of the patients and staff in acute mental health services.

REFERENCES

Banerjee S, Bingley W, Murphy E. 1995 Deaths of Detained Patients: A Review of Reports to the Mental Health Act Commission. London: Mental Health Act Foundation

Carmel H, Hunter M. 1990 Compliance with training in managing assaultative behaviour and injuries from inpatient violence. Hosp and Community Psychiatry 41: 558–560

Carmel H, Hunter M. 1991 Psychiatrists injured by patient attack. Bull Am Acad Psychiatry Law 19: 309–316

College Research Unit. 1998 Management of Imminent Violence: Clinical Practice Guidelines to Support Mental Health Services. Occasional Paper 41. London: Royal College of Psychiatrists

Department of Health. 2002 Mental Health Policy Implementation Guide. National Minimum Standards for General Adult Services in Psychiatric Intensive Care Units (PICU) and Low Secure Environments. London: Department of Health

Folstein MF, Folstein SE, McHugh PR. 1975 'Mini-Mental State': a practical method for grading the cognitive state of patients for the Clinician. J Psychiatr Res 12: 189

Hodgkinson P, McIvor L, Phillips M. 1985 Patient assaults on staff in a psychiatric hospital. A two year retrospective study. Med Sci Law 28: 288–294

James DV, Fineberg NA, Shah AK, Priest RG. 1990 An increase in violence on an acute psychiatric ward: a study of associated factors. Br J Psychiatry 156: 846–852

Katz P, Kirkland FR. 1990 Violence and social structure on mental hospital wards. Psychiatry 53: 262–277

Mortimer A. 1995 Reducing violence on a secure ward. Psychiatr Bull 19: 605–698

Neal LA, Watson D, Hicks T et al. 2004 Root cause analysis applied to the investigation of serious untoward incidents in mental health services. Psychiatr Bull 28: 75–77

Palmstierna T, Huitfeldt B, Wistedt B. 1991 The relationship of crowding and aggressive behaviour on a psychiatric intensive care unit. Hosp Community Psychiatry 42: 1237–1240

Pereira S, Beer D, Paton C. 1999 Good practice issues in psychiatric intensive care units: findings from a national survey. Psychiatr Bull 23: 397–404

Rick J, Perryman S, Young K. 1998 Workplace Trauma and its Management. London: HSE Books

Shugar G, Rehaluk R. 1990 Continuous observation for psychiatric inpatients: a critical evaluation. Compr Psychiatry 30: 48–55

Taylor D, Paton C, Kerwin R. 2005. The Maudsley Prescribing Guidelines. London: Martin Dunitz

The Royal College of Psychiatrists. 1995 Strategies for the Management of Disturbed and Violent Patients in Psychiatric Units. Council Report CR41. London: Royal College of Psychiatrists

Turner T. 1996 Commentary on 'Guidelines for the Management of Acutely Disturbed Patients'. Adv Psychiatr Treat 2: 200–201

Walker Z, Seifert R. 1994 Violent incidents in a Psychiatric Intensive Care Unit. Br J Psychiatry 164: 826–828

Wykes T, Mezey G. 1994 Counselling for victims of violence. In: Wykes T (ed) Violence and Healthcare Professionals. London: Chapman & Hall

Recommended further reading

National Institute for Clinical Excellence. 2005 Violence. The short term management of disturbed/violent behaviour in inpatient psychiatric settings and emergency departments. Clinical Guideline 25. Available online at www.nice.org.uk

3

De-escalation

Roland Dix and Mathew J. Page

The United Kingdom is beginning to see the development of systematic approaches to the prevention and management of violence and aggression. The Mental Health Policy Implementation Guide for Developing Positive Practice to Support the Safe and Therapeutic Management of Aggression and Violence in Mental Health In-patient Settings was published by the National Institute for Mental Health in England (NIMHE) (2004). The Guide places an emphasis on the recognition, prevention and de-escalation of aggressive behaviour and adds that this is best achieved through organisational, environmental and clinical risk assessment and management. One of the key standards set by the Guide is that all staff must be trained in recognition, prevention and de-escalation skills awareness.

Such a programme has been developed by the NHS Security Management Service (SMS) (2004). The National Syllabus for Conflict Resolution training is a generic course for all NHS frontline staff. The SMS is developing a programme specifically to meet the needs of those who work in mental health and learning disability care. This course lasts two days and includes the following modules (Nyberg-Coles 2005):

- Recognising violence and understanding causes
- Raising awareness of staff and service-user perspectives
- The impact of the social and physical environment
- Cultural awareness, diversity and racial equality
- De-escalation and communication
- Problem-solving and risk assessment
- Legal and ethical issues
- The importance of post-incident reviews and learning the lessons

De-escalation must form part of a hierarchy of responses to aggression in inpatient care. Guidance is continually being developed and evaluated. The then National Institute for Clinical Excellence (2005) produced its own suggested techniques, however this chapter aims to describe one model of de-escalation in detail that has been used in clinical practice for several years.

Stevenson (1991) defined de-escalation as a 'complex, interactive process in which a patient is redirected towards a calmer personal space'. Becoming competent at de-escalation is in itself a sophisticated activity requiring much more than just a theoretical understanding of aggression. It cannot be considered in purely academic terms. The practitioner must undertake a developmental process, resulting in highly evolved self-awareness, enabling the skills of de-escalation to become instinctive. Put simply, the practitioner of de-escalation must use their own personality and sense of self to actively engage the person they wish to de-escalate.

The Psychiatric Intensive Care Unit (PICU) and the Low Secure Unit (LSU) have an unavoidable role in setting limits to disturbed behaviour, and therefore require team members to develop a high standard

Psychiatric Intensive Care, 2nd edn., eds. M. Dominic Beer, Stephen M. Pereira and Carol Paton.
Published by Cambridge University Press. © Cambridge University Press 2008

of de-escalation skills. Authors such as Boettcher (1983), Kaplan and Wheeler (1983), McHugh and West (1995), Turnball *et al.* (1990) and NHS SMS (2004) have proposed models of de-escalation. These models have much to offer the PICU/LSU although they do not specifically address the PICU/LSU patient.

The model proposed was specifically designed for use in PICUs and LSUs, and was largely developed from practice experience in such facilities.

Experience in the PICU/LSU suggests three basic components for effective face-to-face de-escalation. They are: assessment of the immediate situation, communication skills designed to facilitate cooperation and tactics aimed at problem-solving. This chapter will attempt to bring together all these components and to demonstrate their practical value within the context of the PICU/LSU. The model for de-escalation offered here is in daily use in several inpatient facilities and has shown good efficacy.

Component 1: assessment of the aggressive incident

Before considering how best to assess an episode of aggression, it is essential that ward staff have a shared understanding of what constitutes aggressive or unacceptable behaviour. This is particularly important for services that operate 24 h a day across a number of shifts. Failure to share an agreed definition of aggressive or unacceptable behaviour may result in an incident being responded to with humour by one shift and PRN (whenever necessary) medication by another. Rating scales such as the Assaultive Rating Scale described by Lanza and Campbell (1991) provide a useful framework.

Assaultive Rating Scale (ARS) (Lanza and Campbell 1991):
1. Threat of assault but no physical contact
2. Physical contact but no physical injury
3. Mild soreness/surface abrasion/scratches/small bruises
4. Major soreness/cuts/large bruises

5. Severe lacerations/fractures/head injury
6. Loss of limb/permanent physical disability
7. Death

The scale described above helps to focus the minds of staff when considering the level of risk or actual aggression they are dealing with. Such scales are helpful in adding objectivity to potential or actual incidents of aggression.

Many studies have considered inpatient violence in terms of a behavioural expression of underlying psychopathology (Betempts *et al.* 1993). Correlations between aggression with symptom profiles, diagnosis and other demographic details have been suggested (Davis 1991; Webster *et al.* 1997). An understanding of these factors is useful to the practitioner of de-escalation, but it does not provide the most practical theoretical framework. Situational analysis is a much more useful basis from which to consider de-escalation. This line of reasoning is supported by Cheung *et al.* (1997), who concluded that 69.9% of inpatient assaults ($n = 332$) were precipitated by interaction with staff. There is also good evidence that issues such as administering medication, prevention of absconding and limit setting, all common in the PICU/LSU, are often the start of aggressive escalation (Blair 1991; Bensley *et al.* 1995). The realities of inpatient life will provide many situations that can result in a sense of injustice, real or perceived provocation and reason for discharge of aggression.

Frude (1989) suggested a model for the situational analysis of an aggressive incident. The model describes a progression of five factors through which aggression can result. This is illustrated in Figure 3.1. Within the context of the PICU/LSU, a common example of the model's application is as follows.

Situation

A detained patient requests to leave the PICU/LSU unescorted to go to the local shop. The clinical assessment and conditions of Section 17 leave require a nurse escort. This is communicated to the patient.

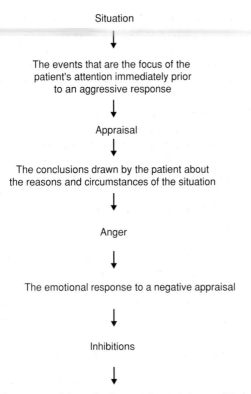

Situation

↓

The events that are the focus of the
patient's attention immediately prior
to an aggressive response

↓

Appraisal

↓

The conclusions drawn by the patient about
the reasons and circumstances of the situation

↓

Anger

↓

The emotional response to a negative appraisal

↓

Inhibitions

↓

The content of the patient's mental state in terms of their
altitudes, values and personal controls against aggression

↓

Aggression

↓

The behavioral result of the progression to the model's
other components

Figure 3.1. Situational analysis of an aggressive incident

Appraisal

The patient appraises this as punitive action by the staff in which his or her freedom is being restricted without therapeutic reason.

Anger

Frustration results from an inability to control this situation. The emotional result is a feeling of anger.

Inhibitions

The patient is suffering with mild manic symptoms resulting in a degree of grandiosity. He or she has a poor tolerance to his or her needs not being immediately met.

Aggression

He or she is verbally abusive to the staff member and kicks the unit entrance several times.

The above is an example of the model's application to a common PICU/LSU event. It can also be applied to many other situations that occur in the PICU/LSU, for example offering unwanted medication, etc. When interacting with the potentially aggressive patient, the practitioner of de-escalation should attempt to make a rapid assessment of the incident's components. During handovers and at other times when aggressive incidents are discussed, the incident in the example could have been simply described as, 'the patient became aggressive because he could not go to the shop'. The application of Frude's model allows this situation to be more thoroughly interrogated resulting in a superior level of description. Through a comprehensive understanding of the incident, intervention may be applied at each point attempting to de-rail the journey from event to aggression. This may be achieved by the use of specific communication skills in combination with de-escalation tactics.

Component 2: communication

It is not possible to set out a list of communication skills the cold application of which will de-escalate an aggressive patient. The communication skills set out here are merely tools that are to be used by the practitioner and moulded by their individual style and personality. The content of communication with an aggressive patient needs to appear genuine and sincere and not just a regurgitation of artificial techniques. A successful de-escalation will be firmly based within the principles of the therapeutic relationship.

Non-verbal communication principles

- Position your body so that you are communicating at an angle that is not confronting.
- Be aware of your body posture. Avoid postures that may appear authoritarian or defensive, e.g. folded arms or hands on hips.
- Attempt to communicate at the same height as the patient, i.e. standing or sitting. Being seated during de-escalation is sometimes useful in appearing non-threatening. However, this may place the staff member at increased risk if physical assault actually occurs.
- Be aware of your facial expression, ensuring that it reflects what you are saying verbally.
- Comfortable proximity between individuals during communication may be approximately one metre. This may need to be increased at least threefold in response to escalating verbal aggression (Lanza 1988). As the intensity of the aggressive responses diminishes then the distance can be reduced accordingly.
- Avoid the temptation to use reassuring touch early in the de-escalation process. As the situation calms, look for non-verbal and verbal cues suggesting permission to touch.
- Be aware of the use of eye contact. Maintain eye contact in the same way as if you were communicating with a non-aggressive person. Avoid intimidating stares; good use of eye contact will communicate genuineness and confidence.

Verbal communication principles

- Use a calm, warm and clear tone of voice as a general principle. Voice tone may be altered as appropriate to reflect energy in the conversation (see mood matching below).
- If a rapport is not already present, personalise yourself as quickly as possible, e.g. appropriate self-disclosure. This will help to increase inhibitions against assault.

- In the early phase of de-escalation, ask for specific acts, avoiding long complicated statements, e.g. 'Let's sit down and discuss what you need'.
- Avoid personal confrontation by remaining focused on the issues at hand, ignoring personally directed attack.
- In the early phase of de-escalation avoid being selective with your attention to the issues the patient is verbalising. Deal with what appears to be the main problem, even if this is uncomfortable.
- Avoid 'passing the buck'. Show yourself to be someone in a position to problem-solve, even if this means after initial de-escalation others are needed to resolve the issue.
- Avoid using jargon.
- Highlight the impact of the patient's behaviour, showing they are being listened to, e.g. 'you are scaring people with your shouting'. Statements of this kind can help to demonstrate that the patient is making an impact and thus diminish the need for further escalation.
- Reinforce your position as a helper rather than a restricter.
- Keep the communication fluid and attentive to the content of the problem. Mood matching is useful in achieving this. This is where the energy in the discussion is temporarily matched by the staff member, e.g. by facial expression or raising the energy in your voice (for further explanation see Davis 1989).
- There are limits to what can be achieved verbally. Remain astute to the progress made towards de-escalation. It may not be possible to return the patient to a complete state of calm. If the expressed aggression has significantly reduced, then be prepared to disengage rather than risk re-escalation. Avoid the need to have the last word.

Component 3: de-escalation and negotiation – the tactics

To suggest that the activity of de-escalation involves the use of tactics may be inappropriately interpreted as a lack of genuineness. However, many aggressive

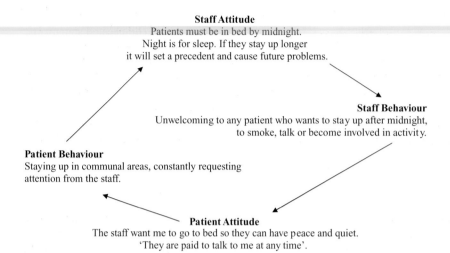

Staff Attitude
Patients must be in bed by midnight.
Night is for sleep. If they stay up longer
it will set a precedent and cause future problems.

Staff Behaviour
Unwelcoming to any patient who wants to stay up after midnight,
to smoke, talk or become involved in activity.

Patient Behaviour
Staying up in communal areas, constantly requesting
attention from the staff.

Patient Attitude
The staff want me to go to bed so they can have peace and quiet.
'They are paid to talk to me at any time'.

Figure 3.2. The attitude and behaviour cycle

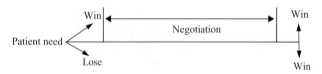

Figure 3.3. The win–lose/win–win equation

responses have areas of commonality, thus it is useful to hold a set of general de-escalating tactics that may be modified to suit the situation.

The attitude and behaviour cycle

This is probably one of the most difficult areas of de-escalation to develop. Many staff within inpatient mental health settings across the full spectrum of services will have fixed attitudes towards institutional rules and patient behaviour. These attitudes may exist at a conscious or subconscious level. These attitudes will affect the practitioner's behaviour and this will subsequently affect the attitude of the patient and in turn their behaviour. It is also fair to suggest that many patients will have preconceived attitudes towards hospitals and their staff, based on previous experience and stereo-typing.

This may be illustrated by the following example given in Figure 3.2.

It is clear from this illustration that in the hospital environment it is very easy to see the behaviour one is expecting, if one does not have a highly developed sense of self-awareness towards one's own attitudes and their effects on others. A positive attitude from staff is more likely to induce positive behaviour and interactions with patients.

The win–lose equation

Many of the situations that may lead to aggression involve a perceived conflict of interests between the patient and staff member. A drama is often enacted where one part is left with a feeling of loss and frustration. This general issue has been tackled by management theorists and has been described by Le Poole (1987) as the win–lose equation. In essence a win or lose scenario is created. It is the objective of the de-escalator to, as far as it is possible, negotiate a win–win situation. Figure 3.3 illustrates that basic situation.

A common situation in which a PICU patient may enter into the win or lose scenario is when negotiating with a patient to accept unwanted medication. If the patient is given the medication against his or her will, then he or she feels he has lost and the staff have won and aggression may result. Through the process of negotiation, a win–win is sought. One method of achieving this is during the process of negotiation, offer the patient choices over which he or she has control. In the case of the unwanted medication, an example would be to offer the patient time to consider the benefits of medication, and then to return to you with his or her decision. This is usually employed in the latter stages of de-escalation. The overall tactic is to create a feeling of empowerment (real or perceived) for the patient. Experience of using this tactic shows that in many cases the patient will return with a statement to the effect of, 'OK I will take it this time, but I want to speak to the doctor again before I take any more'.

Debunking

This is the process of debunking the need of the patient to make his or her point by the use of aggression. This may be achieved by unconditionally accepting the content of the patient's grievance (Maier 1996). For example, a patient makes that statement, 'I am bloody sick of being locked up here, just let me go home'. A debunking response may be, 'I don't blame you, I would feel frustrated too, let's sit down and discuss what is needed for you to go home'. The general principle here is to shift the patient's focus from confrontation to discussion. This tactic is particularly usefully in the early stages of de-escalation as a means of grabbing the patient's attention and confidence.

Aligning goals

A frequent precipitant to aggressive escalation is perceived as a state of affairs where the patient feels he or she has completely different goals to the staff. Examples of this include preventing a patient from leaving, the need to take medication and limit-setting with disturbed behaviour. It is very easy to

reinforce this perception by maintaining a linear focus on the issue of confrontation. If we look at the wider issues there may be far more common ground than there first appears. For example, the patient wishing to leave may feel in confrontation with the staff who are preventing him or her from doing so. During the de-escalation the staff may align these goals by saying, 'I want you to go home too, success for us is when you have no need for hospital, we are working towards this from the day you are admitted'.

Transactional analysis

The use of Berne's (1964) Transactional Analysis can be a useful strategy for de-escalating aggression (Farrell and Grey 1992). This involves a detailed understanding of three different contexts within which interaction takes place. These are defined by Berne as 'ego states' and during social intercourse they are in the form of the Parental, the Adult or the Child context. During the course of de-escalation the principle is to ensure that the ego state within which the de-escalator is interacting is complementary to the patient's ego state. Transactional Analysis is a large area of study in itself and courses in its use are recommended.

Conclusion

The model of de-escalation offered here comprises three separate but interdependent components, they are: assessment, communication and tactics (ACT). The ACT model should be considered as cyclical, requiring the de-escalator to remain fluid during de-escalation. During the course of de-escalation, it is necessary to continually revisit each component and ensure they all remain complementary to one other. This is illustrated in Figure 3.4.

Under each of the headings, tools have been suggested which experience has shown to be effective in the PICU setting. The list is by no means exhaustive, and each practitioner can modify the suggested tools to suit their own individual styles.

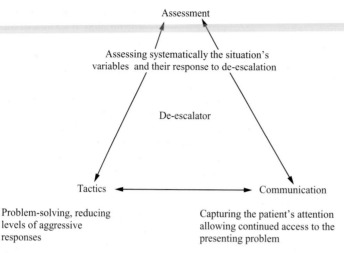

Figure 3.4. The ACT model

During this chapter the focus of de-escalation has been on the content of situations, rather than the psychopathology of the patient. There is good evidence that many aggressive responses are indeed precipitated by situations rather than being driven by purely psychiatric symptoms (Poyner and Warne 1986; Whittington and Patterson 1996; McDougall 1997). In many situations, psychotic and other psychiatric phenomena no doubt play a part in the aggressive responses of patients. However, in many cases these can be considered as one of many variables that need to be incorporated into the ACT model of de-escalation.

Training in the prevention of violence and aggression is finally being prioritised, but it must form part of a complete hierarchical system of responses that have to be regulated and evaluated centrally.

The nature of PICU and LSU care causes potential confrontation between those being cared for and those who provide care. The use of a model of de-escalation provides opportunity to avoid physical aggression, but it must be accepted that sometimes people detained against their will may use violence to facilitate their wants, and this must not routinely be viewed as a failure of the care-giver in the technique of de-escalation – it was ever thus.

REFERENCES

Bensley L, Nelson N, Kaufman J, Silverstein B, Shield J. 1995 Patient and staff views of factors influencing assaults on psychiatric hospital employees. Issues Mental Health Nursing 16: 433–446

Berne E. 1964 Games People Play: The Psychology of Human Relationships. Harmondsworth: Penguin

Betempts E, Somoza E, Buncher C. 1993 Hospital characteristics, diagnoses, and staff reasons associated with the use of seclusion and restraint. Hosp Community Psychiatry 44: 367–361

Blair D. 1991 Assaultive behaviour: does provocation begin in the front office? J Psychosoc Nursing Mental Health Serv, 29 (5): 21–26

Boettcher E. 1983 Preventing violent behaviour: an integrated theoretical model for nursing. Perspect Psychiatr Care 21 (2): 54–58

Cheung P, Schweitzer I, Tuckwell V, Crowley K. 1997 A prospective study of assaults on staff by psychiatric in-patients. Med Sci Law 37 (1): 46–52

Davis W. 1989 The prevention of assault on professional helpers. In: Howells K, Hollin C (eds) Clinical Approaches of Violence. Chichester: Wiley, pp. 311–328

Davis S. 1991 Violence by psychiatric in-patients: a review. Hosp Community Psychiatry 42 (6): 585–589

Farrell G, Gray C. 1992 Aggression: A Nurse's Guide to Therapeutic Management. London: Scutari Press

Frude N. 1989 The physical abuse of children. In: Howells K, Hollin C (eds) Clinical Approaches to Violence. Chichester: Wiley, pp. 155–181

Kaplan S, Wheeler E, 1983 Survival skills for working with potentially violent clients. J Contemp Social Work 339–346

Lanza M. 1988 Factors relevant to patient assault. Issues Mental Health Nursing 9: 259–270

Lanza M, Campbell R. 1991 Patient assault: a comparison of reporting measures. Qual Assur 5: 60–68

Le Poole S. 1987 Never Take No For An Answer: A Guide to Successful Negotiation. London: Kogan Page

Maier G. 1996 Managing threatening behaviour. The role of talk down and talk up. J Psychosoc Nursing 34 (6): 25–30

McDougall T. 1997 Coercive interventions: the notion of the 'last resort'. Psychiatr Care 4: 19–21

McHugh I, West M. 1995 Handle with care. Nursing Times. 91 (6): 62–63

National Institute for Clinical Excellence. 2005 Violence: The Short-Term Management of Disturbed/Violent Behaviour in Psychiatric Inpatient Settings and Emergency Departments. London: NICE

National Institute for Mental Health in England. 2004 Mental Health Policy Implementation Guide: Developing Positive Practice to Support the Safe and Therapeutic Management of Aggression and Violence in Mental Health Inpatient Settings. London: NIMHE

NHS Security Management Service. 2004 Conflict Resolution Training: Implementing the National Syllabus. London: NHS

Nyberg-Coles M. 2005 Promoting safer and therapeutic services. Mental Health Practice 8 (7): 16–17

Poyner B, Warne C. 1986 Violence to Staff: A Basis for Assessment and Intervention. London: HMSO

Stevenson S. 1991 Heading off violence with verbal de-escalation. J Psychosoc Nursing Mental Health Serv 36: 6–10

Turnball J, Aiken I, Black L, Patterson B. 1990 Turn it around: short-term management for aggression and anger. J Psychosoc Nursing 28 (6): 7–10

Webster C D, Douglas K S, Eaves D, Hart S D. 1997 HCR-20 Assessing Risk of Violence, Version 2. Burnaby: Simon Fraser University and Forensic Psychiatric Services Commission of British Columbia

Whittington R, Patterson P. 1996 Verbal and non verbal behaviour immediately prior to aggression by mentally disordered people: enhancing assessment of risk. J Psychiatr Mental Health Nursing 3: 47–54

4

Rapid tranquillisation

Caroline L. Holmes and Helen Simmons

Introduction

Violence is a continuing problem in both inpatient and outpatient psychiatry. Past authors have concluded that violence is no more likely in the psychiatric population than in the general population, but there is an increasing consensus that people with psychotic illnesses are more likely to exhibit violence in the community (Mullen 1988; Monahan 1992; Mulvey 1994; Swanson *et al.* 1996).

Violence in the psychiatric setting may be acute, as seen in a severely disturbed patient with paranoid schizophrenia or mania, or ongoing, as seen inpatients who are chronically psychotic or those with personality disorders. In the UK, the acutely violent patient should ideally be treated in a Psychiatric Intensive Care Unit (PICU) until more settled. In the context of acute violence on the ward, the primary concern is to ensure the safety of patients and staff and any intervention should be the minimum required to calm the patient. However, in many cases medication is needed.

Rapid tranquillisation (RT) has been defined as 'the use of psychotropic medication to control agitated, threatening or destructive psychotic behaviour' (Ellison *et al.* 1989). The NICE guidelines describe RT as drug treatment used to achieve a, 'reduction in agitation or aggression without sedation' (National Institute for Clinical Excellence; NICE 2005).

It should not be confused with rapid neuroleptisation (RN), which entails giving high loading doses of neuroleptics to achieve an early remission. There is no evidence that RN offers any therapeutic advantages over the use of standard doses while side-effects are significantly greater. It has been suggested that in the confusion between RN and RT, concerns about excessive doses and side-effects of antipsychotic medication have, in part, led to the introduction of different classes of drugs for RT such as benzodiazepines (Dubin 1988).

Several reviews of RT have been published (Dubin 1988; Sheard 1988; Ellison *et al.* 1989; Goldberg *et al.* 1989; Kerr and Taylor 1997). Goldney *et al.* (1986) looked at the use of high-dose neuroleptics in the PICU but did not look specifically at RT. It wasn't until Pilowsky's audit of RT that anyone made an attempt to systematically examine the use of RT in clinical practice (Pilowsky *et al.* 1992). It was noted that patients requiring RT tend to fall into two groups: those who require repeated injections due to persistent refusal of oral medication and resulting aggressive behaviour and those who require only one or two injections early on in their treatment (Pilowsky *et al.* 1992). This study and others that followed helped to inform the process towards the formation of a consensus of sorts regarding a hospital RT policy.

A hospital policy for RT should include a discussion of the indications for its use; namely, that patients are acutely disturbed and at high risk of

Psychiatric Intensive Care, 2nd edn., eds. M. Dominic Beer, Stephen M. Pereira and Carol Paton.
Published by Cambridge University Press. © Cambridge University Press 2008

harming themselves or others in the very near future, and that non-pharmacological interventions have been considered (these will be discussed later). According to the Royal College of Psychiatrists' paper on the Management of Imminent Violence (Royal College of Psychiatrists 1998), training for RT should involve assessment and monitoring of the risks associated with the procedure. These include the cardiorespiratory effects, knowledge of the need to prescribe within therapeutic limits and the need to titrate dose to effect. Training should also include working and training as a team using cardiopulmonary resuscitation techniques as well as being familiar with the use of flumazenil (NICE 2005). Ideally, violence should be anticipated and the use of alternative management strategies optimised. This will minimise the need for RT.

The use of RT

Staff should be aware of the procedures for RT before difficulties arise (Royal College of Psychiatrists 1998). NICE published guidelines for RT in 2005 that recommended, 'staff who use rapid tranquillisation should be trained in the assessment and management of service users specifically in this context'.

We will first focus on the practical steps and pitfalls which need to be faced when restraining an individual and giving them RT, and then a more detailed discussion of the choices of medication available. This section also includes a suggested template for a hospital RT policy.

Practical RT

The first step is to assess the situation with the multidisciplinary team. Safety is of paramount importance. Ensuring the patient, staff and other patients on the ward are safe allows further assessment to take place and may involve the need for physical restraint. Staff should be called in to help if needs be. There should be enough staff available so that a staff member is free to review with the doctor events leading up to the use of restraint, and to prepare medication. The doctor is present to manage the situation and to diagnose underlying conditions leading to disturbed behaviour, not to get involved in the restraining procedure itself. If there are not enough staff available, then either the patient should be allowed to leave and then the police called, or immediate assistance from the police should be requested.

Restraint

Voluntary application of restraint may be possible, e.g. by explaining to the patient that it is necessary to restrain them for their own protection and to prevent others from getting hurt. Ideally, there should be five nurses restraining: one person for each limb and one person to give orders and hold the head (Jacobs 1983). The patient should be held gently but firmly, on their back with one arm above their head and one arm by their side. They should be reassured, all procedures being explained during restraint, and should be able to respond to spoken messages throughout the period of sedation (Royal College of Psychiatrists 1998). If the patient appears to be asleep then 'more intensive monitoring is required' (NICE 2005). In this instance the Maudsley guidelines recommend the use of a pulse oximeter (Figure 4.1; Taylor *et al.* 2005; see below). Restraints should be checked to ensure good circulation to the limbs (Jacobs 1983). Staff should continue to observe the patient to see if they are continuing to struggle against restraint or whether the nurses have been able to relax their hold without the use of medication. Restraint on the floor should be avoided (NIMHE 2004), as should restraint in the prone position (Norfolk, Suffolk and Cambridgeshire Strategic Health Authority 2003).

A review of case notes is necessary to check for contraindications to medication or any organic complications that may be contributing to the present situation (NICE 2005). However, although establishing a differential diagnosis is extremely important, it should not delay intervention in a dangerous situation. If the patient does have an organic condition, further violence will worsen their physical health. In

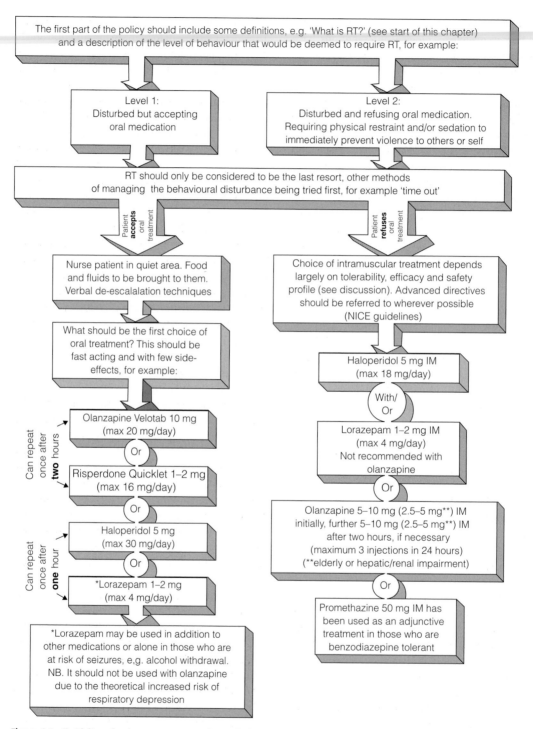

Figure 4.1. Guidelines for the management of acute behavioural disturbance and safe rapid tranquillisation. Adapted from the Maudsley Guidelines and intended as guidance only (Taylor *et al.* 2005)

situations leading up to restraint, non-verbal signals may be necessary, e.g. to indicate when to restrain, and these should be decided beforehand wherever possible.

If the patient is still aroused in spite of restraint, and staff members are unable to escort them to a safe environment without risk of injury to themselves or other patients, then RT is clearly necessary. Choice of drugs will depend on whether the patient has had antipsychotic medication previously and whether there is a history of severe extrapyramidal side-effects. The presence of complicating physical factors and the current physical and mental state of the patient will also be important. Clearly it will be impossible to examine a restrained patient adequately but, once the patient is calm, their physical state should be reviewed.

Monitoring

During and just before the administration of medication, vital signs should be measured including blood pressure, pulse and respiratory rate. Ideally, a pulse oximeter should be used to measure oxygen saturation. This is a non-invasive method for measuring oxygen saturation in arterial blood via a transmitter and detector placed on either side of a peripheral tissue such as a digit or earlobe. The tissue here is thin enough to allow visible red and infrared light transmission and it is the ratio between these two detected signals which is used to calculate oxygen saturation; oxygenated blood absorbing different amounts of light than deoxygenated (Jones 1995). Readings may be affected by tight clothing or tight restraint, which may affect blood flow. Nail varnish can interfere with digit readings and smokers can have raised carboxyhaemoglobin levels for up to 4 h after smoking, resulting in false readings (Sims 1996). At the start of RT, the oximeter is attached usually to a digit and the machine switched on. A baseline oxygen saturation is recorded. While treatment is given, the monitor shows continuously the oxygen saturation in the blood and should be observed closely. Blood pressure, pulse and respiratory rate should be recorded

every 5–10 min for the first hour, then half-hourly until the patient is back on their feet (Taylor et al. 2005). If a pulse oximeter is not available, respiratory rate should be monitored more closely (Taylor et al. 2005).

Facilities for mechanical ventilation and cardiac resuscitation should be readily available as should the benzodiazepine antagonist flumazenil. If the patient's oxygen saturation starts to drop then the attachment of the oximeter should be checked and the patient closely observed for falling respiratory rate, rising pulse and cyanosis. A sudden drop in saturation is an immediate indication to stop tranquillisation, as is a fall in systolic blood pressure to less than 80 mmHg, or diastolic to less than 60 mmHg. If the respiratory rate drops below 10 breaths per minute then 200 μg of flumazenil should be given intravenously (Taylor et al. 2005). It should be emphasised that the above are recommendations based on clinical practice and are suggestions only.

Choice of medication

Dubin, in his review of RT, suggested that the choice of drugs for RT should be in part dictated by the diagnosis of the underlying cause of the disturbed behaviour (Dubin 1988). He advised that schizophrenic patients should be given primarily neuroleptics possibly with the addition of a benzodiazepine to lower the dose of the neuroleptic required, but that manic patients should be given mainly benzodiazepines, and neuroleptics should only be used if these fail to control the situation. Patients with a history of substance abuse should receive benzodiazepines if the degree of agitation and violence is mild to moderate, but neuroleptics should be used in severe violence.

However, more recent opinion is that RT primarily controls behaviour (Ellison et al. 1989; Swanson et al. 1996) and hence there is no reason why benzodiazepines should not be used preferentially to achieve behavioural control, even if the patient has schizophrenia. A few studies have supported the use of benzodiazepines alone for RT (Bick and Hannah

1986; Modell 1986; Salzman 1988; Salzman *et al.* 1991), more recently for safety reasons (McAllister-Williams and Ferrier 2001).

The NICE guidelines state that the drugs of choice for RT should have a rapid onset and have few side-effects and hence advise using IM olanzapine, haloperidol or lorazepam (NICE 2005). They go on to say that such drugs should be used with caution because of the risk of loss of consciousness, oversedation with 'loss of alertness', possible damage to the therapeutic relationship and 'issues in relation to diagnosis' which are not specified. The risk of loss of consciousness is not to be taken lightly and is the reason why RT should always be the treatment of last resort and also that it should be carefully monitored. Monitoring and regular review will also allow for vigilance regarding revision of diagnosis, e.g. awareness of organic factors. However, surely if patients have become sufficiently disturbed to require RT such that they are presenting an immediate risk to themselves or others, some degree of mild sedation in the immediate aftermath would not be unexpected or unreasonable and would probably aid in the safe management of those patients in the ensuing hours. This does not mean of course that patients should be unconscious after RT. Pilowsky recommends the use of small bolus doses of medication titrated to the effect on the target symptoms, e.g. overt aggression, in order to minimise the risks of the procedure (Pilowsky *et al.* 1992).

The idea that one would worry about the therapeutic relationship between the patient and clinician in such a situation where RT is required is also unlikely, given that RT should only be given in the emergency situation where all other treatment options have been tried.

Benzodiazepines

Benzodiazepines were introduced as an alternative to neuroleptics for controlling acutely disturbed behaviour, as it was becoming clear that the use of neuroleptics in a dose necessary for sedation can result in severe extrapyramidal side-effects and postural hypotension.

Benzodiazepines, classically lorazepam IM or diazepam IV, are the drugs of choice in cases where organic factors have caused the disturbed behaviour, e.g. acute confusional states secondary to alcohol/drug withdrawal, infection, cerebral upset and epilepsy. They are widely used in conjunction with neuroleptics in RT to reduce the neuroleptic requirement.

Benzodiazepines should be administered very slowly and hence are better given IV to allow for titration of the dose. Generally, diazepam 10 mg IV (as Diazemuls®) or lorazepam 2 mg IM is used. Diazepam should never be given IM due to its prolonged and erratic absorption. The IV route is safe and effective (Lerner *et al.* 1979), and should be achieved via a large vein to minimise the risk of painful extravasation into the tissues and thrombophlebitis. Some concern however has been expressed about using the IV route in isolated units (Silva 1999).

Lorazepam has a short half-life with no active metabolites and is safer in liver impairment than diazepam, which has a longer half-life and has active metabolites, hence tending to accumulate with frequent administration. Clonazepam is used as maintenance treatment in epilepsy, but has also been found to be helpful in the treatment of agitation and arousal not responding to other treatment. Clonazepam also has a long half-life of (19–60 h compared with 8–24 h for lorazepam and 14–70 h for diazepam). From recent studies it appears that benzodiazepines, particularly clonazepam, are more useful than previously thought for the management of drug-induced agitation, for mania in combination with lithium and when used alone in mania without psychotic symptoms (Freinhar and Alvarez 1985).

Intramuscular lorazepam has been used alone in the management of the violent patient, even when psychosis is present, and found to be at least as effective as neuroleptics in controlling violent behaviour (Pilowsky *et al.* 1992). Arana *et al.* (1986) looked at fourteen psychotic patients treated with lorazepam alone and compared their progress with patients treated with lorazepam and haloperidol. They concluded that lorazepam is a useful treatment in the first 48 h, but that the initial improvement in psychotic symptoms is temporary and does not improve with increasing doses. Modell (1986) also found that lorazepam alone has limited use in maintaining improvement. However, Salzman *et al.* (1991) compared IM lorazepam with IM haloperidol and concluded that 2 mg of lorazepam may be better in RT than 5 mg of haloperidol. Midazolam, a rapid-acting benzodiazepine, has been used in doses of 1–3 mg IM in RT. It has a low incidence of side-effects and its intramuscular absorption is predictable (Mendoza *et al.* 1987).

Neuroleptics

Traditionally, sedative drugs such as chlorpromazine have been used for agitated patients but Kane's review of the treatment of schizophrenia points out that there is no evidence to show they are more effective in controlling aggressive behaviour than non-sedating drugs (Kane 1977). There are also many difficulties with their parenteral use in that IV administration is not always possible, due to problems titrating the dose and because of the numerous side-effects of sedating neuroleptics such as phenothiazines, some potentially fatal.

Haloperidol has been used most commonly in RT because its use in RT has been best evaluated. Droperidol was previously recommended for RT, then a study by Reilly *et al.* (2000) identified an association between droperidol, thioridazine and QT prolongation, which although appeared to be dose related occurred within the normal therapeutic dosing range. As a result droperidol has been withdrawn. This has up to very recently left only haloperidol to use for RT. In 2006 the Medicines and Healthcare Regulatory Authority (MHRA) reviewed the cardiovascular safety of all antipsychotic drugs. They concluded that there was good evidence that haloperidol prolonged the cardiac QTc interval; this is a known risk factor for arrhythmias and sudden cardiac death. Consequently, the requirement to conduct a baseline ECG was added to the Summary of Product Characteristics (SPC; product licence) for haloperidol. Although the situation with the use of haloperidol in RT is still evolving, it may be wise to use benzodiazepines alone if this is clinically acceptable. Promethazine is an alternative in benzodiazepine-tolerant patients.

If the potential benefit is thought to outweigh the risk, haloperidol can be given IV or IM; IV administration is more rapid and between 5 and 10 mg is given initially, and may be repeated after 10 min (IV) or 30 min (IM) if it has had no effect. The NICE guidelines recommend the IM route over the IV route as it is seen as safer. The guidelines state that the IV route should only be used in 'exceptional circumstances' (NICE 2005). Minimum doses of neuroleptics should be used and this is facilitated by concomitant use of benzodiazepines. The combination of haloperidol and diazepam has been particularly recommended due to its synergistic effect (Dubin 1988), although haloperidol and lorazepam are also highly effective. Small bolus doses should be given and there should be at least a 10-min wait between IV boluses or a 30-min wait if the IM route has been used. If there is concern about the possibility of extra pyramidal symptoms (EPS), either because the patient has a history of EPS or the patient is neuroleptic naive, then IM procyclidine (5–10 mg) should also be given.

Combined therapy with both neuroleptics and benzodiazepines has been successful. There has been no evidence of a higher incidence of adverse effects with this approach, and it may have therapeutic advantages. Kerr and Taylor (1997) have suggested two points in favour of a combination of benzodiazepines and neuroleptics. Firstly, the use of benzodiazepines allows a lower dose of the more toxic neuroleptic to be used and secondly, through their anticonvulsant effect, benzodiazepines may offset the lowering of the seizure threshold caused by neuroleptics. It has been shown in one survey that, when the combination is used, a second administration of medication is less likely and serious adverse effects are rare (Pilowsky *et al.* 1992). More recently IM lorazepam has been compared to IM haloperidol and promethazine in a randomised trial on 200 patients presenting to the emergency services, promethazine being used because of its sedating properties and its role in preventing dystonic reactions with haloperidol. Lorazepam 4 mg IM was found to be as effective in controlling agitated and aggressive behaviour as 10 mg haloperidol plus promethazine 25 or 50 mg mixed in the same syringe. However, the combination treatment resulted in a more rapid onset of tranquillisation and more individuals were rated as 'clinically improved'. As the authors themselves point out, one of the weaknesses of the study was that assessments at 2 h were not blind and because there were many raters inter-rater reliability may not be high (Alexander *et al.* 2004). But this study is yet another example of the positive effect of a combination treatment in RT.

However, the NICE guidelines advise that, wherever possible, a single drug should be used in preference to a combination in RT, yet somewhat confusingly they go on to state that where RT is 'urgently needed' a combination of IM haloperidol and IM lorazepam should be considered (NICE 2005). Since RT is by definition an urgent treatment, the advice on single treatment or combination treatment is by no means clear. It is possible that some confusion has been introduced between the use of RT for a psychiatric emergency and the use of medication to prevent the further deterioration of an agitated but not acutely disturbed or violent individual when by definition RT is not needed. However, as discussed above, the evidence for the benefits of combination treatment in RT remains.

With the increased spotlight on the QTc interval, the focus has turned to the new antipsychotics. Intramuscular olanzapine has potentially replaced droperidol and provided an alternative to haloperidol that is free of extrapyramidal side-effects. But how effective is it in RT? Studies appear to reveal a rapid onset of action, behavioural control without sedation and few side-effects (Wright *et al.* 2001; Meehan *et al.* 2001; Breier *et al.* 2002). However, it should be noted that the study group were acutely psychotic and agitated, but did not necessarily present with the degree of disturbance of those ordinarily requiring RT. Indeed, informed consent was required. A dose–response relationship was noted for IM olanzapine and a steady-state plasma con-

centration similar to oral, hence a maximum daily dose of 30 mg is advised for both oral and IM (Breier *et al.* 2002). However, a study looking at 'rapid initial dose escalation' found that individuals tolerated doses of up to 40 mg/day orally and that this achieved 'tranquillisation without sedation' (Baker *et al.* 2003). In this study the group were given 20 mg of olanzapine orally for 4 days, then for the next 2 days an additional 10 mg as required up to 40 mg/day was prescribed. Finally, for the next 2 days an extra 10 mg as required up to 30 mg/day was prescribed (Baker *et al.* 2003). Once again the study group was selected; in this case they all had been in hospital at least 5 days and a history of substance misuse was excluded. Some authors noted the limitations of oral olanzapine in RT, since patients remained alert although this has been described as an advantage in the NICE guidelines (NICE 2002 1.5.2). It was postulated that olanzapine provided rapid neuroleptisation, not RT. However it was suggested that oral olanzapine's apparent ineffectiveness may be because of its then lack of an intramuscular formulation and the 'inability to dose aggressively' (Karagianis *et al.* 2001). This especially since the *British National Formulary* (BNF) daily maximum for oral olanzapine remains at 20 mg. The intramuscular formulation is advised to be given as a 10-mg dose initially and a further 5–10 mg can be given in 2 h to remain within the BNF maximum of 20 mg/day whether oral or IM. Quite how this maximum can be maintained in an individual who is on regular olanzapine 20 mg orally who may require RT is not addressed. However, overall it is clear that olanzapine appears to be safe, fast acting and well tolerated.

Intramuscular ziprasidone has also been favourably compared to haloperidol in the treatment of 'acute agitation and psychosis' (Brook *et al.* 2000; Lesem *et al.* 2001). Once again a selected group was studied and there were many exclusions such as substance misuse or 'imminent risk of suicide or homicide'. As this is likely to be the population who are most at risk of requiring RT, it poses questions as to the validity of such studies. As with olanzapine, the studies provide a preliminary indication that the drug may be helpful, but its use in RT needs to be evaluated in a PICU setting and it is not available in the UK.

Clopixol Acuphase (zuclopenthixol acetate) has been purported to be useful in RT and has the advantage that its effect lasts for 2–3 days, thus avoiding repeated injections and further confrontations with a disturbed individual. It is an intermediate acting neuroleptic, lasting 72 h (peak 24–36 h). Dosage is between 50 and 150 mg. However, it can take up to 3 h to have an effect and the few controlled clinical studies available have given equivocal results (Coutinho *et al.* 1997) although three studies have suggested more intense and earlier sedation (Coutinho *et al.* 2000). Bourdouxhe *et al.* (1987) compared twenty patients given acuphase to thirteen patients given IM haloperidol, but found no difference with respect to effectiveness and side-effects between both groups. Baastrup *et al.* (1993) compared Acuphase with oral and IM haloperidol and conventional zuclopenthixol. They noted increased rigidity and hypokinesia in the first 24 h in the haloperidol group, but otherwise no differences between the treatments. However, they observed that Acuphase had an equal rapidity of action to the other treatments. Chouinard *et al.* (1994) also found Acuphase as effective as IM haloperidol, but observed an increase in dyskinesia in the Acuphase group.

These studies confirm Acuphase as an effective alternative to conventional IM medication. However, there is little evidence to suggest that it has fewer side-effects, although Fitzgerald (1999) makes the point that there are several advantages to Acuphase as a result of the reduced number of injections: less muscle injury, less psychological trauma because of less restraint, less physical injury and fewer breakthrough symptoms. The drug seems to have been evaluated in acute psychotic relapse, but not in the control of acute behavioural disturbance. A common problem with studies in this area is that many are conducted in 'acutely disturbed and disruptive individuals' without a clear definition of what constitutes such behaviour (Royal College of Psychiatrists 1998).

Overall Acuphase is not recommended for use in RT because its onset and length of action cannot always be predicted. For this reason it should never be given to a highly aroused, struggling patient because of potential adverse effects on the myocardium (see below). In addition, because the drug may have an onset of action between 20 min and 3 h after administration, it limits the safe use of further medication. It should also not be given to the neuroleptic-naive patient.

Both loxapine and thiothixene have been evaluated in RT. Tuason (1986) found 25 mg loxapine IM to be at least as effective as haloperidol 5 mg IM in the initial treatment of aggressive patients with schizophrenia and there was no difference between the two with regard to side-effects. Loxapine (25 mg IM) was compared to haloperidol (5 mg IM) and has also been compared to 10 mg IM thiothixene (Dubin and Weiss 1986). Both were found to be comparable in terms of efficacy and side-effect profile, but response to IM loxapine was faster. Molindone has also been used in RT. Thiothixene, IM loxapine and molindone are not available in the UK.

Chlorpromazine has been used extensively in the past to control agitated and aggressive patients due to its sedative properties. Cunnane's (1994) survey of consultant psychiatrists looked at their suggestions for medication, having been given the clinical vignette of a young schizophrenic patient in his first admission. The most frequent suggestion was chlorpromazine 100 mg IM (above BNF limits) repeated 1–6 hourly. This is no longer recommended. Man and Chen (1973) compared IM chlorpromazine with IM haloperidol and concluded that the incidence of hypotension with chlorpromazine was higher than reported and suggested using a test dose of 10 mg to test sensitivity, although suggesting that overall haloperidol was the safer drug to use in RT.

Following RT

The patient should be given an opportunity to discuss his/her experiences afterwards and should be

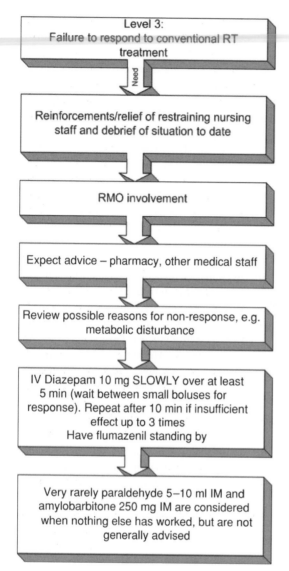

Figure 4.2. Guidelines for the management of acute behavioural disturbance refractory to conventional RT treatment. Adapted from the Maudsley Guidelines and intended as guidance only (Taylor *et al.* 2005)

given an explanation for the decision to use RT, both being documented (NICE 2005).

Unless the patient remains highly sedated, oral medication should be resumed. If oral medication is refused, then the patient can be managed on an oral/IM regime where, if oral dose is refused, the equivalent dose is given IM. This could be haloperidol. For example, 10 mg of haloperidol orally is equivalent to 5 mg IM. Olanzapine has been found to be well tolerated when making the transition from 10 mg IM to 5–20 mg oral per day. Incidentally, it has been noted that clinicians appear to have poor knowledge of equivalent doses and tend to overestimate the dose (Mullen *et al.* 1994).

Clopixol Acuphase can also be used following RT, although it should never be administered to a neuroleptic-naive patient. It is important to determine the patient's underlying diagnosis and also their legal status before giving an antipsychotic that could last up to 72 h. The efficacy of lithium and other mood stabilizers as acute antimanic agents should not be forgotten in the aftermath of RT. Short-term use of anxiolytics can also be helpful.

Dangers of rapid tranquillisation

As with any pharmacological intervention, RT is not without its hazards, and the clinician must assess the risk–benefit ratio of treatment. It is important not to underestimate the risks of inadequate tranquillisation, which in the violent patient can lead to harm to self and others. Other factors to consider include the patient's current treatment regimen and possible drug interactions, their age and physical state, and the proposed route of administration. RT, if administered with care and if there is good aftercare, is generally very safe, particularly when balanced against the risks of not medicating the patient.

To reduce risks inherent in the procedure, the patient should be securely restrained. Injecting a struggling patient can lead to inadvertent intra-arterial injection, nerve damage, and a higher than expected blood level of the drug due to increased bioavailability from IM or IV use (up to five times) and increased blood flow to the muscles (Thompson 1994). Highly aroused patients are also more sensitive to adrenergic and noradrenergic effects on the myocardium. Even restraint alone is not without risks, and it has been suggested that restraint in the prone position with tying of the ankles and hands leads to splinting of the respiratory apparatus. This can result in respiratory muscle fatigue and death due to positional asphyxia (Bell *et al.* 1992). David Bennet died as a result of his inability to breathe when he was restrained in the prone position for 25 min with no one to check the position of his head. The report recommended that the prone position should be avoided and whenever necessary should be no longer than 5 min (Norfolk, Suffolk and Cambridgshire Strategic Health Authority 2003). Following administration of medication, close monitoring including measurement of saturation with pulse oximetry gives early indication of hypoxaemia secondary to oversedation (Charlton 1995).

RT can cause both minor and major systemic complications. In Pilowsky's survey of 102 incidents of rapid tranquillisation, 70% of patients had no or only minor local complications with 30% reporting minor bruising, pain or extravasation. Cardiovascular or respiratory complications were seen in four cases, with only one of these being serious (Pilowsky *et al.* 1992). It was felt that the complications that did occur were related primarily to idiosyncratic drug reactions, predictable side-effects and interactions, and overmedication, of which the majority could have been prevented by adequate training in RT.

Goldberg *et al.* (1989) have also reviewed fully the other side-effects of rapid tranquillisation, which include local complications (bruising, pain or extravasation in up to 30% of patients), respiratory complications in 2%, cardiovascular complications in 3% (again particularly with phenothiazines) and seizures due to lowering of the seizure threshold.

Chlorpromazine is no longer recommended for parenteral administration as IV intravenous administration is not licensed and IM injection is painful. As mentioned above, parenteral chlorpromazine can also cause profound hypotension, particularly dangerous in the elderly and those with coronary artery disease, and has been associated with prolonged unconsciousness (Quenstedt *et al.* 1992).

Even where neuroleptics such as haloperidol have been found to be relatively safe to use in RT,

problems of sudden cardiac death and neuroleptic malignant syndrome have been reported (Konikoff *et al.* 1984; Huyse and van Schijndel 1988), emphasising the need for good aftercare of the patient, to ensure prompt intervention when necessary. Antipsychotics should not be used in a suspected case of phencyclidine (PCP) psychosis as they may precipitate anticholinergic psychoses.

Benzodiazepines are a recommended choice for RT in psychiatric emergencies due to their low toxicity, with diazepam and lorazepam being the two most frequently employed. However, withdrawal seizures can occur and benzodiazepines are associated with confusion, nausea, vomiting and oversedation, particularly in the elderly. In Modell's study of the use of lorazepam for behavioural control in 75 agitated patients, 50% of patients developed ataxia, and 25% experienced nausea and vomiting (Modell 1986). Benzodiazepines should only be used in the acute phase, and not for long-term management, as there is a high risk of dependence. In the practice of RT, the most serious complication of benzodiazepine use is respiratory depression due to sedation. All benzodiazepines are contraindicated in patients with pulmonary disease, as they depress hypoxic respiratory drive. As previously noted, respiratory depression can be reversed by the use of the benzodiazepine antagonist flumazenil. Flumazenil is not an easy drug to use and clear instructions should be easily accessible. For example, the half-life of flumazenil is short compared to the benzodiazepines used in RT and repeated doses may be required. Flumazenil may also precipitate withdrawal seizures in those with significant prior exposure to benzodiazepines (De la Fuente *et al.* 1980).

Other drugs previously used in psychiatric emergencies are no longer recommended. These include the barbiturates, which are associated with dependence, tolerance, hazardous drug interactions, profound hypotension and irreversible respiratory depression. Paraldehyde may be used where all other methods have failed, but it is painful when given intramuscularly and may cause profound respiratory depression. Its use is also associated with sterile abscesses and nerve damage. Paraldehyde should not be administered via plastic syringes. It should never be administered intravenously in the psychiatric setting.

The QTc debate

The QT interval varies with heart rate and so a drug that increases heart rate will decrease the QT interval and one that slows heart rate will lengthen the QT interval (Taylor 2003). Absolute QT intervals are difficult to interpret and, for this reason, QT is corrected for heart rate and called QTc. The normal QTc interval is less than 440 ms in males and 470 ms in females and varies with various factors including time of the day (Welch and Chue 2000; Taylor *et al.* 2005). Although it has been proposed that prolongation of the QTc interval is responsible for the rare appearance of torsade de pointes (TDP) (Wilson and Weiler 1984), a potentially fatal cardiac arrhythmia, there is no evidence for a direct link between QTc lengthening and the risk of TDP. Although the absolute relationship between drug-related lengthening of the QTc, the risk of TDP and sudden death is unclear (Glassman and Bigger 2001; Reilly *et al.* 2000; Taylor *et al.* 2005), TDP is a plausible mechanism for sudden death in the context of antipsychotic treatment (Reilly *et al.* 2000). In addition, not all drugs that lengthen the QTc interval cause TDP and not all drugs that cause fatal cardiac events lengthen the QTc interval (Glassman and Bigger 2001; Taylor *et al.* 2005). However, a large retrospective cohort study showed 'large relative and absolute increases in the risk of sudden cardiac death' in those on moderate doses of neuroleptics (Ray *et al.* 2001).

What drugs used in RT affect the QTc interval? Together with other phenothiazines, chlorpromazine has a quinidine-like effect on the myocardium and cardiac conduction system. However, chlorpromazine is not the only neuroleptic implicated in cardiac conduction abnormalities. Droperidol and thioridazine have been withdrawn because of their effects on prolonging the QT interval but many other neuroleptics currently in use have effects on the QTc interval; for example, haloperidol prolongs it but not to the same degree as thioridazine.

More is known about the cardiorespiratory effects of the newer antipsychotics because of the increased regulatory requirements (Taylor 2003). Sertindole was found to have a significant effect on the QTc interval such that it was implicated in a number of unexplained deaths and hence was withdrawn. However, it has been postulated that other new antipsychotics may be just as likely to prolong the QTc interval but the risk that sertindole presents may be a product of its effects on the QTc interval and on the heart rate (causing tachycardia; Taylor 2003). Olanzapine, quetiapine and risperidone are also known to prolong the QTc interval and ziprasidone rather more so, but there is no evidence that torsade de pointes is likely to be a serious problem (Glassman and Bigger 2001). Intramuscular olanzapine was compared to placebo with respect to its effect on the QTc interval and was not found to have any extra effect over placebo (David *et al.* 2002). However, the message is, 'at this point in time, an atypical antipsychotic without concern does not exist' (Glassman and Bigger 2001).

Current use of RT

Several studies have looked at the use of RT in everyday practice. Surveys of trainees (Ellison *et al.* 1989, Mannion *et al.* 1997) and of Consultants and Senior Registrars (Cunnane 1994; Simpson and Anderson 1996) have revealed worrying discrepancies. Generally, although most senior psychiatrists advised sensible drug regimes, 10% advised the use of Clopixol Acuphase in a neuroleptic-naive patient (Simpson and Anderson 1996), a practice not advised by the Royal College of Psychiatrists Consensus Statement (Thompson 1994). Only 15% of psychiatrists reported that their units had protocols for RT and only 48% reported that their juniors had received training in the use of RT.

Nearly 50% of psychiatrists felt that the BNF was unhelpful in providing advice about RT and that maximum doses stated in the BNF were not relevant to RT (Simpson and Anderson 1996). Mannion *et al.* (1997) found that 39% of trainees surveyed used doses within the high range and 24% prescribed more than one neuroleptic. The study also suggested that trainees tended to prescribe the same dose whether given orally or intramuscularly and had little knowledge of dose equivalents. Simpson and Anderson (1996) point out that the BNF does not report RT as an indication for the use of benzodiazepines. Moreover, it does not indicate clearly the best drugs to use in RT. Although the BNF cites tranquillisation as an indication for haloperidol, it does not give a consensus view and does not specify which drugs are *not* suitable for RT.

A recent study has looked at patient satisfaction in a PICU and found there was no significant association between patient dissatisfaction and experiencing side-effects of medication and receiving RT. However, patients who received RT at least once during their stay had significantly higher total side-effects than those who did not. In the group who received RT, patients who had a number of different antipsychotics experienced more side-effects than those who had monotherapy, and those who had Clopixol Acuphase had fewer side-effects than those given haloperidol (Hyde *et al.* 1998).

Alternatives to RT

Although psychotropic medication in the form of RT remains the mainstay of treatment for the aggressive patient, it should always be used in conjunction with psychological and behavioural techniques. Some patients may be amenable to psychological and behavioural strategies alone, although this has not been examined in a controlled manner. McLaren *et al.* (1990) have shown that even after other strategies have been used, up to 20% of patients in a locked ward setting still need enforced medication. However, a broad psychotherapeutic approach should still be encouraged.

Psychological and behavioural approaches to the aggressive patient include: decelerative/de-escalation techniques (Corrigan *et al.* 1993) (also known as talking-down), time out from reinforcement, and seclusion and restraint. Basic techniques

can be found in any textbook of nursing skills with a fuller discussion in Kidd and Stark (1995). Even if these skills do not prevent the administration of RT, they can help to preserve the therapeutic relationship and the safety of all involved.

De-escalation, also described as 'defusing' or 'talking down', has been defined as a set of verbal and non-verbal responses, which, if used selectively and appropriately, reduce the level of a person's hostility by reducing anger and the predisposition to assaultative behaviour (Leadbetter and Paterson 1995). It assumes a proactive approach to manage anger or aggression before a violent incident occurs. Unfortunately, there is not a standard method and little systematic research on the content of the current approaches.

In addition to de-escalation techniques, behavioural interventions may also be useful with the aggressive client (Corrigan *et al.* 1993). These include self-controlled time out, a technique based on operant principles. Patients undergo short-term removal for a few minutes from over stimulating situations, the emphasis being on their control over the process. A similar method involves the use of a low-stimulus environment, where staff support and counsel patients for a 15-min period in a specifically allocated quiet area. The successful use of such an area within a PICU has been described in the literature (Hyde and Harrower-Wilson 1994). Continuous observation may be another useful method for managing patients representing an acute risk. A continuous observation protocol provides several elements that may be important in reducing violent episodes including reduced stimulation, protection, intensive observation and an opportunity for therapeutic contact. It is also less restrictive than seclusion or restraints. Shugar and Rehaluk (1990) evaluated a continuous observation protocol and found brief episodes of observations for less than 72 h to be effective and practical. Clinical review should take place if more than 72 h of observation is required.

Physical restraint has also been advocated as a therapeutic procedure, with several authors discussing clinical guidelines for its use (Bursten 1975; Rosen and DiGiacomo 1978). Restraint may be applied by mechanical means (e.g. by leather straps) as described by Jacobs (1983). In the UK, physical restraint is most often seen in the form of 'control and restraint' (C&R), a term referring to a set of intervention skills involving wrist locks used by a team of trained staff to facilitate control of an assaultative patient. These techniques have been endorsed by professional nursing bodies in accordance with the Mental Health Act Code of Practice, which advises the use of 'the minimum necessary restraint to deal with the harm that needs to be prevented' (Department of Health and Welsh Office 1993). Thus, C&R is not perceived as a therapeutic procedure, although clinical experience suggests that it can sometimes act as one. The most important criterion for its use is that it must be performed by staff who are fully trained to apply it in a safe, rapid and effective manner.

The most restrictive of alternatives to RT is the use of seclusion, a topic fully discussed elsewhere in this book. It should not be confused with time out, which occurs with the patient's agreement and understanding as part of their care plan. Instead, seclusion is often an emergency measure used to contain or deal with a situation on a short-term basis. It differs from restraint in that all social contact and interaction is removed. The Mental Health Act Code of Practice defines seclusion as 'supervised confinement of a patient alone in a room which may be locked for the protection of others from significant harm' (Department of Health and Welsh Office 1993). The Code of Practice also gives guidelines for its use suggesting that this should be as infrequently as possible, for the smallest possible duration and only when alternative methods have failed. It does not advise use for those with a risk of self-harm or suicide. Surveys show that seclusion is used for a wide variety of conditions and behaviours (Mattson and Sacks 1978; Plutchik *et al.* 1978; Russell *et al.* 1986). It may also serve to contain staff anxiety as well as patient disturbance (Russell *et al.* 1986). However, there is little evidence to suggest that seclusion results in any long-term changes in behaviour, and the Code of Practice is careful to state that its use may be damaging to staff–patient relationships (Soliday 1985) and to the patient's mental state (Plutchik *et al.* 1978; Binder and McCoy 1985; Wadeson and Carpenter 1976).

Electroconvulsive therapy (ECT) may be another alternative to RT in the management of the acutely aggressive patient, particularly when the patient is only responding slowly to pharmacological methods. It has previously been described as an effective treatment of the positive symptoms of schizophrenia (Taylor and Fleminger 1980), although its principal benefit appears to be in speeding up the response to antipsychotics (Taylor 1993). ECT is also effective in mania; however, now it is recommended only for the treatment of severe depression, a prolonged or severe manic episode or catatonia (catatonic stupor or excitement being the reduction or increase in muscle tone and activity associated with schizophrenia or affective disorders) (NICE 2003). ECT cannot act as a replacement for RT in the emergency situation.

Legal considerations and advanced directives

The use of RT clearly involves infringement of an individual's civil liberties and hence the giving of medication to someone against their will is a decision not to be taken lightly. One has to consider the protection of patients' rights against the safety of others. An important issue is the patient's right to refuse treatment, debated in *Rogers* v. *Commissioner* in the USA (Gutheil 1985). The opinion of the court was that a committed mental patient is considered competent and has the right to refuse treatment until declared incompetent by a judge. If the patient is incompetent, then the judge decides the patient's most likely choice regarding medication, if the patient had been competent. The court stated that the only instance where antipsychotic drugs can be given without consent is in an emergency to prevent 'immediate, substantial and irreversible deterioration of a serious mental illness'. In all other situations, then the psychiatrist has to take the patient to court before compulsory treatment can be given.

Gutheil (1985) criticised the court's view of antipsychotic medication as 'extraordinary treatment' and also pointed out that the court's ruling assumed and could create an adversarial relationship between patient and doctor. In addition, the ruling would result in unnecessary delay in a patient's treatment and a longer stay in hospital. Other concerns were that the restriction of involuntary medication to severe behavioural emergencies would actually put others at risk because it would not allow medical staff to give treatment to avoid such incidents (Gutheil 1985; Moldin 1985). The court also suggested that in the case of 'predictable crises' the consent of the patient for treatment with antipsychotic drugs should be obtained when the patient is 'competent and calm' (Gutheil 1985).

Here then we see the appearance of the advance directive. Preparation of advance directives for RT specifically may be problematic in that a 'competent and calm' patient may find it difficult to accept that they might need RT (the possibility of violence seeming a remote event) and the discussion itself may be damaging to the therapeutic relationship. Also when an advance directive is prepared and violence occurs some time later, how valid is the consent given weeks or months previously? In some jurisdictions, consent can be given by a prearranged substitute, but this may result in undue delay (Fitzgerald 1999). The NICE guidelines, however, recommend the use of advance directives in the treatment of schizophrenia (NICE 2002) and some effort has been made to evaluate their impact (Papageorgiou *et al.* 2002; Henderson *et al.* 2004). Papageorgiou *et al.* (2002) found that the use of advance directives had no impact on subsequent compulsory admissions of fifteen patients when compared to a control group of sixteen. This was put down to lack of understanding of or ability to concentrate on the advance directive at recruitment, lack of insight and denial of the illness or simply failure to remember details of the advance directive one year down the line at follow-up (Papageorgiou *et al.* 2002). A later study comparing fourteen patients with advance directives with thirty-one controls did find that the use of advance directives reduced the number readmitted over the 15-month follow-up and also the number requiring compulsory admission (Henderson *et al.* 2004). Although the numbers involved are small, both studies seem to support the use of advance directives. However, Papageorgiou *et al.*'s study makes it clear that advance directives are not enough. There needs to be an appropriate level of staffing to be able to provide an ongoing dialogue about the patient's wishes, needs and understanding with respect to their illness (Papageorgiou *et al.* 2002).

Fortunately in the UK, few legal restraints on RT have been introduced and reasonable clinical judgement is accepted. Certain constraints do have to be kept in mind. Occasionally, RT may have to be given to a patient who is informal, hence treatment is given under common law. In this case, it is inadvisable to give longer-acting neuroleptics such as Clopixol Acuphase. Fitzgerald discusses the ethical issues of using an intermediate acting neuroleptic for RT such as Clopixol Acuphase and points out that although Acuphase acts beyond the time necessary for restraint, one could argue that it maximises the individual's autonomy by reducing the need for multiple injections (Fitzgerald 1999). However, at the pivotal point of the discussion is the discrimination between restraint and treatment. Short-acting IM medication could be considered as a form of 'chemical restraint' but Acuphase would certainly not fall into this category (Fitzgerald 1999).

Generally, a section of the Mental Health Act should be instituted as soon as possible. The same applies to a patient on Section 5(2) since this section is a holding order only. Close relatives should be informed about the giving of forced medication at the appropriate time and told why it was necessary.

Lord Donaldson clarified the indications for medical treatment under common law. Firstly, the doctor needs to assess the capacity to give informed consent; if the patient is unable to give consent, then the duty of the doctor is to treat the patient in his or her best interests, e.g. to save life. The doctor is deemed to have acted in the best interests of the patient if he or she acts in accordance with current practice by a responsible body of medical opinion.

The following statements cover RT under common law:

• That it is permissible to give treatment to a non-consenting capable patient who is suffering from 'a mental disorder which is leading to behaviour that is an immediate serious danger to himself or to other people' (Department of Health and Welsh Office 1993).

- 'Any patient whose mental disorder leads to such behaviour is unlikely to possess the high level of mental capacity that is required' (Jones 1996).

The ability to give informed consent obviously presents a problem for the assessing doctor.

A disturbed aggressive patient will not be able to cooperate in the assessment of competence, but could be assumed to be incompetent as above. But arguably, even if aroused and actively psychotic, the patient may be capable of giving consent.

Clearly, in RT, assessment of capacity presents a problem, although even if a patient is capable of giving consent, medication can be given if he or she is mentally ill and presenting a danger to others.

Rapid tranquillisation is a procedure that should not be carried out without consideration of alternatives. But as long as strict guidelines are followed with respect to a patient's rights, choice of medication and physical monitoring, then it remains a safe, acceptable procedure for controlling disturbed, potentially dangerous behaviour in mental illness.

Dedication

This chapter is dedicated to the memory of Professor Lyn Pilowsky. Lyn made outstanding contributions in the study of the psychopharmacology of schizophrenia, and was excellent at using her knowledge in the clinical setting, as well as imparting it to others. The practical approach in this chapter results from knowledge gained in a PICU setting under the direct supervision of Lyn Pilowsky.

REFERENCES

Alexander J, Tharyan P, Adams C, John T, Mol C, Philip J. 2004 Rapid tranquillisation of violent or agitated patients in a psychiatric emergency setting. Pragmatic randomised trial of intramuscular lorazepam v. haloperidol plus promethazine. Br J Psychiatry 185: 63–69

Arana GW, Ornsteen ML, Kanter FF, Friedman HL, Greenblatt DJ, Shader SI. 1986 The use of benzodiazepines for psychiatric disorders: a literature review and preliminary clinical findings. Psychopharmacol Bull 22(1): 77–87

Baastrup PC, Alhfors UG, Bjerkenstedt L et al. 1993 A controlled Nordic multicentre study of zuclopenthixol acetate in oil solution, haloperidol and zuclopenthixol in the treatment of acute psychosis. Acta Psychiatr Scand 87: 48–58

Baker RW, Kinon BJ, Maguire GA, Liu H, Hill AL. 2003 Effectiveness of rapid initial dose escalation of up to forty milligrams per day of oral olanzapine in acute agitation. J Clin Psychopharmacol 23(4): 42–348

Bell MD, Rao VJ, Weitli C, Rodriguez RN. 1992 Positional asphyxia in adults: 30 cases. Am J Forensic Med Pathol 13: 101–107

Bick PA, Hannah AL. 1986 Intramuscular lorazepam to restrain violent patients. Lancet 1(8474): 206

Binder RL, McCoy SM. 1985 Patients' attitudes towards placement in seclusion. J Nervous Mental Dis 173: 273–286

Bourdouxhe S, Mirel J, Denys W, Bobon D. 1987 L'acetate de zuclopenthixol et l'haloperidol dans la psychose aigue. Acta Psychiatr Belg 87: 236–244

Breier A, Meehan K, Birkett M et al. 2002 A double-blind, placebo-controlled dose-response comparison of intramusular olanzapine and haloperidol in the treatment of acute agitation in schizophrenia. Arch Gen Psychiatry 59: 441–448

Brook S, Lucey JV, Gunn KP for the Ziprasidone IM Study Group. 2000 Intramuscular ziprasadone compared with intramuscular haloperidol in the treatment of acute psychosis. J Clin Psychiatry 61(12): 933–941

Bursten B. 1975 Using mechanical restraints on acutely disturbed psychiatric patients. Hosp Community Psychiatry 30: 48–55

Charlton JE. 1995 Monitoring and supplemental oxygen during endoscopy. Br Med J 310: 886–888

Chouinard G, Safadi G, Beauclair L. 1994 A double-blind controlled study of intramuscular zuclopenthixol acetate and liquid oral haloperidol in the treatment of schizophrenic patients with acute exacerbation. J Psychopharmacol 14(6): 126–129

Corrigan PW, Yodufsky SC, Silver JM. 1993 Pharmacological and behavioural treatments for aggressive psychiatric inpatients. Hosp Community Psychiatry 44: 125–133

Coutinho E, Fenton M, Campbell C, David A. 1997 Details of studies of zuclopenthixol are needed (letter). Br Med J 315: 884

Coutinho E, Fenton M, Adams C, Campbell C. 2000 Zuclopenthixol acetate in psychiatric emergencies: looking for evidence from clinical trials. Schizophr Res 46: 111–118

Cunnane JG. 1994 Drug management of disturbed behaviour by psychiatrists. Psychiatr Bull 18: 138–139

David SR, Beasley CM Jr, Alaka K. 2002 QTc intervals during treatment with olanzapine in acutely agitated patients. Schizophr Res Suppl 53: 164

De la Fuente JR, Rosenbaum AH, Martin HR Niven RG. 1980 Lorazepam-related withdrawal seizures. Mayo Clin Proc 55(3): 190–192

Department of Health and Welsh Office. 1993 Code of Practice – Mental Health Act 1983. London: HMSO

Dubin WR. 1988 Rapid tranquillization: antipsychotics or benzodiazepines? J Clin Psychiatry Suppl 49: 5–12

Dubin WR, Weiss KJ. 1986 Rapid tranquillization: a comparison of thiothixene with loxapine. J Clin Psychiatry 47(6): 294–297

Ellison J, Hughes D, White K. 1989 An emergency psychiatry update. Hosp Community Psychiatry 40(3): 250–260

Fitzgerald P. 1999 Long-acting antipsychotic medication, restraint and treatment in the management of acute psychosis. Aust N Z J Psychiatry 33: 660–666

Freinhar JP, Alvarez WH. 1985 Use of clonazepam in two cases of acute mania. J Clin Psychiatry 46(1): 29–30

Glassman AH, Bigger JT Jr. 2001 Antipsychotic drugs: prolonged QTc interval, torsades de pointes and sudden death. Am J Psychiatry 158: 1774–1782

Goldberg RJ, Dubin WR, Fogel BS. 1989 Review. Behavioural emergencies, assessment of psychopharmacologic management. Clin Neuropharmacol 12(4): 233–248

Goldney RD, Spence ND, Bowes JA. 1986 The safe use of high-dose neuroleptics in a psychiatric intensive care unit. Aust N Z J Psychiatry 20: 370–375

Gutheil TG. 1985 Rogers v. Commissioner. Denouement of an important right-to-refuse-treatment case. Am J Psychiatry 142(2): 213–216

Henderson C, Flood C, Leese M, Thornicroft G, Sutherby K, Szmukler G. 2004 Effect of joint crisis plans on use of compulsory treatment in psychiatry: single blind randomised controlled trial. Br Med J 329:136–138

Huyse F, van Schijndel RS. 1988 Haloperidol and cardiac arrest. Lancet ii: 568–569

Hyde CE, Harrower-Wilson C. 1994 Psychiatric intensive care: principles and problems. Hosp Update May: 287–295

Hyde CE, Harrower-Wilson C, Morris J. 1998 Violence, dissatisfaction and rapid tranquillisation in psychiatric intensive care. Psychiatr Bull 22: 477–480

Jacobs D. 1983 Evaluation and management of the violent patient in emergency settings. Psychiatr Clin North Am 6(2): 259–269

Jones R. ed. 1996 Mental Health Act Manual, 5th edn. London: Sweet & Maxwell

Jones SE. 1995 Getting the balance right. Professional Nurse 368–373

Kane JM. 1977 Treatment of schizophrenia. Schizophr Bull 13(1): 133–156

Karagianis JL, Dawe IC, Thakur A, Begin S, Raskin J, Roychowdhury SM. 2001 Rapid tranquillization with olanzapine in acute psychosis: a case series. J Clin Psychiatry 62(2): 12–16

Kerr IB, Taylor D. 1997 Acute disturbed or violent behaviour: principles of treatment. J Psychopharmol 11(3): 271–277

Kidd B, Stark C (eds). 1995 Management of Violence and Aggression in Health Care. London: Gaskell

Konikoff F, Kuritzky A, Jerushalmi Y, Theodor E. 1984 Neuroleptic malignant syndrome induced by a single injection of haloperidol [letter]. Br Med J 289: 1228–1229

Leadbetter D, Paterson B. 1995 De-escalating aggressive behaviour. In: Kidd B, Stark C (eds) Management of Violence and Aggression in Health Care. London: Gaskell, pp. 49–84

Lerner Y, Lwow E, Levitin A, Belmaker RH. 1979 Acute high-dose parenteral haloperidol treatment of psychosis. Am J Psychiatry 136: 1061–1064

Lesem MD, Zajecka JM, Swift RH, Reeves KR, Harrigan EP. 2001 Intramuscular ziprasidone, 2 mg versus 10 mg, in the short-term management of agitated psychotic patients. J Clin Psychiatry 62(1): 12–18

Man PL, Chen CH. 1973 Rapid tranquillization of acutely psychotic patients with intramuscular haloperidol and chlorpromazine. Psychsomatics 14: 59–63

Mannion L, Sloan D, Connolly L. 1997 Rapid tranquillisation: are we getting it right? Psychiatr Bull 21(7): 411–413

Mattson MR, Sacks MH. 1978 Seclusion: uses and complications. Am J Psychiatry 135: 1210–1213

McAllister-Williams R, Ferrier IN. 2001 Rapid tranquillisation: time for a reappraisal of options for parenteral therapy. Br J Psychiatry 179: 485–489

McLaren S, Browne FWA, Taylor PJ. 1990 A study of psychotropic medication given as required in a regional secure unit. Br J Psychiatry 156: 732–735

Meehan K, Zhang F, David S *et al.* 2001 A double-blind, randomized comparison of the efficacy and safety of intramuscular injections of olanzapine, lorazepam, or placebo in treating acutely agitated patients diagnosed with bipolar mania. J Clin Psychopharmacol 21(4): 389–397

Mendoza R, Djenderedjian AH, Adams J, Ananth J. 1987 Midazolam in acute psychotic patients with hyperarousal. J Clin Psychiatry 48(7): 291–292

Modell JG. 1986 Further experience and observations with lorazepam in the management of behavioural agitation. J Clin Psychopharmacol 6(6): 85–387

Moldin SO. 1985 The effect of Rogers on forensic, emergency psychiatry. Am J Psychiatry 142(12): 1521–1522

Monahan J. 1992 Mental disorder and violent behaviour. Am Psychologist April: 511–521

Mullen P. 1988 Violence and mental disorder. Br J Hosp Med 40: 460–463

Mullen R, Caan AW, Smith S. 1994 Perception of equivalent doses of neuroleptic drugs. Psychiatr Bull 18(6) 335–337

Mulvey EP. 1994 Assessing the evidence of a link between mental illness and violence. Hosp Community Psychiatry 45(7): 663–668

National Institute for Clinical Excellence. 2002 Schizophrenia: Core Interventions in the Treatment and Management of Schizophrenia in Primary and Secondary Care. Clinical Guideline1. www.nice.org.uk

National Institute for Clinical Excellence. 2003 Guidance on the Use of Electroconvulsive Therapy. Technology appraisal 59. www.nice.org.uk

National Institute for Clinical Excellence. 2005 Violence. The Short Term Management of Disturbed/Violent Behaviour in Inpatient Psychiatric Settings and Emergency Departments. Clinical Guideline 25. www.nice.org.uk

National Institute for Mental Health in England. Mental Health Policy Implementation Guide: Developing Positive Practice to Support the Safe and Therapeutic Management of Aggression and Violence in Mental Health Inpatent Settings. 2004. London: Department of Health

Norfolk, Suffolk and Cambridgeshire Strategic Health Authority. 2003 Independent Inquiry into the Death of David Bennett. Cambridge: Norfolk, Suffolk and Cambridgeshire Strategic Health Authority. Available online at www.irr.org.uk/pdf/bennett_inquiry.pdf

Papageorgiou A, King M, Janmohamed A, Davidson O, Dawson J. 2002 Advance directives for patients compulsorily admitted to hospital with serious mental illness.

Randomised controlled trial. Br J Psychiatry 181: 513–519

Pilowsky LS, Ring H, Shine PJ, Battersby M, Lader M. 1992 Rapid tranquillisation. A survey of emergency prescribing in a general psychiatric hospital. Br J Psychiatry 160: 831–834

Plutchik R, Karasu TB, Conte HR, Siegal B, Jerret I. 1978 Toward a rationale for the seclusion process. J Nervous Mental Dis 166(8): 571–579

Quenstedt M, Ramsey R, Bernadette M. 1992 Rapid tranquillisation. Br J Psychiatry 161: 573

Ray WA, Meredith S, Thapa PB, Meador KG, Hall K, Murray KT. 2001 Antipsychotics and the risk of sudden cardiac death. Arch Gen Psychiatry 58: 1161–1167

Reilly JG, Ayis SA, Ferrier IN, Jones SJ, Thomas SHL. 2000 QTc-interval abnormalities and psychotropic drug therapy in psychiatric patients. Lancet 355: 1048–1052

Rosen H, DiGiacomo JN. 1978 The role of physical restraint in the treatment of psychiatric illness. J Clin Psychiatry 39: 228–232

Royal College of Psychiatrists. 1998 Management of Imminent Violence. Clinical Practice Guidelines to Support Mental Health Services. Occasional Paper OP41 March. London: Royal College of Psychiatrists

Russell D, Hodgkinson P, Hillis T. 1986 Time out: are disturbed patients secluded for purely clinical reasons? Nurs Times 82(9): 47–49

Salzman C. 1988 Use of benzodiazepines to control disruptive behaviour inpatients. J Clin Psychiatry 49(12) [suppl]: 13–15

Salzman C, Soloman D, Miyawaki E *et al.* 1991 Parenteral lorazepam versus parenteral haloperidol for the control of psychotic disruptive behaviour. J Clin Psychiatry 52(4): 177–180

Sheard MH. 1988 Review: clinical pharmacology of aggressive behaviour Clin Pharmacol 11: 483–492

Shugar G, Rehaluk R. 1990 Continuous observation inpatients: a critical evaluation. Compr Psychiatry 31(1): 48–55

Silva E. 1999 Rapid tranquillisation in isolated units, i.m. medication preferable to i.v. J Psychopharmacol 13: 200–201

Simpson D, Anderson I. 1996 Rapid tranquillisation: a questionnaire survey of practice. Psychiatr Bull 20(3): 149–152

Sims J. 1996 Making sense of pulse oximetry and oxygen dissociation curve. Nursing Times 92(1): 34–35

Soliday SM. 1985 A comparison of patient and staff attitudes towards seclusion. J Nervous Mental Dis 173: 273–286

Swanson JW, Borum R, Swatrz MS, Monahan J. 1996 Psychotic symptoms and disorders and the risk of violent behaviour in the community. Criminal Behav Mental Health 6: 309–329

Taylor D, Paton C, Kerwin R. 2005 The South London and Maudsley NHS Trust Prescribing Guidelines, 8th edn London: Martin Dunitz

Taylor DM. 2003 Antipsychotics and QT prolongation. Acta Psychiatr Scand 107: 85–95

Taylor P, Fleminger JJ. 1980 ECT and schizophrenia. Lancet, 1(8183): 1380–1382

Taylor PJ. 1993 Mental illness and violence. In: Taylor PJ (ed) Violence in Society. London: Royal College of Physicians

Thompson C. 1994 Consensus statement: the use of high-dose antipsychotic medication. Br J Psychiatry 164: 448–458

Tuason VB. 1986 A comparison of parenteral loxapine and haloperidol in hostile and aggressive acutely schizophrenic patients. J Clin Psychiatry 47(3): 126–129

Wadeson H, Carpenter WT. 1976 Impact of the seclusion room experience. J Nervous Mental Dis 163: 318–328

Welch R, Chue P. 2000 Antipsychotic agents and QT changes. Rev Psychiatr Neurosci 25(2): 154–160

Wilson WH, Weiler SJ. 1984 Case report of phenothiazine induced torsade de points. Am J Psychol 141: 1265–1266

Wright P, Birkett M, David S *et al.* 2001 Double-blind placebo-controlled comparison of intramuscular olanzapine and intramuscular haloperidol in the treatment of acute agitation in schizophrenia. Am J Psychiatry 158(7): 1149–1151

5

Pharmacological therapy

Chike I. Okocha

General principles

In the past few decades, drugs have become the cornerstone of treatment for mental disorders. With the refinement of diagnostic categories and the development of newer drugs it has become important to have guidelines underpinning such treatments.

These guidelines are largely based on assumptions such as the existence of:

- clear-cut diagnostic categories
- effective drug treatments
- disorders that are either life-long or represent life-long vulnerabilities

A further important assumption is that exacerbations and recurrences are unfavourable for patients, their families and society.

In intensive care psychiatry, treatment goals are generally short-term although, where appropriate, long-term goals can also be set. These goals are to reduce symptoms as rapidly as possible; build an alliance for long-term management; educate the patient and their families about the illness, its treatment, and its course (treated and untreated); and lay the groundwork for a return to premorbid levels of functioning.

Effective strategies for achieving these goals include:

- the use of medication in adequate doses for adequate durations before abandoning a drug trial
- avoiding polypharmacy where possible

- optimising long-term drug treatment regimes
- combining drug treatment with psychological treatment strategies, and providing systematic psycho-education for patients and their families

Although the ideal duration of treatment for mental disorders remains debatable, it is generally accepted that almost all acute treatments should continue for at least 6 months, and with disorders such as schizophrenia it may take 18 months, until symptom remission. Furthermore it is recommended that a discrete 6-month period of remission passes before tapering of therapeutic medication commences.

In the longer term, the primary goals of treatment are to aid return to premorbid levels of functioning and prevent relapse, as this results in symptom exacerbation as well as impairment in social and occupational functioning. In patients where the benefits of continuing long-term medication outweigh the risks, it is important to aim for the minimal effective dose while continuously monitoring side-effects and life circumstances. It is also beneficial to maintain contact with families and carers to maximise compliance and reduce the burden of living with someone with a chronic psychiatric illness.

Use of neuroleptics

The term 'neuroleptic' was originally coined to describe drugs that had the capacity to alter neuronal

Psychiatric Intensive Care, 2nd edn., eds. M. Dominic Beer, Stephen M. Pereira and Carol Paton.
Published by Cambridge University Press. © Cambridge University Press 2008

activity, but the term is now used almost exclusively to describe drugs with antipsychotic potency. The modern era of the use of such drugs started in the 1950s with the introduction of chlorpromazine. Since that serendipitous discovery, a number of other drugs have also been discovered. More recently, however, drugs with more clearly defined receptor sites of action and, as a consequence, better adverse effect profiles have been manufactured.

Although the biochemical effects of antipsychotics are known in some detail, the relationship between these effects and therapeutic properties is often unclear. Their use is largely, therefore, empirical rather than wholly evidence based. They are not generally curative but accelerate recovery and prevent or postpone relapse in the course of major illnesses.

Antipsychotics are now classified into two groups: older or so-called classical, conventional or typical antipsychotics and the newer atypicals. The atypicals are distinguished from typicals, at least clinically, by lacking extrapyramidal motor side-effects. They are also arguably more efficacious in the treatment of negative, affective and cognitive symptoms.

In using antipsychotics, it is important to remember that their pharmacokinetic properties determine their bioavailability. Orally administered drugs are influenced by factors such as gastric motility and emptying and first-pass metabolism in the liver. For example, only 30%–60% of orally administered chlorpromazine reaches the general circulation compared to parenteral administration. Other factors influencing bioavailability are frequency of administration, lipophilicity and protein binding. The breakdown of drugs can be influenced by genetic factors – as is the case with the oxidative metabolism of risperidone, which is subject to genetic polymorphism – or the drug itself, as with chlorpromazine which induces its own metabolism.

Antipsychotic drugs have a number of uses, which can broadly be grouped as follows:

- calming of disturbed patients ('tranquillisation') with a range of diagnoses, such as schizophrenia, mania and organic mental disorders
- treatment of acute symptoms of psychotic illnesses (of various aetiologies)

- treatment of mood disorders
- provision of maintenance treatment in psychosis
- treatment of symptoms of anxiety disorders

They are also used in the management of personality disorders such as emotionally unstable personality disorder (borderline personality disorder). These indications are described individually below.

Tranquillisation

This refers to the practice of rapidly loading medication to decrease behavioural agitation when other non-drug strategies have failed. Patients with psychosis do sometimes become acutely disturbed for a variety of reasons, including their abnormal experiences, and may endanger themselves or others at such times. This practice does not in any way refer to an attempt to rapidly 'treat' the underlying cause of psychosis, e.g., schizophrenia.

Antipsychotics alone, or in combination with benzodiazepines, are typically administered parenterally to patients for their calming effects (Chapter 4). The choice of antipsychotics and benzodiazepines varies and depends to a large extent on local policy. The butyrophenone haloperidol is now commonly used, since the withdrawal of droperidol; note that haloperidol too has been associated with QTc prolongation necessitating an electrocardiogram (ECG) prior to prescribing. It is used alone or in combination with diazepam or lorazepam. The use of chlorpromazine has been limited because of its potential to cause postural hypotension. Olanzapine Velotab® alone or in combination with a benzodiazepine is used sometimes when oral administration is preferred or judged clinically appropriate. It is likely that the introduction of the intramuscular formulation of olanzapine in 2004 will result in its use in most patients especially those who are very sensitive to the unpleasant side-effects of conventional or typical antipsychotics (Meehan *et al.* 2001; Breier *et al.* 2002). Although not available in the UK, the intramuscular formulation of ziprasidone is also used for rapid tranquillisation.

In patients with an established history of antipsychotic treatment, zuclopenthixol acetate with or without a benzodiazepine should be considered. This short-acting depot lasts for up to 72 h and may reduce the need for repeated confrontation with reluctant or struggling patients.

Acute psychosis

Psychosis is characterised by loss of touch with reality which may manifest as hallucinations, delusions, bizarre behaviour and disorders of thought. Its underlying causes include detectable brain disease, such as may result from a head injury, dementia, or psychoactive substance abuse, and psychiatric disorders such as schizophrenia, affective disorder and various other brief disorders.

The use of antipsychotic drugs in the treatment of acute psychosis aims to alleviate psychotic symptoms and shorten the acute episode of illness. Several 'typical' and 'atypical' antipsychotics are now available. The antipsychotic potency of the typical antipsychotics was thought to depend entirely on dopamine-2 (D_2) receptor blockade in the mesolimbic and cortical areas of the brain. Similar blockade of basal ganglia dopamine receptors in excess of about 75% results in extrapyramidal symptoms especially parkinsonism. The newer 'atypicals', however, do not have such a high affinity for D_2 receptors but appear to have affinity for other receptor types, particularly serotonin receptors. They all share a high 5-HT_{2A}: striatal D_2 receptor blockade ratio (Kapur and Remington 2000).

Irrespective of mode of action, there is no convincing evidence that any one drug or class of drugs, except clozapine, is more effective than another. Despite this equal efficacy across classes of drugs, patients do not respond equally to all classes and it is difficult to predict to which drug a patient will respond. This differential response is thought to be genetically determined and is the subject of intense research by pharmacogeneticists and pharmacogenomists (visit www.pharmgkb.org for more information). The choice of drugs seems to be determined largely by side-effects, which differ from drug to drug or class to class. Equally important is a previous history of response to a particular antipsychotic.

Therapeutic response with lessening of symptoms is observed in up to 3–4 weeks following the onset of treatment.

Treatment of mood disorders

The role of antipsychotics in the treatment of severe depressive disorder with psychosis is well established. Also, antipsychotics are often used as adjunctive treatment of bipolar disorder. These patients often have psychotic symptoms and manic patients, in particular, present with delusions, irritability, agitation or aggressive and violent behaviour. The use of antipsychotics in these patients can, in a proportion of patients, reduce the delay between the onset of treatment and response to it. In addition to their antipsychotic potency, clinical trials and open label studies suggest that atypical antipsychotics such as risperidone, olanzapine, ziprasidone (not available in the UK) and quetiapine are effective for the treatment of mania and have mood-stabilising effects (Lakshmi and Yatham 2003). Olanzapine and quetiapine are of course licensed for the treatment of acute mania associated with bipolar disorder.

Maintenance treatment in psychosis

The use of antipsychotics in the maintenance treatment of psychosis is aimed at the prevention of relapse or worsening of psychotic symptoms and disability. About 80% of untreated patients with schizophrenia relapse. Maintenance treatment is, therefore, indicated but it raises issues about antipsychotic dosage and the length of time patients should be exposed to antipsychotics to minimise the risk of long-term side-effects, especially tardive dyskinesia.

Two commonly adopted strategies are:
- the intermittent or targeted approach where antipsychotics are withdrawn and then reintroduced at the first symptomatic signs of psychosis;
- the fixed low-dose approach where treatment is continuous with a low dose of medication in combination with close follow-up (Schooler 1991; Kane and Marder 1993)

Both strategies have their critics and are not thought to be very successful at preventing relapse (Schooler 1991; Kane and Marder 1993). Studies on patients with schizophrenia have shown that 75% of patients who switched to placebo after a year of being symptom-free relapsed within 6–24 months. This is in contrast to a relapse rate of 23% in patients receiving continuous antipsychotic medication (Hegarty *et al.* 1994). The strategy used will depend largely on the patient's history but close collaboration with the patient over medication strategies and doses may enhance their engagement.

The advantages and disadvantages of oral medication are well rehearsed as are those for depot antipsychotics. It is argued that the use of low-dose depot medication, as opposed to oral medication, may have additional benefits in terms of relapse prevention (Davis *et al.* 1994). The use of atypical antipsychotics for long-term maintenance has not yet been fully validated but there are no reasons to suggest that they are not effective. Early observations with Risperdal Consta®, the first injectable atypical antipsychotic, has shown that only half of the sample of patients in our study achieved some improvement on the clinical global impression scale (change) at 6 months. Although half of these patients improved at 3 months it is possible that further improvements will occur over time with this injection (Paton and Okocha 2004). Drug treatment must be combined with appropriate psycho-socio-educational strategies to achieve maximum benefits (Bellack and Mueser 1993; Mortimer 1997).

Alleviation of symptoms of anxiety

Some antipsychotics, in much smaller doses than are used in psychoses, are useful as sedatives particularly in patients who are likely to become dependent on benzodiazepines (Okocha 1996). Thioridazine (Mellaril®), which was particularly favoured in this regard, is no longer widely used because of cardiac side-effects. Small doses of flupenthixol hydrochloride (Fluanxol®), up to 3 mg a day, and chlorpromazine 50–100 mg are also effective. Although these drugs do not pose the same problem of dependence as benzodiazepines, they can cause acute side-effects such as akathisia and dystonia and, in the longer-term, dyskinesias. The benefits of using them should therefore be weighed against these risks. The use of sedative atypical antipsychotics such as olanzapine that are not licensed for anxiety disorders and do not cause these side-effects may increase.

Alleviation of symptoms in personality disorders

Personality disorders are generally considered to represent the extremes of normal variation in personality traits and not illness per se. Borderline personality disorder, as currently defined, is perhaps the nearest to illness of all the personality disorders. It has been described as bordering psychotic illness, affective illness, impulse control disorders and post traumatic disorder. It is characterised by affective instability, chronic feelings of emptiness, transient stress-related paranoid ideas, suicidal and self-harming behaviours, inappropriate intense anger, impulsivity, unstable intense interpersonal relationships, identity disturbance and frantic efforts to avoid abandonment (American Psychiatric Association 1994).

Borderline personality disorder is common amongst psychiatric inpatients with a prevalence rate of 15% or so (Winston 2000) and a suicide rate of 10% (Paris 2000). Many of these patients are referred to the intensive care unit as a result of their challenging behaviour. Treatment guidelines such as those of the American Psychiatric Association recommend psychotherapy as first-line tratment. However, psychotropic medications are often prescribed off-license for these patients, mostly for the control of three common symptom clusters: transient psychotic symptoms, affective instability and impulsivity. In reviewing the evidence that underpins the use of psychotropic drugs, Paton and Okocha (2005) found that polypharmacy is likely to be high due to a high initial placebo response that is often short-lived. Patients usually respond to a range of antipsychotic drugs but low-dose flupenthixol seemed to help patients with multiple suicide attempts and clozapine those who are aggressive and repeatedly engage in self-harming behaviour. Divalproex and lithium are more promising than carbamazepine for mood-related symptoms.

Choice and adverse effects of antipsychotics

As there are no significant differences between antipsychotics in terms of efficacy, the choice of drug in clinical practice depends to a large extent on the anticipated side-effect profile of the drug and the previous response to treatment. Other factors of importance are patient characteristics, diagnosis and the clinician's knowledge of available drugs. Considering the prevalence of side-effects in patients prescribed antipsychotics, it is important that these are discussed. Side-effects, particularly akathisia, weight gain, sexual dysfunction and the unpleasant feeling of dysphoria, tend to reduce compliance.

Typical antipsychotics consist of drugs in a number of chemical groups:
- the phenothiazines, which are grouped on the basis of the side-chain, e.g. aliphatic (chlorpromazine), piperidene (thioridazine) and piperazine (fluphenazine, trifluoperazine)
- the thioxanthenes, e.g. flupentixol and thiothixene
- the butyrophenones, e.g. haloperidol
- the diphenylbutylpiperidines, e.g. fluspirilene and pimozide

These drugs cause a range of side-effects: those that are predictable from the pharmacology of the drugs and those resulting from an allergic or idiosyncratic response. Dopamine-blocking effects underlie some adverse effects and blockade of other receptors most of the others.

Extrapyramidal syndromes

These consist of a range of reactions that are mostly well defined although occasionally atypical. They occur at different times during treatment: some early, others later.

Acute dystonia develops within 1–2 days of exposure to antipsychotics or on increasing the dose. Approximately 10% of patients are affected. With depot formulations, it may take 3 days to develop. It usually affects young males and may involve the tongue, lip and jaw although the trunk and limbs can also be affected. Treatment is by parenteral anticholinergic medication.

Akathisia is a subjective sense of restlessness accompanied by ceaseless movements of the hands or feet with repeated standing or pacing. It occurs in 20%–25% of patients taking antipsychotic drugs. To the inexperienced, it can be mistaken for increasing agitation. Akathisia has been associated with aggression, both towards others and self directed. Benzodiazepines, cyproheptadine or a beta-adrenoceptor blocker such as propranolol may provide relief. Anticholinergic drugs are not particularly beneficial.

Parkinsonism is perhaps the most common extrapyramidal side-effect and ranges from bradykinesia in its mildest form, to akinesia with rigidity, festinant gait, crouched posture, coarse tremor, hypersalivation and seborrhoea. It is more common in women and the elderly and can be confused with apathy, depression or dementia. Its onset is usually in the first month of treatment and it tends to lessen with time, after dose reduction or anticholinergic drug administration. The common practice of concomitant administration of an anticholinergic drug with an antipsychotic, in the absence of this side-effect, is not advisable as it worsens the anticholinergic side-effects of the antipsychotic such as dry mouth and constipation, and is liable to abuse for its euphoriant effects.

Tardive dystonia and dyskinesia are long-term extrapyramidal side-effects of antipsychotic use. Tardive dystonia is relatively rare, with a prevalence of about 2%, and typically presents as a craniofacial syndrome in younger patients. Tardive dyskinesia, however, is more common with a prevalence of 15%–25% or more, and starts months or years following antipsychotic medication although non-drug-related cases in the elderly have been reported. Relevant risk factors for its development are female sex, affective disorder, organic brain disease, parkinsonian side-effects during acute treatment, alcohol abuse, negative symptoms of schizophrenia and increasing age. It usually presents as choreoathetoid movements of the mouth and face but the trunk and limbs can also be affected. Its precise aetiology is unclear and theories abound. It is thought that using the smallest possible dose of antipsychotics and treating for short periods, if practicable, are likely to minimise the risk of developing tardive dyskinesia. The treatment of tardive dyskinesia is difficult and strategies that have been tried include dose reduction, benzodiazepines such as clonazepam as muscle relaxants, tetrabenazine (a dopamine-depleting agent), vitamin E (a free radical scavenger) and lithium. In severe cases, switching to clozapine should be considered. It is wise to examine for abnormal movements before prescribing antipsychotic drugs and to review patients every 6 months. If necessary, use of the Abnormal Involuntary Movement Scale (AIMS) should be considered.

Neuroleptic malignant syndrome

This is perhaps the most dangerous neuromuscular adverse effect of typical and atypical antipsychotics. There are case reports of neuroleptic malignant syndrome (NMS) following the use of clozapine, risperidone, olanzapine and quetiapine. In moderate to severe cases, the incidence in antipsychotic-treated patients is in the range of 0.2%–1%, although milder cases are often unrecognised. Symptoms often develop early in treatment or are associated with rapid upward dosage titration.

The key clinical features are:
- hyperthermia
- muscle rigidity
- varying degrees of unconsciousness
- labile hypertension
- sweating
- tachycardia
- elevated creatinine phosphokinase (CPK)

The hyperthermia is thought to be mediated by dopaminergic systems in the striatum and hypothalamus and is fatal in 20% or so of patients. More serious cases can result in death from shock, renal failure (with myoglobinuria), respiratory failure, or disseminated intravascular coagulation. The treatment of this condition is by cooling, rehydration and specific drug treatments to counter muscle stiffness and promote dopamine activity. Dopamine agonists such as bromocriptine and amantadine and the antispasticity drug, dantrolene, are useful specific treatments although the precise regimen for use in this condition remains to be established.

Other side-effects of antipsychotics

- Anticholinergic effects, e.g. blurred vision, dry mouth, constipation and difficulty with micturition
- Sedation, which varies between drugs
- Postural hypotension, reflex tachycardia, and delayed ejaculation result from α_1-adrenergic antagonism
- Endocrine effects such as an increase in prolactin level due to dopaminergic blockade may cause galactorrhoea (and amenorrhoea), and loss of libido in men
- Neuropsychological effects include impairment of coordination, attention and memory, and the emergence of secondary negative symptoms or antipsychotic-induced deficit syndrome, which is sometimes indistinguishable from depression. This can cause patients' compliance to falter
- Granulocytopenia and other blood dyscrasias
- Cardiac irregularities and a lowering of epileptic fit threshold are other less common side-effects

Increased weight gain associated with atypical antipsychotic therapy deserves special mention as it is distressing for patients and can lead to discontinuation of treatment. It occurs in up to 60% of patients and has implications for cardiovascular health. Obesity is associated with the development of type II diabetes mellitus, hypertension and hyperlipidemia, all of which increase the risk of coronary heart disease (Fontaine *et al.* 2001).

Clozapine appears to present the greatest risk for increased weight, with olanzapine following closely. Risperidone appears to be associated with less weight gain and quetiapine a modest increase. Ziprasidone, which is not available in the UK is not associated with significant weight gain (Allison *et al.* 1999). The mechanisms underlying antipsychotic-mediated weight gain remain elusive. Affinity for the $5-HT_{2C}$ receptor, which is involved in the modulation of hunger and satiety, has been implicated as has the dysregulation of the polypeptide hormone leptin, which modulates eating behaviour and energy metabolism.

There is a ninefold higher incidence of type II diabetes in patients with schizophrenia and bipolar disorder compared to the general population. The reasons for this increase are not clear but may include the use of antipsychotics, with atypicals resulting in a 9% greater incidence of diabetes than typical antipsychotics (Sernyak *et al.* 2002). Although weight gain is implicated in the aetiology of diabetes, atypical antipsychotics may also have direct effects on glucose metabolism.

Use of 'high-dose' antipsychotics

High-dose antipsychotic treatment can be defined as the use of a dose in excess of the upper limit recommended by the *British National Formulary* (BNF) or the product data sheet produced by the manufacturers of the antipsychotic (Thompson 1994). There remains some uncertainty about whether low- or high-dose antipsychotics are the most appropriate treatment for psychosis (McEvoy *et al.* 1991). Studies with high doses have shown little evidence of superior effectiveness in the treatment of psychosis, with a similar proportion of patients responding to high and standard doses (McCreadie and MacDonald 1977; McCreadie *et al.* 1979; Kane and Marder 1993). It is thought, however, that about 10%–20% of schizophrenic patients may require higher than recommended doses of medication but there is no effective way of identifying this subgroup (Little *et al.* 1989).

Indiscriminate use of higher than necessary doses of antipsychotics, which will have initial sedative benefits, may produce more potentially bothersome side-effects of dystonia, extrapyramidal syndrome and general dysphoria that correlate with poor compliance and, therefore, poor long-term outcome (Barnes and Bridges 1980; King *et al.* 1995). Other serious adverse effects include cardiac arrhythmias (Fowler *et al.* 1976) and sudden death (Mehtonen *et al.* 1991; Jusic and Lader 1994).

The Royal College of Psychiatrists' consensus statement on the use of high-dose antipsychotic medication (Thompson 1994) notes that there are three main circumstances in which high doses are commonly used and advises alternatives to the use of such high doses.

These circumstances are:
- psychiatric emergencies
- acute treatment
- long-term treatment

In the latter, high-dose use seems to be largely driven by treatment resistance, polypharmacy, where two or more drugs are prescribed concurrently, and limited resources in inpatient units.

In a recent national audit of antipsychotic prescribing in the UK (the author was the psychiatrist member of the audit team of the Research Unit of the Royal College of Psychiatrists) we found that of a total of 3132 patients receiving antipsychotics on the audit date, 47% were receiving more than one antipsychotic drug concurrently (polypharmacy). Approximately 20% were receiving antipsychotic medication in doses exceeding the BNF upper limit (high dose). In 6% of these patients the high-dose prescription was due solely to a single antipsychotic and in the remaining 14% it was due to polypharmacy (Harrington *et al.* 2002a; 2002b). We found that the three most common reasons, which were not mutually exclusive, advanced for multiple prescribing (polpharmacy) were:
- a single antipsychotic drug failed to control the patient's symptoms (76% of cases)
- two or more drugs were needed to treat an acute exacerbation (38)
- the patient was being switched from one antipsychotic drug to another (27%)

As these reasons were not mutually exclusive, it follows in some patients that two or more of these reasons were present (Lelliott *et al.* 2002).

Although the use of high doses is to be discouraged, they may be necessary in some patients (Hirsch and Barnes 1994). In such cases, high doses should be used with caution and under specialist guidance. The Royal College of Psychiatrists has set out guidelines and suggestions for such prescribing. These guidelines are considered good practice and should minimise the risk of litigation. They include the need to:

- seek consent from the patient
- discuss the treatment with a specialist colleague
- undertake investigations before initiating treatment and review these as appropriate, and check vital signs regularly

Dose increases should be slow and regular reviews of the treatment must be instituted so that the dose can be reduced to an acceptable level as soon as possible (Hirsch and Barnes 1994; Thompson 1994).

Atypical antipsychotics

There is no consensus view about the definition of an atypical antipsychotic (Meltzer 1991). This group of drugs has become important over the last decade, although the prototype, clozapine, was first synthesised in 1959.

Atypical antipsychotics have been described as:

- Producing an antipsychotic action at doses that do not cause significant acute or subacute extrapyramidal side-effects, such as parkinsonism and akathisia. Using this definition, it follows that substituted benzamides such as remoxipride and sulpiride are atypicals
- Being associated with a reduced risk of tardive dyskinesia
- Having low dopamine receptor occupancy in clinically effective doses
- Having a high $5HT_2:D_2$ affinity
- Failing to increase serum prolactin levels (except substituted benzamides, zotepine and risperidone)

- Having improved efficacy in negative symptoms and treatment-refractory patients. Only clozapine has proven efficacy in refractory illness

Apart from clozapine, which remains the most efficacious treatment in otherwise refractory patients, there are no clear clinical differences between the atypicals. Clozapine is effective in at least 30% of schizophrenic patients who had failed to respond to at least two trials of antipsychotic drugs of different classes (treatment-resistant) when given for 6 weeks (Kane *et al.* 1988). After 1 year, up to 60% respond.

Despite the above definition of atypical antipsychotics, there is emerging evidence of adverse effects such as extrapyramidal symptoms, tardive dyskinesia and neuroleptic malignant syndrome. Further, many have metabolic adverse effects such as weight gain, hyperlipidemia, hyperglycemia and diabetes mellitus. It is important therefore that patients are monitored for these adverse effects and continuation of treatment balanced against these risks.

The following is a brief account of atypical antipsychotics, based on chemical grouping and in vitro receptor binding profile, and covers relevant prescribing information, side-effects and precautions.

Clozapine is a dibenzapine tricyclic and is chemically related to loxapine. It has a spectrum of action across a range of receptor types: D_1, $5HT_2$, $5HT_6$, $5HT_7$, adrenergic α-1 and α-2, H_1 and ACH. It has a low D_2 receptor occupancy of 30%–60%. Clozapine is licensed for the treatment of people with schizophrenia who are intolerant of conventional antipsychotics due to adverse effects or who fail to respond to them. Clozapine should be started at a low dose and ideally be used as monotherapy. The dose should be increased gradually and ideally administered in two divided doses because the half-life is 12–16 h. The maximum daily dose is 900 mg. Response to clozapine in antipsychotic-resistant patients may not be evident until after 6 months or more has elapsed (Meltzer 1992). Blood levels may be useful in optimising therapy if no response occurs. A good response is more likely when the level is above 350 ng/ml (Taylor and Duncan 1995; Cooper 1996; Perry *et al.* 1998).

Clozapine causes agranulocytosis in up to 1% of patients, a rate higher than that found with standard antipsychotics (about 1:2000). The great majority of these cases occur between 1 and 5 months into therapy (Atkin *et al.* 1996). Regular blood monitoring through the manufacturers (Novartis, Ivax or Denfleet) aims to reduce this risk. Weekly blood counts are required in the first 18 weeks of treatment, followed by 2-weekly counts until 1 year and then monthly checks thereafter.

Clozapine causes sedation, sialorrhoea and postural hypotension. It can cause epilepsy (Wilson and Claussen 1994) especially in doses of over 600 mg a day where the risk is approximately 5% (Devinsky *et al.* 1991). It has been proposed that patients on such doses should be routinely commenced on the anticonvulsant drug sodium valproate.

Some patients who may benefit from clozapine treatment refuse to cooperate with blood tests, oral medication or both. It is important to fully explore reasons for refusal and work with the patient to encourage adherence to treatment (Pereira *et al.* 1999).

Risperidone is a benzisoxazole derivative and, like clozapine, is a potent antagonist of $5HT_{2A}$, $5HT_7$, α-1 and 2 adrenergic, and histamine H_1 receptors. It does, however, have a higher D_2 receptor affinity than clozapine but its potency as an antagonist at D_1 receptors is low. Because it produces hyperprolactinaemia, extrapyramidal side-effects (EPSEs) at higher doses (Marder and Meibach 1994), and a somewhat inconsistent benefit in negative symptoms, some have disputed its place as an atypical (Cardoni 1995).

Risperidone is metabolised in the liver to an active metabolite, 9-hydroxyrisperidone, which has a half-life of 17–22 h. In doses of 4–8 mg/day, it appears to be at least equivalent and possibly superior to haloperidol, 10–20 mg/day, in decreasing positive and negative symptoms (Castelao *et al.* 1989; Claus *et al.* 1992; Chouinard *et al.* 1993; Marder and Meibach 1994). Common adverse effects of risperidone are insomnia, anxiety, agitation, sedation, dizziness, rhinitis, hypotension, weight gain and menstrual disturbances. It has been reported to

cause neuroleptic malignant syndrome and careful observation is therefore advised (Sharma *et al.* 1995). Unlike clozapine, no special monitoring is required with risperidone. Further, risperidone is now available in an injectable form with dosages of 25 mg, 37.5 mg and 50 mg administered every fortnight.

Olanzapine is a thienobenzodiazepine similar in structure to clozapine. It has a high affinity for several of the 5HT receptor subtypes, α-1 adrenoreceptors, histaminergic and muscarinic receptors. It has a weak affinity for D_2 receptors compared to typical antipsychotics but more than clozapine (Reus 1997).

Olanzapine is well absorbed after oral administration and reaches peak blood levels in 5–8 h. It is metabolised to inactive metabolites by the liver mostly via CPY1A2. In a number of studies, it was at least as effective as haloperidol, in a range of doses (5–20 mg), and caused a similar frequency of EPSE to placebo (Beasley *et al.* 1996a, 1996b, 1997; Tollefson *et al.* 1997). Serum level measurements are now readily available and may be necessary in patients for whom there may be a problem with compliance.

Apart from use in pregnant or breast-feeding women and patients with narrow-angle glaucoma there are no contraindications to the use of olanzapine. Common side-effects are drowsiness and weight gain which can be significant. Others are anticholinergic effects such as dry mouth and constipation, dizziness, peripheral oedema and postural hypotension. Asymptomatic elevation of liver enzymes has been reported (Beasley *et al.* 1996b) and it may therefore be necessary to perform a baseline liver function test and re-check this after treatment with olanzapine has started.

Quetiapine has a broad receptor binding profile with low to moderate affinity for D_1, D_2, $5HT_{1A}$ and $5HT_{2A}$ receptors, moderate affinity for α-1 and α-2 adrenoceptors, and high affinity for histamine-1 receptors. A number of double-blind randomised trials have shown it to be as effective as conventional antipsychotics in the treatment of schizophrenia (Hirsch *et al.* 1996; Markowitz *et al.* 1999). Trials have shown that the incidence of EPSEs in patients taking quetiapine was similar to those taking placebo across the full dosage range (150–750 mg). The most frequent side-effects reported from short-term controlled trials included sedation (17.5%), dizziness (10%) and constipation (9%). Quetiapine does not raise serum prolactin levels. It is contraindicated in breast-feeding mothers. Quetiapine has been associated with the development of cataracts in laboratory animals and there have been a small number of reports in humans (causality has not been determined).

Treatment dosage is usually in the range of 300–450 mg a day in two divided doses with a maximum dosage of 800 mg. However, the average dose for the treatment of mania is 600 mg/day with a higher therapeutic dose range of 400–800 mg/day compared to schizophrenia.

Substituted benzamides, e.g. sulpiride, amisulpride and remoxipride, comprise a group of drugs classified as atypicals because of their selectivity for limbic or cortical dopamine receptors rather than striatal dopamine receptors. They therefore have a considerably reduced potential for EPSEs but do, however, raise serum prolactin.

Sulpiride is a very well established drug in the UK, having been around for about a decade. It is specific for dopamine D_2, D_3 and D_4 receptors. Maximum dosages differ for patients depending on whether they present with positive or negative symptoms. Positive-symptom patients should be treated with doses of up to 2.4 g a day; negative symptom patients, 800 mg a day.

Amisulpride also has a high affinity for D_2 and D_3 receptors predominantly at limbic sites. It is commonly prescribed in France and seems to be effective against negative symptoms when used in low doses such as 100 mg a day (Boyer *et al.* 1995; Loo *et al.* 1997), although no more effective than low-dose haloperidol. EPSEs and raised prolactin are dose-dependent.

Zotepine is also available in the UK. It has a complex pharmacology. Zotepine causes hyperprolactinaemia, EPSEs at higher doses and precipitates epilepsy.

Ziprasidone is a potent D_2 and $5HT_2$ receptor antagonist which is not yet available in the UK. It is reported to have an effect on comorbid anxiety

and depression (Tandon *et al.* 1997) and has a low propensity to cause weight gain. It, however, causes somnolence in 20% of patients.

Aripiprazole was launched in the UK in 2004. In terms of the pharmacodynamics it is reported to have a high affinity for dopamine D_2 and D_3 receptors, serotonin $5HT_{1A}$ and $5HT_{2A}$ receptors, and moderate affinity for dopamine D_4, serotonin $5HT_{2C}$ and $5HT_7$, α-1 adrenergic and histamine H1 receptors. Its antipsychotic effect is thought to result from a combination of partial agonist activity at D_2 and $5HT_{1A}$ receptors and antagonistic activity at $5HT_{2A}$ receptors. This unique receptor affinity profile is thought to be responsible for its reported efficacy against positive and negative symptoms of schizophrenia and the low rates of side-effects. The incidence of movement disorders, weight gain and general adverse side-effects was low in clinical trials. Also, reductions in plasma prolactin, glucose and lipids were reported in clinical trials. Nausea and postural hypotension seem to be the most problematic side-effects (Goodnick and Jerry 2002). Drug interactions with other agents used in psychiatric populations can occur due to induction or inhibition of cytochrome enzymes in the liver. These include elevation of blood levels with fluoxetine, which inhibits CYP2D6, and reduced blood levels with carbamazepine due to induction of CYP3A4. The effective treatment dose ranges from 10 to 30 mg/day.

Paliperidone ER is the newest atypical antipsychotic that was launched in the UK in 2007. It differs from the atypical antipsychotic risperidone by the addition of a hydroxyl group and has a high affinity for $5HT_{2A}$ receptors and D_2 receptors from which it rapidly dissociates after binding. This rapid dissociation from D_2 receptors is thought to permit antipsychotic effect without movement side-effects or hyperprolactinaemia (Kapur and Seeman 2001). Given by mouth, paliperidone ER uses the osmotic-release oral system (OROS) technology that steadily delivers the drug over a 24-h period thereby reducing peaks and troughs in plasma level and making single daily dosing possible. In double-blind placebo-controlled studies lasting 6 weeks, paliperidone ER reduced psychotic symptoms (Davidson *et al.* 2007; Kane *et al.* 2006) with side-effects occurring in 2% or more patients. These side-effects included headache (13%), akathisia (6.5%), extrapyramidal disorder (5.4%), somnolence (4.9%), dizziness (4.8%) and sedation (4.2%). Continued use of paliperidone ER in stabilised patients also improved their ability to maintain symptom control and delayed their time to relapse (relapse rate, 48.5% for paliperidone vs 77.9% for placebo). All patients had previously received paliperidone during an 8 week initiation period (3–15 mg flexibly dosed, with a 9 mg starting dose) and stabilised with an additional 6 weeks of therapy at the same dose. The trial was terminated early because of findings from an interim analysis that demonstrated the drug's long-term therapeutic efficacy (Kramer *et al.* 2007).

Paliperidone ER has limited first-pass metabolism through the cytochrome P450 pathway and as such is likely to have little interaction with drugs metabolised by this route. Furthermore, no dose adjustment is required in patients with mild to moderate hepatic impairment. It is available in 3, 6, and 9 mg tablet strengths with a recommended dosing of 9 mg.

Treatment resistance

There is no firm agreement about the definition of treatment resistance. It is, however, accepted by most to mean a lack of satisfactory clinical improvement despite the use of at least two antipsychotics from different chemical classes prescribed at an adequate dose for an adequate duration (Brenner *et al.* 1990). A much stricter criterion, proposed by Kane (1992), requires the patient to have had several treatment trials for over 6 weeks with different antipsychotics in doses of over 500 mg chlorpromazine equivalents per day. Daniel and Whitcomb (1998) argue for a multi-axial classification of treatment resistance that focuses attention on specific target problems in the belief that this may be more helpful in directing treatment. They suggest the following target problems: misdiagnosis or comorbidity; positive symptoms,

negative symptoms, and agitation; treatment intolerance due to side-effects; and poor compliance.

About one-third of patients with schizophrenia do not respond to conventional or classical antipsychotics. This non-response, by which is meant the continuation of symptoms with considerable functional disability and or behavioural disturbance (Brenner *et al.* 1990), is commoner in patients with negative symptoms, aggressive behaviour, cognitive impairment and comorbid mood symptoms.

Strategies for the management of treatment resistance include ensuring compliance and increasing insight into dose–response relationships, dosage adjustment, change of antipsychotics and augmentation with other drugs or treatment methods (Daniel and Whitcomb 1998).

Compliance issues

It is important to ensure that patients are compliant with their medication as poor compliance contributes significantly to poor response and prognosis (Kemp *et al.* 1996). It appears to be perpetuated by lack of insight, psychosis and intolerable side-effects. Two other important factors are a complicated drug regimen and poor follow-up. It may be necessary to measure the plasma level of some drugs to check compliance and, where applicable, therapeutic levels. A review of the patient's diagnosis, drug regimen and follow-up programme may be required.

High-dose antipsychotics

The use of high doses of conventional or typical antipsychotics is discussed above. This is arguably the most common treatment approach for the treatment-resistant patient (Hirsch and Barnes 1994). There have been a number of anecdotal and controlled reports supporting such an approach although not all studies favour high doses (Ital *et al.* 1970; Rifkin *et al.* 1971; Quitkin *et al.* 1975). The use of high doses must be guided by the patient's response and should be reviewed on a regular basis. In the absence of clinical improvement, a medication review is needed.

Atypical antipsychotics

Atypical antipsychotics are worth trying, particularly clozapine which is licensed in treatment-resistant illness. A number of open design studies suggest that risperidone in modest doses of 4–8 mg/day is effective in treatment-resistant patients. However, studies that have compared risperidone to clozapine have reported inconsistent findings: some reported similar efficacy, others significantly less (Bersani *et al.* 1990; Chouinard *et al.* 1994; Cavallero *et al.* 1995; Sharif 1998).

Clozapine is an established treatment for this group of patients. About 30% of patients improve after 6 weeks of treatment and up to 60% improve after 1 year. It has been suggested that a clozapine plasma level of over 350 ng/ml distinguishes responders from non-responders (Perry *et al.* 1991; Hasegawa *et al.* 1993; Lieberman and Kane 1994; Potkin and Bera 1994). There is no evidence for a therapeutic window and some patients respond at plasma levels below 350 ng/ml. It may, however, be prudent to exceed the recommended maximum daily dose of 900 mg if the plasma level of clozapine is less than 350 ng/ml and the patient is free of major side-effects (Hasegawa *et al.* 1993). Closer monitoring will, of course, be required.

The usefulness of combination treatments is being researched in patients who do not respond to clozapine. Of particular interest are combinations of clozapine with electroconvulsive therapy or risperidone. No robust data are currently available in favour of either combination. The primary literature must always be consulted before using such combinations, as additional side-effects have been reported.

Adjunctive treatments

Adjunctive treatments have been in use in treatment-resistant patients for some time. Most of these strategies were in use before the availability of drugs such as clozapine, for the treatment of this recalcitrant population. They are, however, useful in a number of patients.

Antidepressants

Research into the aetiology and treatment of post-psychotic depression, negative symptoms, and antipsychotic-induced akinesia indicates that a small group of patients responds to adjunctive tricyclic antidepressants (Siris *et al.* 1991; Meltzer 1992). Newer selective serotonin-reuptake inhibitors (SSRIs) are also beneficial (Geoff *et al.* 1990). It is suggested that the $5HT_{1A}$ agonist buspirone may also be beneficial (Brody *et al.* 1990). However, further research is needed to establish the role of buspirone in the treatment of these patients. In practice antidepressants are recommended if significant symptoms of depression exist.

Lithium

Lithium has been used for over two decades for the effective treatment of patients with manic-depressive psychosis. A number of studies have reported a reduction in symptoms in patients who have been given lithium in addition to conventional antipsychotics (Carman *et al.* 1981). Patients with significant affective symptoms or those diagnosed as suffering from schizoaffective disorder seem to particularly benefit (Biederman *et al.* 1979; Hirschowitz *et al.* 1980). The combination of lithium with high doses of haloperidol should be avoided as neurotoxicity may result (Cohen and Cohen 1974).

Propranolol

Some studies have examined the usefulness of propranolol in addition to antipsychotics in treatment-resistant schizophrenia. Some report improvement (Yorkston *et al.* 1977; Lindstrom and Persson 1980) whereas others do not (Myers *et al.* 1981). Dosages in these studies are large and range from 400 to 2000 mg a day. It is, however, difficult to predict which patients will respond or indeed what dose of propranolol to use. Furthermore, propranolol increases the plasma levels of antipsychotics and may therefore lead to considerably more side-effects (Peet *et al.* 1980).

Carbamazepine

Carbamazepine in combination with antipsychotics may be beneficial to some patients with schizophrenia, particularly those with EEG abnormalities, a history of violence or aggression, or manic symptoms (Hakola and Laulumaa 1982; Klein *et al*. 1984; Luchins 1984). The risk of lowering antipsychotic plasma levels, probably through induction of hepatic enzymes, should be borne in mind as this may require an increase in the dose of the antipsychotic. Carbamazepine should not be combined with clozapine as it may increase the risk of bone marrow depression.

Electroconvulsive therapy

The use of ECT in schizophrenia is a long-established practice although available evidence indicates that it is not as effective as medication (Salzman 1980). In treatment-resistant patients, it may improve symptoms in about 5%–10% of cases, but the response is usually short lived and maintenance treatments may be required. Response is better in patients with a long history of illness, significant affective symptoms, or catatonia (Meltzer 1992).

Others

Benzodiazepines are other agents proposed for the treatment-resistant patient. Benzodiazepines have not resulted in consistent improvement and can produce violent behaviours in some patients (Karson *et al*. 1982). Advocates suggest modest improvement (Wolkowitz *et al*. 1992). Their use should, however, be limited to the anxious patient who has not responded to other management strategies. The risk of abuse and dependence should always be borne in mind.

Anxiolytics and other medications

Anxiety is a commonly used word which is defined as 'uneasiness of the mind and concern about imminent danger' (The Concise Oxford Dictionary 1995).

It is common in the day-to-day life of virtually everyone. Anxiety disorder, however, implies excessive, severe and prolonged anxiety, which compromises normal functioning. The prevalence of moderate to severe anxiety in the general population ranges from 2.5% to 6.5% depending on definition and gender (Weissman and Merikangas 1986; Kessler 1994). This pathological anxiety, which occurs in a range of clinical states, often requires treatment.

Range of anxiety disorders

Although most psychiatric disorders, such as schizophrenia and organic brain syndromes, may be associated with pathological anxiety requiring treatment, only the group of disorders that share the subjective, physiological and behavioural features of anxiety are grouped under the term 'anxiety disorders'. The tenth edition of the International Classification of Diseases (ICD10) groups these disorders under 'neurotic, stress-related, and somatoform disorders' (F40-F48). They include:
- phobic anxiety disorders such as agoraphobia, social and specific phobias
- panic disorder
- generalised anxiety disorder (GAD)
- obsessive-compulsive disorder (OCD)
- post-traumatic stress disorder (PTSD)
- adjustment disorder with anxiety (and depression)

Management

The treatment of anxiety disorders depends on the type and severity of the disorder as well as other associated factors, which will be evident from the assessment of the patient. Non-pathological anxiety and panic attacks rather than panic disorder, which are attributable to an identifiable stress, can effectively be treated with reassurance about symptoms, counselling, and relaxation techniques.

Patients with anxiety disorders typically require both psychological treatment, aimed at addressing any underlying problems, and drug treatment for the relief of symptoms. For a significant number of these patients, drug treatment may be indicated initially before the patient can participate effectively in psychological treatment, especially when depression is present (Okocha 1996).

Drug treatments

Available drugs for the treatment of anxiety disorders include: benzodiazepine and non-benzodiazepine anxiolytics, antidepressants, beta-blockers and antipsychotic drugs.

Benzodiazepines

These drugs, which are very effective anxiolytics, were for many years the mainstay of treatment but the risk of dependence has now greatly limited their use (Okocha 1995). They do, however, still have a role in the management of some patients. The benefits of treatment must be weighed against the risk of dependence in individual cases. Patients with incapacitating GAD, panic disorder or PTSD may benefit from an initial course of a benzodiazepine, e.g. diazepam (6 mg in divided doses) or lorazepam (1–4 mg a day), to control their symptoms until longer-term drug treatment and psychological therapy become effective.

The triazolobenzodiazepine, alprazolam, which has a different chemical structure to typical benzodiazepines such as diazepam, is effective in the treatment of generalised anxiety (and panic) disorder. However, it is also associated with dependence, which may be worse than with typical benzodiazepines. Furthermore, it is not available for prescription on the National Health Service in the UK.

Whenever possible, intermittent use of benzodiazepines, rather than regular use, must be encouraged and the risk of dependence discussed with patients before and during use.

Buspirone hydrochloride

This drug, unlike the benzodiazepines which act on the GABA-chloride complex, acts via 5HT receptors. It is indicated in the short-term management of anxiety disorders and appears to have moderate efficacy in this regard. Unlike benzodiazepines, however, buspirone has a slow onset of action but does not appear to impair psychomotor function or cause dependency problems. Nausea, dizziness, headache and fatigue can be bothersome for patients, such that up to 10% default from treatment. Patients who have previously been treated with benzodiazepines respond poorly to buspirone and may suffer more side-effects.

Antidepressants

The use of antidepressants in the treatment of anxiety disorders is well established. Antidepressants are effective even in the absence of depression and this has led to the suggestion that the two conditions may share a common underlying biological cause.

The three main groups of antidepressants that are used in the treatment of anxiety disorders are:
- tricyclic antidepressants (TCAs)
- selective serotonin-reuptake inhibitors (SSRIs)
- monoamine oxidase inhibitors (MAOIs)

As with the treatment of depression, there is no consensus among specialists on whether a TCA or an SSRI should be used as first-line therapy in the treatment of anxiety disorders. Some drugs in each of these groups are, however, licensed for the treatment of particular disorders or have shown significantly more efficacy. Once good effect has been achieved, antidepressant treatment should be continued for about 6–8 months and then tapered to minimise the likelihood of symptom recurrence on withdrawal.

Tricyclic antidepressants

These drugs act by blocking the neuronal uptake of catecholamines and serotonin thus increasing the effective concentrations of these monoamines at central receptor sites (monoamine reuptake inhibition). Their effectiveness varies in different conditions. For example, clomipramine, which inhibits reuptake of serotonin and to some degree noradrenaline through its metabolite methylclomipramine, is reputed to be effective in OCD. Tricyclics with weak serotonergic activity, such as imipramine, appear to be ineffective in OCD. Both clomipramine and imipramine are, however, effective in panic disorder, although the doses must be increased gradually as their side-effects can be bothersome. The common side-effects are dry mouth, blurred vision, constipation, sedation, weight gain, sexual dysfunction and urinary retention. They are also dangerous when taken in overdose and are slow in onset of action, taking up to 3 weeks to produce an effect.

Selective serotonin-reuptake inhibitors

With the evidence that serotonin may be implicated in the pathogenesis of anxiety has come an increased interest in these drugs. They do not bind to any specific neuroreceptors but selectively block serotonin reuptake through inhibition of the reuptake 'carrier'. This inhibition results in an increase of serotonin in the synapse. It is thought that the lack of clinical efficacy for at least 2 weeks or so is due to the stimulation of presynaptic autoreceptors resulting in a reduction in serotonergic turnover in the synaptic cleft. Eventual desensitisation of the presynaptic autoreceptors results in increased serotonin release and enhancement of serotonergic transmission. This process takes about 2 weeks to occur. Although other explanations have been put forward for the delay in onset of action, this is perhaps the most favoured, as the reduction in serotonergic turnover from stimulation of the autoreceptors is thought to be responsible for the exacerbation of anxiety that occurs soon after these drugs are started.

These drugs are preferred to TCAs because of their relative safety in overdose although some deaths have been attributed to citalopram (Ostrom *et al.* 1996). Their common side-effects are nausea, headache, agitation and sexual dysfunction. Advising patients of these and starting treatment at a low dose will minimise these problems. A benzodiazepine can be added for a short period.

All SSRIs have been used in the treatment of various anxiety disorders. However, they are not all licensed for the treatment of these disorders.

Monoamine oxidase inhibitors

These drugs inhibit the intracellular enzyme monoamine oxidase (MAO) thereby increasing the concentration of noradrenaline, dopamine and serotonin. MAOIs such as phenelzine have been found to alleviate generalised anxiety, panic and phobic disorders. Phenelzine is, however, not licensed for the treatment of panic disorder. Their use is limited by dietary restrictions and dangerous interactions with a range of other drugs such as pethidine and cold remedies. They also have troublesome side-effects, e.g. weight gain, oedema, postural hypotension, sexual dysfunction and urinary retention. The reversible and selective MAOI moclobemide has fewer side-effects and minimal dietary restrictions but has not been used extensively in the treatment of these disorders.

Beta-blockers

Propranolol has long been used to treat anxiety, particularly where autonomic symptoms such as palpitations, tremor and gastrointestinal upset are prominent. Patients with performance anxiety may also respond well. Propranolol does not, however, have any effect on the subjective or behavioural manifestations of anxiety such as impaired concentration and avoidance. Its effectiveness in relieving a patient's anxiety disorder depends, to some extent, on the significance of the bodily symptoms in the maintenance of the disorder.

Mood stabilisers

Mood stabilisers are drugs that lower and maintain mood at euthymic levels in patients with mania or hypomania. They also sustain euthymic mood in patients with unipolar depression when combined with an appropriate antidepressant. These drugs, which are particularly useful in the treatment of patients with bipolar-affective disorder, include lithium, carbamazepine and sodium valproate.

Lithium

Lithium is an alkali earth element, similar to sodium and potassium. It is an established treatment in patients with bipolar-affective disorder. Its precise mode of action is uncertain but it is known to reduce the neurotransmitter-induced activation of adenylate cyclase at certain postsynaptic receptors. Adenylate cyclase is required for the formation of cyclic adenosine monophosphate (cAMP), which mediates changes in most neurotransmitter target cells. This inhibition of adenylate cyclase also occurs in other organs, such as the thyroid gland and the kidneys. In the thyroid, it results in hypothyroidism due to a poor response of the gland to thyroid-stimulating hormone. In the kidneys, nephrogenic diabetes insipidus with the typical symptom of polyuria occurs as a result of poor response to anti-diuretic hormone.

Lithium is effective in acute mania although some studies have indicated that 30%–60% of patients do not respond well (Kukopulos *et al.* 1980; Small *et al.* 1988, 1991). Poor response is commoner in patients with mixed mania, i.e. presence of manic symptoms with dysphoria, and rapid or continuous cycling patients (Faedda *et al.* 1991; Bauer *et al.* 1994). Clinical improvement with lithium is relatively slow, with an initial response generally occurring 1–2 weeks after commencing treatment. Initial improvement may not occur for up to 4 weeks in some patients. Antipsychotic medication is often required during this lag period due to the aggressive and disruptive behaviour of the acutely manic patient. The combination of lithium with high doses of haloperidol should be avoided because of the risk of neurotoxicity (Cohen and Cohen 1974).

Lithium has also been shown to markedly reduce the risk of recurrence of manic and depressive episodes in patients with bipolar-affective disorder (Baastrup *et al.* 1970; Coppen *et al.* 1971; Fieve *et al.* 1976). Its protective effect against subsequent episodes appears, however, to be lower for depressive episodes than for manic episodes (Dunner and Fieve 1974). Maintenance lithium appears to be most effective in patients with an uncomplicated manic episode, good functioning between episodes and a family history of bipolar illness (Goodwin and Jamison 1990). As with acute treatment, mixed mania and rapid cycling mania respond poorly to maintenance treatment with lithium. Other predictors of poor response are severe or chronic depression, mood-incongruent psychotic symptoms, significant substance abuse and personality disorder.

Before commencing lithium, thyroid and kidney function should be tested. Hypothyroidism due to lithium is common and occurs in up to 20% of women (Lindstedt *et al.* 1977). Lithium should be discontinued or thyroxine treatment commenced. The effects on the kidneys are twofold: nephrogenic diabetes insipidus, which is largely reversible, and persistent impairment of concentrating ability, which occurs in 10% of cases. Reversible ECG changes due to the displacement of potassium in the myocardium have been described. These look like those of hypokalaemia, with T-wave flattening and inversion or widening of the QRS.

A suitable starting dose of lithium carbonate is 400 mg daily. Plasma levels need to be monitored 12 h after the last dose and at weekly intervals initially. Plasma levels of between 0.4 and 1.0 mmol/l should be aimed for. Levels above 1.5 mmol/l lead to lithium toxicity.

Patients on lithium may complain of side-effects such as:

- nausea
- metallic taste in the mouth
- excessive thirst and polyuria
- tremor
- weight gain

These side-effects are worse with higher plasma levels. Lithium interacts with a number of drugs including non-steroidal anti-inflammatory drugs, which are known to delay its clearance. Lithium should be avoided in pregnant women especially in the first trimester: it is known to increase cardiovascular anomalies (Kallen and Tandberg 1983). In such patients, antipsychotics should be used if manic symptoms occur following discontinuation of lithium.

Symptoms of lithium toxicity are:

- coarsening tremor
- nausea
- vomiting and dizziness
- ataxia
- dysarthria
- drowsiness

- confusion
- epileptic fits
- coma

Carbamazepine

Carbamazepine has been established as being effective in both the acute and prophylactic treatment of mania, mixed states, rapid cycling bipolar illness and other lithium-non-responsive patients (Ballenger and Post 1980). There is evidence that it is superior to placebo and as effective as lithium and antipsychotics in the treatment of acute mania (Klein *et al.* 1984; Post *et al.* 1987, 1989; Small *et al.* 1991). The addition of lithium to the regimen of poor responders appears to lead to clinical improvement (Kramlinger and Post 1989). Carbamazepine does, however, produce a less robust response in acute bipolar depression than it does in mania (Ballenger and Post 1980; Post *et al.* 1986).

For prophylactic and maintenance treatments, carbamazepine is superior to placebo and at least as effective as lithium although there is evidence that patients on carbamazepine relapse earlier than those on lithium (Ballenger and Post 1980; Okuma 1983; Placidi *et al.* 1986; Watkins *et al.* 1987).

Carbamazepine has a number of side-effects, for example drowsiness, ataxia and diplopia, which develop when the plasma concentrations are too high. Others are erythematous rash, water retention, hepatitis and leucopenia or other blood dyscrasias. Carbamazepine induces liver enzymes and may therefore accelerate the metabolism of other drugs such as contraceptive pills, antidepressants and antipsychotics.

Valproate

Valproate, which is commonly available as sodium valproate, has been shown in well-designed studies to be effective in the treatment of manic patients (Emrich *et al.* 1985; Pope *et al.* 1991; Freeman *et al.* 1992). It is superior to placebo (Emrich *et al.* 1985), and as effective as lithium in acute mania (Pope *et al.* 1991). Freeman *et al.* (1992), found that val-

proate and lithium were both effective in improving manic symptoms, although lithium was slightly more effective overall. Furthermore, they found valproate to be superior to lithium in the management of acute episodes of mania accompanied by coexisting depression, i.e. mixed states or dysphoric mania. Double-blind controlled studies examining the use of valproate for prophylaxis or maintenance treatment of mania are rare. However, open studies show that it is as effective as lithium or carbamazepine (Puzynski and Klosiewicz 1984; Emrich *et al.* 1985; Hayes 1989; Pope *et al.* 1991).

The common adverse effects of valproate are gastrointestinal disturbance, potentiation of the effects of sedative drugs and obesity. Thrombocytopenia, tremor and impairment of liver function tests occur occasionally.

Valproate is a major teratogen and women of childbearing age who are prescribed valproate should be made aware of this.

Electroconvulsive therapy

Meduna first introduced convulsive therapy for schizophrenia using camphor in 1934 but electrical induction of convulsions was not introduced until 1938. At the time, it was thought that schizophrenia and epilepsy never coexisted (Abrams 1992). Convulsive treatments were used widely in the 1940s and 1950s to the extent of being the standard against which new drugs were compared. Interest in ECT died down as new and effective drugs became available, and public concern about its frequency of use increased. It is now used in limited circumstances (American Psychiatric Association Task Force on ECT 1990) and remains a very effective treatment. Real ECT has been shown to be more effective than sham ECT (Freeman *et al.* 1978; Johnstone *et al.* 1980; West 1981; Brandon *et al.* 1984; Gregory *et al.* 1985).

Changes in the use and practice of ECT over recent decades have increased its safety and efficacy. Modified ECT is achieved with the use of short-acting anaesthetics and muscle relaxants. These considerably reduce the frequency of bone fractures and the unpleasant awareness of paralysis of the respiratory muscles during treatments with muscle relaxants only. Modern ECT is given as brief pulse stimulation from a constant-current machine with a stimulus setting that can be altered to take into account the individual's seizure threshold. The aim of treatment is thus to produce a seizure that will lead to amelioration of symptoms whilst minimising adverse cognitive side-effects.

Unilateral ECT, where the two treatment electrodes are placed over the non-dominant hemisphere, produces minimal adverse cognitive effects compared with the more traditional bilateral treatment. The main adverse effect of ECT is post-treatment confusion and variable degrees of anterograde and retrograde amnesia. Patients treated with unilateral ECT suffer these side-effects less (Squire 1986). There does, however, appear to be significant differences in clinical efficacy between the two methods of ECT treatment, with bilateral treatments being more effective (Gregory et al. 1985). Evidence shows that the dose of electricity must be increased several-fold in unilateral treatments to achieve the same clinical efficacy as bilateral treatment (Sackeim et al. 1993).

Although the frequency and number of treatments vary, ECT is commonly administered two or three times a week in courses that range from 4 to 12 treatments (Weiner 1994). More treatments have been proposed in patients with schizophrenia (Salzman 1980). In some patients, maintenance or continuation treatments are given every 2 weeks or monthly for 6 months or more to prevent relapse and maintain improvement (Weiner 1994; Karliner 1994).

Indications

By far the commonest reason for the use of ECT is major depression, particularly if it is life threatening or resistant to treatment (Fink 1994). Other uses are mania especially manic delirium, and catatonic schizophrenia. In developing countries where ECT is an available and inexpensive treatment, schizophrenia continues to be an important indication for the use of ECT (Salzman 1980). The elderly also represent a high percentage of ECT recipients, presumably because ECT has a better safety profile compared to some pharmacological alternatives and because rates of life-threatening depression are probably higher in the elderly. Further, medication resistance and intolerance are commoner in the elderly (Sackeim et al. 1990). Electroconvulsive therapy can be life-saving in cases of neuroleptic malignant syndrome and can be used across all ages. In pregnancy and certain physical illnesses, it may be considered safer than antidepressant medication (Royal College of Psychiatrists 1995).

Mode of action

The exact mode of action of ECT has not yet been determined (Fink 1990). Previous theories have focused largely on psychological factors such as induction of fear, punishment, memory loss for underlying cause of depressive symptoms, and euphoria akin to that seen in some types of brain damage; all have been discarded. There is, to date, no evidence that ECT produces any kind of brain damage as shown by the absence of quantitative or qualitative changes using imaging techniques (Devanand et al. 1994).

Animal and human studies, using a range of techniques, show that ECT causes a variety of neurophysiological changes in the brain. These changes include an increase in cerebral blood flow, oxygen consumption and glucose metabolism; short-lasting reversible inhibition of protein synthesis, which is thought to play a role in the cognitive effects through loss of neuronal plasticity necessary for consolidation of memory; and transient disruption of the blood–brain barrier leading to permeability of larger molecules (Davis and Squire 1984; Sackeim 1994).

Therapeutic benefit from ECT is thought to be associated with enhanced function of the serotonergic, dopaminergic and noradrenergic pathways. There is also an associated increase in gamma aminobutyric acid concentration in specific brain regions and, like most antidepressants, ECT results in increased density of the GABA-B receptor. Cholinergic activity is, however, reduced and this is thought to be partly responsible for the amnestic effects of ECT (Nutt and Glue 1993; Mann and Kapur 1994).

Adverse effects and dangers

The mortality rate associated with ECT is comparable with that of general anaesthesia in minor surgery and is estimated to be about one death per 10 000 patients treated (Abrams 1992; Royal College of Psychiatrists 1995). Complications related to ECT are more likely in the elderly (particularly the oldest age groups), those with other medical conditions (particularly cardiac illnesses) and those receiving medication for medical illnesses.

Patients with any of the following medical conditions are believed to be at considerably higher risk of mortality from ECT:

- space-occupying cerebral lesions or other conditions that increase intracranial pressure
- recent myocardial infarction associated with unstable cardiac function
- recent intracerebral haemorrhage
- unstable vascular aneurysm or malformation
- retinal detachment
- phaeochromocytoma

Although there are no absolute contraindications to the use of ECT, except perhaps raised intracranial pressure, patients with any of the above are best not treated with ECT until the medical condition has stabilised.

Ethical and legal issues

The responsibility for appropriate use of ECT and adoption of guidelines for obtaining informed consent remains that of the psychiatrist. Every patient must give written and valid informed consent before treatment can commence. In life-saving circumstances, one or possibly two treatments can be given under common law but a second opinion, under the Mental Health Act 1983, must be sought for subsequent treatments if consent is unobtainable. In patients under 16 years, the Royal College of Psychiatrists recommends that the opinion of a Child and Adolescent Psychiatrist be sought in addition to the consent of the child and their parents (Royal College of Psychiatrists 1995).

Antilibidinal drugs

Antilibidinal drugs may be of some use in patients who commit sexual offences, in whom they complement psychological and social treatments. Sexual offences refer to a breach of acceptable sexual behaviour. Sexual disorders, which largely fall into dysfunctions such as anorgasmia and problems related to orientation and body image difficulties, do not necessarily result in offences. Paraphilias are perhaps the most likely disorders to lead to offending behaviour. Depending on the findings during assessment, antilibidinal drugs may be used. Their use, however, is often involuntary in that patients are forced to receive them by law as an alternative to imprisonment or an aid to early release from prison or secure hospital. The evidence base underpinning these treatments is poor.

By far the most commonly used drug is cyproterone acetate, a steroidal antiandrogen that has a direct blocking effect at the cellular level but also additional anti-androgen properties, blocking gonadotropin secretion. It reduces sexual interest, drive, arousal and deviant fantasies (Bradford 1983; Cooper 1986). It may take 2–3 weeks to work. Anti-androgens are available in tablet or depot injection forms. It is necessary to explain anticipated effects and side-effects before prescribing antilibidinal drugs. Written consent is desirable, where applicable, and regular liver function tests are required.

The butyrophenone benperidol is also widely believed to be effective for the control of deviant sexual behaviour (Tennent *et al.* 1974). This effect is probably due to hyperprolactinaemia and is unlikely to be different from the sexual dysfunction commonly reported with all antipsychotic drugs.

Conclusion

Almost all patients admitted to psychiatric intensive care units receive pharmacological interventions and for many medication is the major treatment intervention. Staff should be aware of the uses and side-effects of commonly used drugs and be able to access information to assist in planning drug strategies for those patients with more refractory illness.

REFERENCES

Abrams R. 1992 Electroconvulsive Therapy. New York: Oxford University Press

Allison DB, Mentore JH, Heo M *et al.* 1999 Antipsychotic-induced weight gain: a comprehensive research synthesis. Am J Psychiatry 156(11): 1686–1696

American Psychiatric Association. 1994 Diagnostic and Statistical Manual of Mental Disorders, 4th edn. Arlington, VA: American Psychiatric Association

American Psychiatric Association Task Force on ECT. 1990 The Practice of ECT: Recommendations for Treatment, Training, and Privileging. Washington, DC: American Psychiatric Press

Atkin K, Kendall F, Gould D. 1996 Neutropenia and agranulocytosis in patients receiving clozapine in the UK and Ireland. Br J Psychiatry 169: 483–488

Baastrup PC, Paulsen JC, Schou M, Thomsen K, Amidsen A. 1970 Prophylactic lithium: double-blind discontinuation in manic-depressive and recurrent depressive disorders. Lancet ii: 326–330

Ballenger JC, Post RM. 1980 Carbamazepine in manic-depressive illness: a new treatment. Am J Psychiatry 137: 782–790

Barnes TRE, Bridges PK. 1980 Disturbed behaviour induced with high-dose antipsychotic drugs. Br Med J 281: 274–275

Bauer MS, Calabrese JR, Dunner DL. 1994 Multisite data vs analysis: validity of rapid cycling as a course modifier for bipolar disorder in DSM-IV. Am J Psychiatry 151: 506–515

Beasley CM Jr, Tollefson G, Tran P. 1996a Olanzapine versus placebo and haloperidol. Acute phase results of the North American double-blind olazapine trial. Neuropsychopharmacology 14: 11–1123

Beasley CM Jr, Sanger T, Satterlee W. 1996b Olanzapine versus placebo: results of a double-blind, fixed-dose olanzapine trial. Psychopharmacology 124: 159–167

Beasley CM Jr, Hamilton SH, Crawford AM. 1997 Olanzapine versus haloperidol: acute phase results of the international double-blind olanzapine trial. Eur Neuropsychopharmacol 7: 125–137

Bellack AS, Mueser KT. 1993 Psychosocial treatment for schizophrenia. Schizophr Bull 19: 317–336

Bersani G, Bressa GM, Meco G. 1990 Combined 5HT2 and dopamine D2 antagonism in schizophrenia: clinical, extrapyramidal and human neuroendocrine response in a preliminary study with risperidone. Hum Psychopharmacol 5: 225–231

Biederman J, Lerner Y, Belmaker RH. 1979 Combination of lithium carbonate and haloperidol in schizoaffective disorder: a controlled study. Arch Gen Psychiatry 36: 327–333

Boyer P, Lecrucibier Y, Puech AJ. 1995 Treatment of negative symptoms of schizophrenia with amisulpride. Br J Psychiatry 166: 68–72

Bradford JM. 1983 Research on sex offenders. Psychiatr Clin North Am 6(4): 715–731

Brandon S, Cowley P, McDonald C, Neville P. 1984 Electroconvulsive therapy: results in depressive illness from the Leicestershire trial. Br Med J 288: 22–25

Breier A, Meehan K, Birkett M *et al.* 2002. A double-blind, placebo-controlled dose–response comparison of intramuscular olanzapine and haloperidol in the treatment of acute agitation in schizophrenia. Arch Gen Psychiatry 59(5): 441–448

Brenner HD, Dencker SJ, Goldstein M. 1990 Defining treatment refractoriness in schizophrenia. Schizophr Bull 16: 551–561

Brody D, Adler LA, Kim T. 1990 Effects of buspirone in seven schizophrenic subjects. J Clin Psychopharmacol 10: 68–69

Cardoni AA. 1995 Risperidone: review and assessment of its role in the treatment of schizophrenia. Ann Pharmacother 29: 610–618

Carman JS, Bigelow LB, Wyatt RJ. 1981 Lithium combined with neuroleptics in chronic schizophrenia and schizoaffective patients. J Clin Psychiatry 42: 124–128

Castelao JF, Ferrerira L, Gelders YG, Heylen SLE. 1989 The efficacy of the D2 and 5HT2 antagonist risperidone in the treatment of chronic psychoses. An open dose finding study. Schizophr Res 2: 411–415

Cavallero R, Colombo C, Smeraldi E. 1995 A pilot, open study on the treatment of refractory schizophrenia with risperidone and clozapine. Hum Psychopharmacol 10: 231–243

Chouinard G, Jones B, Remington G. 1993 A canadian multicenter placebo-controlled study of fixed doses of risperidone and haloperidol in the treatment of chronic schizophrenic patients. J Clin Psychopharmacol 13: 35–40

Chouinard G, Vainer JL, Belanger MC. 1994 Risperidone and clozapine in the treatment of drug-resistant schizophrenia and neuroleptic-induced supersensitivity psychosis. Prog Neuropsychopharmacol Biol Psychiatry 18: 1129–1141

Claus A, Bollen J, de Cuyper H. 1992 Risperidone versus haloperidol in the treatment of chronic schizophrenic inpatient: a multi-centre double-blind comparative study. Acta Psychiatr Scand 85: 295–305

Cohen NJ, Cohen NH. 1974 Lithium carbonate, haloperidol and irreversible brain damage. J Am Med Assoc 230: 1283–1287

Committee on the Safety of Medicines. 1990 Cardiotoxic effects of Pimozide. Current Problems No. 29

Cooper AJ. 1986 Progestogens in the treatment of male sex offenders: a review. Can J Psychiatry 31(1): 73–79

Cooper T. 1996 Clozapine plasma level monitoring: current status. Psychiatr Q 67: 297–311

Coppen A, Noguera R, Bailey J. 1971 Prophylactic lithium in affective disorders: a controlled trial. Lancet ii: 326–330

Daniel DG, Whitcomb SR. 1998 Treatment of the refractory schizophrenic patient. J Clin Psychiatry 59 [Suppl 1]: 13–19

Davidson M, Emsley R, Kramer M et al. 2007 Efficacy, safety and early response of paliperidone extended-release tablets (paliperidone ER): results of a 6 week, randomised, placebo-controlled study. Schizophr Res 10.1016/j.schres.2007.03.003

Davis H, Squire L 1984 Protein synthesis and memory. Psychol Bull 96: 518–559

Davis JM et al. 1994 Depot antipsychotic drugs: place in therapy. Drugs 47: 120–127

Devanand DP, Dwork AJ, Hutchinson ER, Bolwig TG, Sackeim HA. 1994 Does electroconvulsive therapy alter brain structure? Am J Psychiatry 151: 957–970

Devinsky O, Honigfield G, Patin J. 1991 Clozapin-related seizures. Neurology 41: 369–371

Dunner DL, Fieve RR. 1974 Clinical factors in lithium carbonate prophylaxis failure. Arch Gen Psychiatry 30: 229–233

Emrich HM, Dose M, von Serssen D. 1985 The use of sodium valproate and oxycarbamazepine in patients with affective disorders. J Affect Disord 8: 243–250

Faedda GL, Baldessarini RJ, Tohen M, Strakowski SM, Waternaux C. 1991 Episode sequence in bipolar disorder and response to lithium treatment Am J Psychiatry 148: 1237–1239

Fieve RR, Kumbaraci T, Dunner DL. 1976 Lithium prophylaxis of depression in bipolar I, bipolar II, and unipolar patients. Am J Psychiatry 133: 925–930

Fink M. 1990 How does ECT work? Neuropsychopharmacology 3: 77–82

Fink M. 1994 Indications for the use of ECT. Psychopharm Bull 30(3): 269–280

Fontaine KR, Heo M, Harrigan EP et al. 2001 Estimating the consequences of anti-psychotic induced weight gain on health and mortality rate. Psychiatry Res 101(3): 277–288

Fowler NO, McCall D, Chuan T. 1976 Electrocardiographic changes and cardiac arrhythmias in patients receiving psychotropic drugs. Am J Cardiol 37: 223–230

Freeman CPL, Basson JV, Creighton A. 1978 Double-blind controlled trial of electroconvulsive ttherapy (ECT) and simulated ECT in depressive illness. Lancet i: 738–740

Freeman TW, Clothier JL, Passaglia P, Lesem MD. 1992 A double blind comparison of VPA and LI in the treatment of acute mania. Am J Psychiatry 149: 108–111

Geoff DG, Brotman AW, Waites M, McCormick S. 1990 Trial of fluoxetine added to neuroleptics for treatment resistant schizophrenic patients. Am J Psychiatry 147: 492–494

Goodnick PJ, Jerry JM. 2002 Aripiprazole: profile on efficacy and safety. Expert Opin Pharmacother 3(12): 1773–1781

Goodwin FK, Jamison KR. 1990 Manic-depressive illness. New York: Oxford University Press

Gregory S, Shawcross CR, Gill D. 1985 The Nottingham ECT study: a double blind comparison of bilateral, unilateral, and simulated ECT in depressive illness. Br J Psychiatry 146: 520–524

Hakola HP, Laulumaa VA. 1982 Carbamazepine in treatment of violent schizophrenics [Letter]. Lancet ii: 1358

Harrington M, Lelliott P, Paton C, Okocha C, Duffett R, Sensky T. 2002a The results of a multi-centre audit of the prescribing of antipsychotic drugs for in-patients in the United Kingdom. Psychiatr Bull 26: 414–418

Harrington M, Lelliott P, Paton C, Konsolaki M, Sensky T, Okocha C. 2002b Variation between services in polypharmacy and combined high dose of antipsychotic drugs prescribed for in-patients. Psychiatr Bull 26: 418–420

Hasegawa M, Gutierrez-Esteinou R, Way L, Meltzer HY. 1993 Relationship between clinical efficacy and clozapine plasma concentrations in schizophrenia: effect of smoking. J Clin Psychopharmacol 13: 383–390

Hayes SG. 1989 Longterm use of VPA in primary psychiatric disorders. J Clin Psychiatry 50: 35–39

Hegarty JD et al. 1994 One hundred years of schizophrenia: a meta-analysis of the outcome literature. Am J Psychiatry 151: 1409–1416

Henderson DC, Cagliero E, Gray C et al. 2000 clozpinel, diabetes mellitus, weight gain and lipid abnormalities:

a five-year naturalistic study. Am J Psychiatry 157(6): 975–981

Hirsch SR, Barnes TRE. 1994 Clinical use of high-dose neuroleptics. Br J Psychiatry 164: 94–96

Hirsch SR, Link CGG, Goldstein JM. 1996 ICI204,636: a new atypical antipsychotic drug. Br J Psychiatry 168 [Suppl 29]: 45–56

Hirschowitz J, Casper R, Garver DL. 1980 Lithium response in good prognosis schizophrenia. Am J Psychiatry 137(8): 916–920

Ital T, Keskiner A, Heinemann L. 1970 Treatment of resistant schizophrenics with extreme high dosage fluphenazine. Psychosomatics 11: 496–491

Johnstone EC, Deakin JFW, Lawler P, Frith CD. 1980 The Northwick Park electroconvulsive therapy trial. Lancet ii: 1317–1320

Jusic N, Lader M. 1994 Post-mortem antipsychotic drug concentrations and unexplained deaths. Br J Psychiatry 165: 787–791

Kallen B, Tandberg A. 1983 Lithium and pregnancy – a cohort study of manic-depressive women. Acta Psychiatr Scand 62: 134–139

Kane J, Honigfield G, Singer J, Meltzer HY. 1988 The clozaril collaboration study group. Clozapine for the treatment-resistant schizophrenic: a double-blind comparison with chlorpromazine. Arch Gen Psychiatry 45: 789–796

Kane JM. 1992 Clinical efficacy of clozapine in treatment refractory schizophrenia: an overview. Br J Psychiatry Suppl 17: 41–45

Kane JM, Marder SR. 1993 Psychopharmacological treatment of schizophrenia. Schizophr Bull 19: 287–302

Kane J, Canas F, Kramer M et al. 2006 Treatment of schizophrenia with paliperidone extended-release tablets: A 6-week placebo-controlled trial. Schizophr Res 90: 147–161

Kapur S. Remington G. 2000 Atypical antipsychotics. Patients value the lower incidence of extrapyramidal side effects. Br Med J 321: 1360–1361

Kapur S, Seeman P. 2001 Does fast dissociation from dopamine D2 receptor explain the action of atypical antipsychotics?: a new hypothesis. Am J Psychiatry 158: 360–369

Karliner W. 1994 Maintenance ECT. Convuls Ther 10: 238–242

Karson CN, Weinberger DR, Bigelow L, Wyatt RJ. 1982 Clonazepam treatment of chronic schizophrenia: negative results in a double-blind, placebo-controlled trial. Am J Psychiatry 139: 1627–1628

Kemp R, Hayward P, Applewhaite G, Everitt A, David A. 1996 Compliance therapy in psychotic patients: randomised controlled trial. Br Med J 312: 345–349

Kessler RC. 1994 Lifetime and 12 month prevalence of DSMI-IIR psychiatric disorders in the United States: results from the National Co-morbidity Survey. Arch Gen Psychiatry 51: 8–20

King DJ, Burke M, Lucas RA. 1995 Antipsychotic drug-induced dysphoria. Br J Psychiatry 167: 480–482

Klein E, Bental E, Lerer B, Belmaker RH. 1984 Carbamazepine and haloperidol v placebo and haloperidol in excited psychoses. Arch Gen Psychiatry 41: 165–170

Kramer M, Simpson G, Maciulis V et al. 2007 Paliperidone extended-release tablets for prevention of symptom recurrence in patients with schizophrenia: a randomized, double-blind, placebo-controlled study. J Clin Psychopharmacol 27(1): 6–14

Kramlinger KG, Post RM. 1989 Adding lithium carbonate to carbamazepine: antimanic efficacy in treatment-resistant mania. Acta Psychiatr Scand 79: 378–385

Kraus T, Haack M, Schuld A et al. 1999 Body weight and leptin plasma levels during treatment with antipsychotic drugs. Am J Psychiatry 156(2): 312–314

Kukopulos A, Reginaldi D, Laddomada P, Floric G. 1980 Course of the manic depressive cycle and changes caused by treatment. Pharmacopsych 13: 156–167

Lelliott P, Paton C, Harrington M, Konsolaki M, Sensky T, Okocha, C. 2002 The influence of patient variables on polypharmacy and combined high dose of antipsychotic drugs prescribed for in-patients. Psychiatr Bull 26: 411–414

Lieberman JA, Kane JM. 1994 Predictors of response to clozapine. J Clin Psychiatry 55(9): 126–128

Lindstedt G, Nilsson LA, Walinder J, Skott A, Ohman R. 1977 On the prevalence, diagnosis and management of lithium induced hypothyroidism in psychiatric patients. Br J Psychiatry 130: 452–458

Lindstrom LH, Persson E. 1980 Propranolol in chronic schizophrenia controlled study in neuroleptic treated patients. Br J Psychiatry 137: 126–130

Little KY, Gay TL, Vore M. 1989 Predictors of response to high-dose antipsychotics in chronic schizophrenics. Psychiatr Res 30: 1–9

Loo H, Poirer-Littre MF, Theron M. 1997 Amisulpride versus placebo in the medium term treatment of negative symptoms of schizophrenia. Br J Psychiatry 170: 18–22

Luchins DL. 1984 Carbamazepine in violent non-epileptic schizophrenics. Psychopharmacol Bull 20(3): 569–571

Mann JJ, Kapur S. 1994 Elucidation of the biochemical basis of the antidepressant action of electroconvulsive therapy by human studies. Psychopharmacol Bull 30(3): 445–453

Marder SR, Meibach RC. 1994 Risperidone in the treatment of schizophrenia. Am J Psychiatry 15: 825–835

Markowitz JS, Candace SB, Moore TR. 1999 Atypical antipsychotics: pharmacology, pharmacokinetics, and efficacy. Ann Pharmacother 33: 73–85

McCreadie RG, MacDonald IM. 1977 High-dose haloperidol in chronic schizophrenia. Br J Psychiatry 131: 310–316

McCreadie RG, Flanagan WL, McKnight J. 1979 High-dose flupenthixol decanoate in chronic schizophrenia. Br J Psychiatry 135: 175–179

McEvoy JP, Hogarty GE, Steingard S. 1991 Optimal dose of neuroleptic in acute schizophrenia. A controlled study of the neuroleptic threshold and higher haloperidol dose. Arch Gen Psychiatry 48: 739–745

Meehan K, Zhang F, David S et al. 2001 A double-blind, randomized comparison of the efficacy and safety of intramuscular injections of olanzapine, lorazepam, or placebo in treating acutely agitated patients diagnosed with bipolar mania. J Clin Psychopharmacol 21(4): 389–397

Mehtonen OP, Aranko K, Malkonen L. 1991 A survey of sudden death associated with the use of antipsychotic or antidepressant drugs. Acta Psychiatr Scand 84: 58–64

Meltzer HY. 1991 The mechanism of action of novel antipsychotic drugs. Schizophr Bull 17: 263–287

Meltzer HY. 1992 Treatment of the neuroleptic, nonresponsive schizophrenic patient. Schizophr Bull 18: 515–542

Mortimer A. 1997 Treatment of the patient with long-term schizophrenia. Adv Psychiatr Treat 3: 339–346

Myers DH, Campbell PL, Cooks NM. 1981 A trial of propranolol in chronic schizophrenia. Br J Psychiatry 139: 118–121

Nutt DJ, Glue P. 1993 The neurobiology of ECT: animal studies. In: Coffey CE, ed The Clinical Science of Electroconvulsive Therapy. Washington DC: American Psychiatric Press, pp. 213–234

Okocha CI. 1995 Treating addiction to benzodiazepines. Hospital Update September, pp. 396–401

Okocha CI. 1996 Managing anxiety disorders in general practice. Hospital Update November, pp. 415–419

Okuma T. 1983 Therapeutic and prophylactic effects of carbamazepine in bipolar disorders. Psychiatr Clin North Am 6: 147–174

Ostrom M et al. 1996 Fatal overdose with citalopram. Lancet 348: 339–340

Paris J. 2000 Chronic suicidality among patients with borderline personality disorder. Psychiatr Serv 53: 738–742

Paton C, Okocha CI. 2004 Risperidone long-acting injection: the first 50 patients. Psychiatr Bull 28: 12–14

Paton C, Okocha CI. 2005 Pharmacological treatment of borderline personality disorder. J Psychiatr Intensive Care Psychiatry 1: 105–116

Peet M, Middlemiss DN, Yates RA. 1980 Pharmacokinetic interaction between propronolol and chlorpromazine in schizophrenic patients. Lancet ii: 978

Pereira S, Beer D, Paton C. 1999 When all else fails: a locally devised structured decision process for enforcing clozapine therapy. Psychiatr Bull 23: 654–656

Perry PJ, Miller DD, Arndt SV, Cadoret RJ. 1991 Clozapine and norclozapine plasma concentrations and clinical response of treatment refractory schizophrenic patients. Am J Psychiatry 148: 231–235

Perry PJ, Bever KA, Arndt S, Combs MD. 1998 Relationship between patient variables and plasma clozapine concentrations: a dosing nomogram. Biol Psychiatry 44: 733–738

Placidi GF, Lenzi A, Lazzerini F, Cassano GB, Akiskal HS. 1986 The comparative efficacy and safety of carbamazepine versus lithium: a randomized, double-blind 3-year trial in 83 patients. J Clin Psychiatry 47: 490–494

Pope HG, McElroy SL, Keck P, Brown S. 1991 Valproate in the treatment of acute mania: a placebo controlled study. Arch Gen Psychiatry 48: 62–68

Post RM, Uhde TW, Roy-Byrne PP, Joffe RT. 1986 Antidepressant effects of carbamazepine. Am J Psychiatry 143: 29–34

Post RM, Uhde TW, Roy-Byrne PP, Joffe RT. 1987 Correlates of anti-manic response to carbamazepine. Psychiatr Res 21: 71–83

Post RM, Rubinow DR, Uhde TW. 1989 Dysphoric mania: clinical and biological correlates. Arch Gen Psychiatry 46: 353–358

Potkin SG, Bera R. 1994 Plasma clozaril concentrations predict clinical response in treatment resistant schizophrenia. J Clin Psychiatry 55(9): 133–136

Puzynski S, Klosiewicz L. 1984 Valproic acid amide in the treatment of affective and schizoaffective disorders. J Affect Disord 6: 115–121

Quitkin F, Rifkin A, Klein DF. 1975 Very high dosage versus standard dosage fluphenazine in schizophrenia: a double-blind study of non-chronic treatment refractory patients. Arch Gen Psychiatry 32: 1276–1281

Reus VI. 1997 Olanzapine: a novel atypical neuroleptic agent. Lancet 349: 1264–1265

Rifkin A, Quitkin F, Carrillo C. 1971 Very high-dose fluphenazine for non-chronic treatment refractory patients. Arch Gen Psychiatry 25: 398–403

Royal College of Psychiatrists. 1995 The ECT Handbook. Council Report CR 39. London: Royal College of Psychiatrists

Sackeim HA. 1994 Central issues regarding the mechanisms of action of ECT: directions for future research. Psychopharmacol Bull 30(3): 281–312

Sackeim HA, Prudic J, Devanand DP, Decina P, Kerr B, Malitz S. 1990 The impact of medication resistance and continuation pharmacotherapy on relapse following response to electroconvulsive therapy in major depression. J Clin Psychopharmacol 10: 96–104

Sackeim HA, Prudics, Devonod DP. 1993 Effects of stimulus intensity and electrode placement on the efficacy and cognitive effect of electroconvulsive therapy. N Engl J Med 328: 839–846

Salzman C. 1980 The use of ECT in the treatment of schizophrenia. Am J Psychiatry 137: 1032–1041

Schooler JVR. 1991 Maintenance medication for schizophrenia: strategic for dose reduction. Schizophr Bull 17: 311–324

Sernyak MJ, Leslie DL, Alarcon RD, Losonczy MF, Rosenheck R. 2002 Association of diabetes mellitus with use of atypical neuroleptics in the treatment of schizophrenia. Am J Psychiatry 159(4): 561–566

Sharif Z. 1998 Treatment of refractory schizophrenia: how should we proceed? Psychiatr Q 69(4): 263–281

Sharma R, Trappler B, Ng YK, Leeman CP. 1995 Risperidone induced neuroleptic malignant syndrome. Ann Pharmacother 30: 775–778

Siris S, Bermonzohn PC, Gonzalez A, Manson SE. 1991 Use of antidepressants for negative symptoms in a subset of schizophrenic patients. Psychopharmacol Bull 27: 331–335

Small JG, Klapper MH, Kellams JJ. 1988 Electroconvulsive treatment compared with lithium in management of manic states. Arch Gen Psychiatry 45: 727

Small JG, Klapper MH, Milstein V. 1991 Carbamazepine compared with lithium in treatment of mania. Arch Gen Psychiatry 48: 915–921

Squire LR. 1986 Memory functions as affected by electroconvulsive therapy. Ann N Y Acad Sci USA 462: 307–314

Tandon R, Harrigan E, Zorn SH. 1997 Ziprasidone: a novel antipsychotic with unique pharmacological and therapeutic potential. J Serotonin Res 4: 159–177

Taylor D, Duncan D. 1995 The use of clozapine plasma levels in optimising therapy. Psychiatr Bull 19: 753–755

Tennent G, Bancroft J, Cass J. 1974 The control of deviant sexual behaviour by drugs: a double blind controlled study of benperidol, chlorpromazine, and placebo. Arch Sex Behar 3: 261–271

The Concise Oxford Dictionary. 1995 9th edn. Oxford: Oxford University Press

Thompson C. 1994 The use of high-dose antipsychotic medication. Br J Psychiatr 164: 448–458

Tohen M, Zhang F, Taylor CC *et al.* 2001 A meta-analysis of the use of typical antipsychotic agents in bipolar disorder. J Affect Disord 65(1): 85–93

Tollefson GD, Beasley CM Jr, Tran PV. 1997 Olanzapine versus haloperidol in the treatment of schizophrenia, schizoaffective, and schizophreniform disorders: results of an international collaborative trial. Am J Psychiatry 154: 457–465

Watkins SE, Callender K, Thomas DR, Tidmarsh SF, Shaw DM. 1987 The effect of carbamazepine and lithium on remission from affective illness. Br J Psychiatry 150: 180–182

Weiner RD. 1994 Treatment optimization with ECT. Psychopharmacol Bull 30(3): 313–320

Weissman MM, Merikangas KR. 1986. The epidemiology of anxiety and panic disorders. J Clin Psychiatry Suppl 47: 11–17

West ED. 1981 Electric convulsion therapy in depression: a double blind controlled trial. Br Med J 282: 355–357

Wilson WH, Claussen AM. 1994 Seizures associated with clozapine treatment in a state hospital. J Clin Psychiatry 55: 184–188

Winston M. 2000 Recent developments in borderline personality disorder. Adv Psychiatr Treat 6: 211–218

Wolkowitz OM, Tureksky N, Reus VI. 1992 Benzodiazepine augmentation of neuroleptics in treatment resistant schizophrenia. Psychopharmacol Bull 28: 291–295

Yatham LN. 2003 Acute and maintenance treatment of bipolar mania: the role of atypical antipsychotics. Bipolar Disorders 5(S2): 7–19

Yorkston NJ, Zaki SA, Pitcher DR, Gruzelier JH, Hollander D, Sergeant HGS. 1977 Propranolol as an adjunct to the treatment of schizophrenics. Lancet ii: 575–578

Zanarini MC, Frankenburg FR. 1997 Pathways to the development of borderline personality disoder. J Personal Disord 11(1): 93–104

6

Psychological approaches to the acute patient

Marc Kingsley

Introduction

The aim of this chapter is to highlight some important features of psychological work within the context of acute psychiatric services. The specific focus is on psychological work within Psychiatric Intensive Care Unit (PICU) settings. This offers an important opportunity to expand on the growing literature on multidisciplinary team activities within such contexts.

Psychiatric Intensive Care Unit treatment offers a short-term multidisciplinary intensive treatment plan for patients admitted from a number of referring wards. An important feature of this treatment is the inclusion of psychological work. The role of the psychologist on PICUs may vary, and differences in treatment approaches may be expected.

A psychological perspective on patient admissions in PICU settings offers a valuable opportunity for mental health professions to investigate the holistic experience of ward culture and patient treatment on such wards. Such a holistic approach will be important for the overall management of such patients admitted to acute psychiatric services, and is in line with preferred practice outlined in clinical governance. Clinical governance has been defined as a, 'Framework to ensure that all NHS organisations have proper processes for monitoring and improving clinical quality' (Dewar 1999). It is within the above contextual framework that some important functions the psychologist may offer will be highlighted.

The role of the psychologist within a PICU may include a number of functions:

- Providing a psychological assessment of patients:
  - delineating the link between the patient's current admission and their life history
  - forming a developmental history of the patient
  - providing a description of the underlying personality structure of the patient
    - Contributing towards risk assessment, and providing psychometric assessments when necessary
- Providing psychotherapeutic input to patients
  - providing carers' support
- Providing staff support (supervision and training)
- Contributing to ward activities (ward rounds, staff groups)
- Research studies

Box 6.1. Providing a psychological assessment of the patient

Patients admitted to acute psychiatric wards and PICU settings have a multitude of diagnoses and symptom presentations. The inability for such wards to have a homogeneous group of patients will result in patients with a number of different reasons for admission. A crucial aim of the psychologist in such a setting is to offer a psychological formulation of the patient's difficulties. The major impetus to such formulations is to offer the multidisciplinary team a glimpse into the patient's emotional world and the psychological triggers that may have contributed to the current episode and admission. On acute ward

---

Psychiatric Intensive Care, 2nd edn., eds. M. Dominic Beer, Stephen M. Pereira and Carol Paton.
Published by Cambridge University Press. © Cambridge University Press 2008

admissions, the focus is narrowed to the symptom presentation and medication review, and the rich depth of emotional antecedents may be lost.

One of the key elements through which such psychological formulations are achieved is the provision of a psychological assessment; the format may vary but the following points offer some preliminary outline of the assessment.

Attempting to delineate the link between the patient's current admission and life history

The significance of such links can help the team gain a broader and more detailed recognition of underlying psychological factors that have contributed to the current presentation. Such historical links may be overlooked when patients present with overriding symptom descriptions. A case example may help illustrate this point

Case history

An example is the case of a 30-year-old woman who presented to the PICU with symptoms of agitation and mood lability. The psychiatric history of the patient was extensive and included a family history of bipolar affective disorder. The patient's life history was presented to the ward in short discharge summaries, but little was known of her developmental years. A psychological assessment gauged that the patient had lost her mother to suicide at the age of 5 years. She was cared for by her older sister who became a maternal figure. The patient functioned well until the time of her sister's marriage, shortly after which the patient had her first episode of depression. The patient described feeling like she had 'lost' a mother again. The psychological assessment gathered evidence of times in which the patient relapsed: a common theme seemed to be the patient's experience of loss or abandonment, and her regression to an earlier emotional state.

The above vignette gives recognition to the importance of an extensive developmental history for

the team (Wallace 1983). An investigation into the patient's significant life events and developmental milestones can offer the psychologist the opportunity to formulate an outline for the ward of the patient's emotional life and personality structure. A detailed developmental history does not need to be performed exclusively for the psychologist, but can be used by all team members to expand on the holistic understanding of the patient. For a detailed description of developmental history-taking, see Wallace (1983). However, some important pointers to consider when taking a developmental history are outlined below (and see Box 6.2):

- A patient's life history is integral to the understanding of their subjective experience (Wallace 1983; Gabbard 1994)
- A developmental approach recognises the significance of developmental milestones in the course of life maturity
- Significant life courses include the stages of infancy, early childhood, middle childhood, adolescence and adulthood
- The developmental history will attempt to track the patient's experiences through such a life course
- Detailed recognition will be given to situations in which the patient has been adversely affected emotionally (sometimes termed emotional deprivation)
- The links between such adverse life experiences and later personality development will be traced
- It must be recognised that, for many psychiatric patients, their life history is a history of emotional deprivation, neglect, loss and abuse (Wallace 1983)

Box 6.2. Some important features of a developmental perspective

Good and detailed history-taking will outline the relevant and significant life event that may be of importance to the overall understanding of the patient. An aspect of this may be to consider a model in which the current difficulties are seen as reactions to unresolved life events and difficulties, and not only always the result of a biochemical illness (see Gabbard 1994 for more detail).

Providing a description of the patient's underlying personality structure

An important feature to investigate in the psychological assessment is the personality structure of the patient (Kernberg 1975). The recognition of how the underlying personality structure of the patient makes him/her more vulnerable to admission will be outlined. An important aspect of this work is to differentiate those patients whose personality has been an integral and long-standing factor in their admissions from other patients for whom recovery from episodes of psychiatric illness leaves them reasonably intact (Gabbard 1994). The ability to trace the patient's emotional functioning from developmental histories can help to distinguish between these two groups.

The idea of personality structure has been investigated and outlined by a number of theorists and clinicians (e.g. Kernberg 1975). The outline of such models of personality is beyond the scope of this paper (see Wallace 1983 for more detail). The basic outline, however, is for the psychologist to give the ward a basic formulation of the patient's ego functioning. Ego functioning can be broadly defined as that area of the person's personality that is primarily involved in adapting to internal drives as well as external environmental demands (Kaplan et al. 1994). Basic pointers that indicate weakened ego functioning (Kernberg 1975) include:

- Poor control of basic impulses (sexual and aggressive)
- Difficulties with tolerating frustration or emotional pressure
- Maladaptive coping mechanisms (defences) in the event of stress and anxiety
- Poor/diffuse emotional boundaries
- Poor 'object-constancy', constantly changing experiences of both self and others (Kernberg 1975)

The impact of psychiatric illness can often result in weakened ego functioning, and the observation of the above-mentioned features. However, in some patients, such defects in ego functioning are an aspect of their underlying personality structure and are found even in the absence of psychiatric illness (Kernberg 1975). It can be of use to the team treating the patient to have a clearer understanding of the long-standing ego functioning of patients on the ward. This is particularly important in their management and treatment. Those patients for whom long-standing ego weakness remains an integral part of their personality structure have particular therapeutic needs that will be described later.

Providing an assessment of the patient's family and social dynamics

Providing a psychological profile of the patient should include addressing broader sociocultural issues that have an impact on patient admission and care. An important area is that of family dynamics. Much literature has been written on the role of the family in the lives of psychiatric patients (e.g. Faddon et al. 1987; Ostman et al. 2005); however, within the context of intensive care treatment, we can focus on some particular areas.

The experience of the admission to hospital for the patient's family

Admission on to a PICU is an emotional experience for both the patient and his/her close contacts. Coming to terms with the reality of a psychiatric illness can be an important aspect of the patient's stay on the PICU. This is equally an issue of concern for the patient's family and friends. The need for family members to have the opportunity to engage with staff members about this situation cannot be underestimated. The role of the psychologist on the ward would be to guide the team within this area of treatment.

For many family members, having to face an illness of a loved one is a difficult and painful process to bear (Mervis 1999). This applies to facing mental illness as much as to physical illness. The feelings associated with such a process can be complex and depend on the unique history of each family. However, overall, the experience can often be described as a grieving process in which loss can be a central aspect (Mervis 1999). The team must be aware of the potential for the family to experience loss, or in certain cases to defend against feelings of loss, when the patient becomes ill or is admitted to the hospital. Understanding these feelings can assist the team to cope with the emerging dynamics and reactions experienced when dealing with families (Mervis 1999).

Case history

A 30-year-old woman was admitted on to the unit. The ward soon began to receive phone calls from the mother who was angry and demanding. Letters of complaint often arrived about the quality of care on the ward. Staff members felt defensive and angry in the mother's presence. A psychological formulation uncovered how the patient had had a steady decline in emotional functioning from early adulthood. Prior to the first admission, the patient had been a high achiever and successful. The psychological formulation helped to shed light on how painful the process was for the mother to watch her daughter steadily declining in mental health. The mother's anger helped her ward off feelings of underlying sadness and grief. Furthermore, the projection of 'poor care' on to the ward could have been linked to the mother's own feelings of guilt and her anxieties of not having offered sufficient emotional nourishment for her child.

The above vignette offers an example of how important it is for the ward to be aware of the family's reactions to facing the psychiatric illness of the patient. The case, however, is also found where, rather than loss being the overriding feeling for the family, it may be that feelings of fear and avoidance are prominent. When the family experiences a patient in the grips of acute mental illness this can have a lasting effect on carers. Often, family members witness bizarre or violent behaviour, and are left with feelings that need to be worked through. Without an opportunity for the family to face these feelings, 'acting-out' by family members can occur, such as avoidance of the patient, with missed or short visits.

Family dynamics 'spilling over' onto the ward

It may be important for underlying family dynamics to be assessed, so as to be aware of such dynamics

if they are lived out on the ward. Staff may gain insight into the functioning of the family through observation of various interactions as they unfold on the ward. For example, it is important for staff to assess the patient's mental state following interactions with family or friends. A psychologist may be able to comment on some of the emotional effects on the patients and carers, following family interactions, such as in ward rounds.

Case history

A 37-year-old man with a diagnosis of paranoid schizophrenia was admitted on to the PICU. The patient spent most of his time isolated from the staff and fellow patients. He seemed suspicious and guarded. From the onset of his admission to the unit the patient refused to eat hospital food. Staff queried whether this was due to his diagnosis of paranoia. However, it later unfolded that the patient would eat after cookery groups, and preferred his mother's cooking. The family continually brought in food to the ward, spoke for the patient in the ward rounds, and made decisions on his behalf. An examination of his home life indicated that the patient spent the majority of his time in his room, being brought meals by his mother and making minimal independent decisions. The team considered that there was evidence of an enmeshed family with poor boundaries and it became apparent that this family dynamic was being replayed on the unit. On the unit, this was particularly replayed in the patient's resistance to making decisions and living independently, without his family's constant supervision in ward affairs and activities.

The provision of psychotherapy for patients

A core role of the psychologist on the intensive care unit is to be involved in the provision of psychotherapy for patients. The significance of psychotherapy within the spectrum of acute psychiatry is a debated area (Kaplan *et al.* 1994). It is helpful for the team to have some idea of the variety of psychotherapeutic approaches that prevail, and what form of psychotherapy will be offered to the patient. Without an outline of this, many staff members remain doubtful of the effectiveness of therapy in such a setting (Clinton 2000).

Psychologists will often differ in the type of therapy they offer. This will vary in technique and style. This chapter outlines the use of a particular therapeutic approach. The primary basis of such an approach is that which has been outlined by Winnicott (1971), and later developed by Gabbard (1994) and Wallace (1983). The core features of such an approach are:

- The recognition of how the provision of psychotherapy needs to address the level of emotional development in the patient
- The adjustment of therapeutic technique according to the developmental level of the patient

The importance of the clinician taking into account the level of emotional development of the patient was addressed by Winnicott (1971), in which he described how, for certain patients, the provision of a different experience to that of traditional psychoanalytic therapy was more effective. He termed this *therapeutic management*. These ideas have been expanded upon by Gabbard (1994) and Wallace (1983), who describe the importance of adapting the therapeutic technique to the level of ego development in the patient. This would include those patients whose fragility in ego strength is due to their present psychiatric illness. In terms of what this means for clinical work, the team will need to recognise certain key factors that may be applicable to a psychiatric intensive care setting:

- Psychotherapy should be more *supportive* (Wallace 1983), in the sense of supporting the building up of ego resources in the patient.
- The therapist should be cautious not to unravel the fragile defences the patient is employing, and hence contribute to the patient regressing. (Regression is a term employed to describe a defence mechanism in which, in the face of anxiety, a person returns to an early level of emotional functioning.) (See Wallace 1983 for more detail.)
- The emotional needs of the patient should be taken into account. Some of these needs may not be consciously recognised. One of the key emotional needs that has been outlined in work with such

patients is the need for *containment*. This will be outlined in more detail below.

In terms of the above-mentioned descriptions, an important aspect of the therapeutic work is to keep the notion of *emotional vulnerability* in mind (Gabbard 1994). In a short-term setting, this will assist the therapist to formulate a therapeutic strategy that will be meaningful for the patient. Patients may feel more contained if they have a sense of how long they will be working therapeutically, and that sessions are more directive and structured. It could also be useful for therapists to encourage patients to openly address if they feel the therapeutic material is too emotionally painful or stressful.

Difficulties with forming a therapeutic rapport are part of the challenge for the therapist working with patients on the unit. Many of the difficulties found in therapeutic work in the psychiatric setting are highlighted in Chapter 7. It may be useful to expand on some other concerns that occupy the therapist working on the intensive care unit.

The involuntary patient

Patients admitted on to the PICU should have been detained under powers of the Mental Health Act, or equivalent legislation. Szasz (1998) described how the essence of the process of detention included, '. . . the legal and/or physical ability to restrict another'. Inherent in this process is the experience for the patient of some degree of coercion to take treatment. The recognition of the involuntary basis of treatment and the patient's experience of such a process is essential for treatment care. Further discussion of this can be found in Chapter 7.

Some further considerations

Patients may appear resistant to making emotional contact with the therapist. There may be a refusal to attend sessions, or little initiative taken in therapy. The initial reaction of the therapist may be to see this as linked to the patient's mental illness. However, it is also important for the therapist to consider one explanation for the patient's withholding in the sessions as being a possible reaction to the involuntary basis of the treatment. In a sense, the therapist's difficulty with engaging the patient in treatment may be the patient's only sense of control in the treatment, in which s/he feels disempowered. The patient may also fear that, in revealing these feelings, their stay on the unit may be prolonged. The therapist may need to spend time within the sessions addressing these issues with the patient, and attempting in the process to build therapeutic rapport.

Patients may be in need of the physical holding inherent in the secure environment of the unit. This may leave patients with a belief that their anxieties or inner emotional states are unmanageable by themselves and those around them, and that this is the reason for their admission to the unit. Patients may experience the involuntary basis of the treatment as a 'locking away' due to their inner sense of chaos, or external behaviour. One important aim in psychotherapeutic work is to recognise that, for certain patients, a difficulty in making emotional contact may be due to the patient's deep sense of believing that they cannot be contained (Docker-Drysdale 1991). A central role in psychotherapy would be to offer the patient the emotional space in which s/he may begin to experience his/her feelings and emotional states as bearable and tolerated by the therapist (Winnicott 1971; Docker-Drysdale 1991).

The violent patient

Violent patients may pose a considerable challenge to the team on the intensive care unit. The psychologist working psychotherapeutically with such patients forms an integral role in the treatment of such patients (Goldstein 1999). Violence may be the by-product of severe mental illness that will need particular pharmacological action. However, the psychologist may be able to point out to the team some of the *psychological* factors involved in patients' proneness to violence. Many patients who have admissions to acute psychiatric services have long-standing difficulties with containing their own feelings, which are hence turned into some form of action outside themselves. This action may include aggressive and violent behaviour. From a developmental perspective, an understanding of this would include the idea that, since early development, the patient has given up in despair of believing that their emotional states could be understood or managed by the environment around them (Docker-Drysdale 1991). This breakdown in feeling, as well as the concrete expression of feelings through actions, is important for the therapist to consider in the treatment of such patients.

Another important element of the psychological approach to the management of violent or aggressive patients is to understand their underlying feelings, which may include feelings such as rage and anger (Bradshaw 1991). An investigation of the developmental history of the patient may give an indication of some of the antecedent features in the person's life that have left them feeling so angry and enraged. Such an approach would recognise that the manifestation of violence would constitute a long-term building up of feelings that have their origin in some form of environmental failure and/or abusive experience (Winnicott 1975; Miller 1987, 1995). This approach could possibly help offer alternative considerations to the patient's violent behaviour, so that the aggression is not just viewed as a manifestation and by-product of mental illness.

Psychologists may utilise a number of psychological techniques to contain the patient and prevent the emergence of violence (see Chapter 7). An important element in the employment of interventions to assist patients with the management of violence would be to give patients the opportunity to find ways to manage their own feelings and urges. The significance of this is to strengthen the patients' coping skills, but also in the process to help patients to develop a growing sense of internal capacities and resilience. This is specifically linked to an attempt to reduce impulsivity in those patients with histories of impulsive aggression (Dawson *et al.* 2003). Specifically, certain behavioural techniques, such as anger and anxiety charts, may prove effective in such cases (see Appendix, p. 84 for details).

It should be recognised, however, that the effectiveness of such psychological intervention is dependent partly upon the patients' capacity and willingness to use these interventions (Dawson *et al.* 2005). An example of this would be the patients' willingness to consider managing their own violent urges, rather than relying on external containment such as drugs or control and restraint to manage their violence for them. For those patients who lack the abstract cognitive capacities to think about this, or who may on a deeper emotional level fear their own unmanageable feelings so much, the request of staff for the patients to use such techniques may be premature.

Linked to this is the therapist's and staff's willingness to work with violent patients. The emotional impact on staff members of violence and violent patients is a central element in the treatment of such patients (Goldstein 1999). Staff should feel supported and safe enough when expected to undertake this work, and the constant monitoring of countertransference to the patient is important (Docker-Drysdale 1991).

Suicide and self-harm

Many admissions to PICUs include patients who are actively suicidal, or remain at high risk of suicide (Chapter 1). Other patients may become suicidal as their mental illness is treated and insight returns. PICUs formulate effective and structured treatment plans in the assessment and management of the suicidal patient. This may include the implementation of high levels of observation and the consistent monitoring of patients' behaviour and mental state. An important aspect will be the psychological assessment and management of suicide/self-harming.

Addressing hopelessness and reasons for living

An essential feature in the assessment and management of suicidal ideation and intent, independent of diagnosis, is to closely monitor the degree of hope/hopelessness patients may experience about their life and future (Department of Health 2002). Hopelessness is higher in psychiatric patients who have a history of suicidal behaviour, both during and between episodes (Szanto *et al.* 1998; Mann *et al.* 1999), and is closely associated with whether individuals feel they have any reasons for living (Linehan *et al.* 1983; Mann *et al.* 1999; Malone *et al.* 2000). Hopelessness is a potent predictor of suicidal intent, not only in the short-term, but over a longer period of time as well. For example, Beck *et al.* (1985, 1989, 1990) have shown hopelessness to be a significant predictor of completed suicides up to 10 years later. Furthermore, hopelessness can increase depression and suicidal intent within self-harm populations (Wetzel *et al.* 1980; Salter and Platt 1990). It has also been found to predict repetition of self-harming over varying follow-up intervals (Petrie *et al.* 1988; Sidley *et al.* 1999).

Hopelessness has traditionally been treated as a monolithic entity (Heisel and Marnin 2004). However, researchers have begun exploring the dimensions of hopelessness in order to clarify the association between hopelessness and psychopathology (Flett and Hewitt 1994; Hewitt *et al.* 1998; Heisel *et al.* 2003). Psychological examination of the dimensions of hopelessness, especially anticipated positive and negative future experiences and life events, can be greatly beneficial and is an important component to the psychological work with suicidal patients (MacLeod *et al.* 2005). It would be important to consider the multidimensional components of hopelessness, and particularly to consider domain-specific dimensions of hopelessness, such as social hopelessness (Heisel and Marnin 2004; Hewitt *et al.* 1998) Social hopelessness is described as an interpersonal form of hopelessness, in which negative, pessimistic expectancies regarding the prospect of experiencing satisfying interpersonal relationships is at the fore (Heisel and Marnin 2004). In regard to this, Seager (2006:7) notes that the risk of suicide sharply increases where people, '. . . have lost all current meaningful psychological and social connections'. As mentioned earlier, patients who are admitted within acute psychiatry often have long histories of destructive relationships, including being the victims of emotional neglect and abuse from early life (Wallace 1983). In terms of psychological work with PICU patients, the importance, hence, of considering the role that problematic, failed and or abusive relationships have had on the formation of hopelessness about the future is very significant. Furthermore, re-enactment can occur within the relationship between staff and the patient, particularly with patients who present with challenging behaviour, or are seen as 'manipulative' or 'attention-seeking' (Hinshelwood 1999). This may result in patients re-experiencing negative interactions with staff, such as that ranging from neglect, to abusive experiences. This may intensify the sense of hopelessness the person may feel about their interpersonal relating or trust in others. The toxicity of such destructive relationships and environments is outlined by Seager (2006), in his conceptualisation of psychological safety in mental health services.

Psychologists working on PICUs can help implement psychological mindedness on the ward, in which concepts such as transference, negative countertransference/feelings in staff and an awareness and management of *malignant alienation* (Watts and Morgan 1994), the potentially lethal distancing of patients from staff and other patients, are considered. It would hence be important, in light of this, for psychologically minded ideas about the hospital and ward to be at the forefront of staff awareness. As Seager (2006: 6) notes:

A hospital is much more than a place where an illness gets treated. It is a place where new attachments are sought out and even resisted, where the hope of being listened to, understood, contained and 'reached' is both restimulated and defended against. It is a place where new experience can repeat, reinforce or challenge old experience.

Seager (2006) reiterates the significant role that the hospital, wards and staff working with patients can offer in terms of 'hopeful attachments', and how detrimental 'ruptures of containment and attachment' in staff–patient relationships can be for patients. Work within this area is highly significant clinically, as patients who can begin to experience meaningful, consistent relationships may find their feelings of hopelessness about social relationships beginning to shift. A key area in which this can begin to be established is within the *therapeutic alliance* with staff. Hence, the overall attempt by staff to facilitate and develop supportive 'good enough' relationships with patients (Seager 2006) is a crucial buffer against feelings of social isolation and consequent social hopelessness.

Suicide/self-harm management and staff containment

As with suicidal patients, patients with presentations of self-harming can require complex management (Hawton *et al.* 2003; Harriss and Hawton 2005). For an individual who has engaged in self-harm, the risk of dying by suicide is significantly higher than for the general population (Hawton and Fagg 1988; Owens *et al.* 2002), especially during the first 12 months following self-harm (Hawton *et al.* 2003). Repetition of self-harming increases the risk of further self-harm (Owens *et al.* 1994; Zahl and Hawton 2004) and eventual suicide (Hawton and Fagg 1988). Studies indicate, furthermore, that patients who have engaged in multiple (more than two) episodes of self-harm are at significantly greater risk of suicide (Zahl and Hawton 2004). Hence, the importance of offering a therapeutic management plan for this patient group is an essential aspect of their stay on a PICU. However, as with suicidal patients, the therapeutic management of patients with self-harming behaviour can be challenging for staff (Watts and Morgan 1994; Hinshelwood 1999). The highly stressful nature of this form of patient treatment for the multidisciplinary team is recognised by many staff (Watts and Morgan 1994). Many such patients have had numerous hospital admissions and may evoke a range of emotions in the staff who manage their care (Hinshelwood 1999; Chapter 7). The ability of staff members to feel able to recognise and manage the feelings that the suicidal/self-harming patient evoke will influence the overall treatment of such patients. Generally, these emotions may include negative feelings and a move towards moral judge-ment (Hinshelwood 1999). The capacity to offer such patients a meaningful and therapeutic stay on the ward is challenged by their often difficult-to-manage behaviour. Ongoing staff discussions and feedback about such patients are essential, in an attempt to consider the interpersonal effect such patients have on staff and fellow patients. It is often the role of the psychologist to help monitor the psychological effect such patients may have on the staff work-ing with them, and fellow patients on the ward. It is hence important, then, that staff working with suicidal/self-harming patients are given the oppor-tunity to share their experiences and feelings about this work (Hinshelwood 1999). Psychologists can offer support to staff in the form of support groups or one-to-one supervision sessions. This offers staff the opportunity to talk about the emotional impact that such patients evoke and can hopefully have a containing function for the staff member, who then may feel more able to manage another shift and session with the patient. This can also help man-age staff acting out, such as in negative counter-transference reactions to patients, and even in cer-tain cases reduce high staff turnover via resignations from the unit (Hinshelwood 1999). Staff may also fear allowing themselves to get too close emotionally to the suicidal patient, for fear of the patient's dying, and the emotional consequence of this for the staff member.

Psychologists wanting to include such staff sup-port groups on the ward would need to recognise the possibility of the ambivalence that some staff mem-bers may feel about joining such groups (Hinshel-wood 1999). The necessity for some staff to maintain a particular 'professional' image in front of peers, and the fear that staff may experience feelings of becom-ing too vulnerable in a group should be consid-ered. Furthermore, for those psychologists actively involved on the unit, the capacity to take on such a leadership role in the group may be seen as a possi-ble boundary impingement. Outside facilitation may hence become a viable option.

Furthermore, the amount of time needed to work with such complex presentations may require a longer period of treatment than a short stay on a PICU. Ongoing support and professional contact with patients vulnerable to suicidal ideation/self-harming is necessary, and an investigation into the longer-term support available for such patients is important (Hawton *et al.* 2003). A key feature of the psychologist's role in the treatment of patients with suicide/self-harming is to address the possibility of referrals for psychotherapy post-discharge, though this may be very difficult due to staff shortages and long waiting lists. It is also important for the multi-disciplinary team to be aware of the psychological dangers and risks of patients being discharged with-out ongoing containment and support from health professionals (Seager 2006). Hence, it is essential for staff who meet at patient ward rounds and care pro-gramme approach reviews to consider psychosocial aspects of care, which multidisciplinary team mem-bers may implement in the ongoing treatment plan post-discharge from the PICU.

Reasons for living

Patients who struggle with suicidal urges or feelings may describe reasons for living which help them resist these suicidal feelings (Malone *et al.* 2000). Addressing *protective factors* or buffers which may set in when patients contemplate suicide is as cru-cial as addressing the risk issues linked to the sui-cidal potential in the patient. Treatment strategies that increase awareness of reasons for living and meaningful purpose in life are seen as crucial in psychological work with patients presenting to the PICU. At such a vulnerable point in people's lives, strategies which could strengthen meaning and help patients to hold in mind such reasons for living are crucial elements of a psychosocial approach on the PICU.

The work of Linehan *et al.* (1983) is crucial in this respect. The Reasons for Living Scale (Linehan *et al.* 1983) can help identify the factors associ-ated with reasons for living. It can be used as an assessment technique in the suicide risk battery, as well as a tool to guide the shorter-term thera-peutic work on the PICU. This strategy is advised, independent of diagnosis, and is focused on helping staff to assess potential buffers and protective factors which may 'kick in' when suicidal ideation becomes prominent. The Reasons for Living Scale is a 48-item self-report measure that assesses the beliefs and expectations for not committing suicide. The Scale consists of six subscales and a total scale. The subscales include: Survival and Coping Beliefs (24 items) Responsibility to Family (7 items), Child-Related Concerns (3 items), Fear of Suicide (7 items), Fear of Social Disapproval (3 items) and Moral Objections (4 items). The subscales and total scale are scored by summing the items and dividing by the number of items. The overall objectives are: (1) to measure and assess whether the total score is above or below the cut-off point; and (2) to assess the scores of each of the subscales, and whether they fall above or below the cut-off point for that factor. The Survival and Coping subscale has been noted, in particular, to be an important shield to hopelessness and suicidal ideation, when strengthened. The essential feature of this subscale is the ability to utilise effective coping mechanisms and find effective solutions to problems when despair or hopelessness sets in. Helping patients to strengthen existing and/or find new adaptive coping mechanisms is an essential therapeutic intervention and is closely linked to therapeutic work on problem-solving. Problem-solving deficits are closely associated with hopelessness and increased risk of suicide/self-harming (Townsend et al. 2001), especially in patients with histories of suicide attempts and or self-harming. Hence, helping patients to adaptively find problem-solving techniques as well as strengthen protective buffers, i.e. reasons for living, is a crucial aspect of the brief therapeutic work that can be undertaken on the PICU. An integral element of this may be to help patients to draw up 'crisis cards' (Sutherby et al. 1999), in which they list their most significant reasons for living. These cards can be effective in times of emotional distress/crisis, when it may be more difficult for the person to hold in mind the various reasons for living. It hence becomes an external reminder of those internal factors, and at times may help buffer impulsive acts. However, the efficacy of such crisis cards

in reducing overall repetition rates has in certain studies been found not to be effective (Evans et al. 1999). Psychologists can help with the training of the multidisciplinary team in utilising this assessment tool, as well as drawing up crisis cards. This can become an effective element of PICU interventions, ranging from nursing keyworker sessions to ward rounds.

Coming to terms with admission and illness

As described in the section on 'Providing an assessment of the patient's family and social dynamics', the emotional impact of facing mental illness is crucial for the psychologist to address. For the person admitted on to the unit, the reality of facing a psychiatric diagnosis and admission on to a locked ward can evoke an array of feelings. The psychologist needs to consider the psychological impact of the admission on the individual patient. *This becomes important in terms of how much the patient is able to accept the reality of their mental illness.* Patients may differ in this respect, and an integral role for the psychologist in individual sessions could be to assess the level of this acceptance of the illness. Some reactions the patient may experience in the struggle to come to terms with the diagnosis and treatment can be important to consider in the management of the patient on the intensive care unit and in referral back to the referring ward.

The multidisciplinary team may be faced with patients who seem to have *poor insight* into their condition. They may deny the presence of mental illness, or minimise the extent to which they are ill. This lack of insight may be seen by the team to be a by-product of the illness; the psychological approach would be to consider the possibilities of *denial* and *avoidance*. The patient may utilise defences such as these and it is important to consider how emotionally painful and frightening it can be to face the reality of such an illness.

The psychologist may help uncover some underlying reasons for this reaction by the patient, such as the role which social stigma may play (Szasz 1998).

For patients, such as those who had high levels of social and occupational functioning, the label of psychiatric patient may be very difficult to acknowledge.

An important aspect in facing this label may be the experiencing of feelings of self-loathing or shame. Bradshaw (1991) has described shame as linked to a person's sense of feeling that there is something defective about themselves. The aim for the psychologist may be to examine such feelings, and the impact of the mental illness on self-esteem.

Some patients may go through a period of low mood following admission to the unit and coming to terms with the reality of the mental illness. Rather than denying the extent of the illness, these patients may experience feeling emotionally 'stuck' and unable to move forward. They may be left with a sense of loss and hopelessness (Mervis 1999). The psychologist may need to help the multidisciplinary team become aware of this form of reactive depression, which may at times be confused with the initial presentation, and hence overlooked in the management of the patient.

In other cases, admission to the unit may be one of several psychiatric admissions to acute psychiatric services (Wallace 1983). Patients may respond well to acute management, but may become more vulnerable when the recognition sets in of having been so ill again. This may become a crucial time for psychological work, when the patient is particularly emotionally vulnerable. Patients may feel unable to bear living with another relapse. This is often found in the cases of patients with good premorbid functioning, and in those patients who had assumed that they would not become ill again (Mervis 1999). Patients may have the insight to recognise how much their functioning has declined, and how different they may feel from those around them. The ability for the intensive care unit to offer psychological treatment, in which these issues can be addressed and worked with, is crucial. Patients may be able to do this in their individual therapy sessions, as well as in group therapy sessions. It is also important for the referring wards who have admitted the patient to the unit to have an idea of how best to continue this psychological work after discharge from the intensive care unit.

Conclusion

The aim of this chapter has been to highlight some important features of psychological work in PICU settings. The recognition by the team of psychological factors inherent in the process of patient care has been outlined. The essential aspect of this outline has been the recognition of how patients admitted to and treated on the unit have an emotional experience and reaction to their illness and care. The aim of the psychological work is to bring these features to the fore, and to address them with both the patient and the multidisciplinary team. The psychological work begun on the unit is ideally continued once the patient is back in the referring ward, so that the patient has a sense of continuity in terms of psychological care.

APPENDIX:
Anger management group (example)

Khadija Chaudhry

Introduction

The Anger Management Group (Chaudhry *et al.* 2006) comprises 12 weekly sessions of 40 min duration, each looking at particular aspects of anger. Due to variable lengths of stay and frequently changing group membership, sessions are designed to be self-contained and 'stand alone', each focusing on a small number of key points.

Philosophy

Aggressive and violent behaviour coexist with a multitude of major psychiatric illnesses. Such behaviour tends to be more persistent in patients admitted to Psychiatric Intensive Care Units. These patients often have long-standing difficulties with managing their anger. The main focus of an Anger Management Group is to help the patients deal with their anger more appropriately and effectively, also to gain better understanding of some of the causes of their aggression as well as deeper feelings underlying the anger, such as hurt, resentment and disappointment.

Aims and objectives

The main aims and objectives of an Anger Management Group are as follows.

Psycho-education

- To educate patients regarding the negative effects, both internal (mental health) and external (consequences), of poorly expressed anger
- To increase understanding about anger as a normal human emotion

Strategies and skills

- To empower patients with the choice to control their anger
- To explore strategies allowing patients to cope more easily with angry feelings (e.g. relaxation exercises)
- To teach practical skills in assertive behaviour and problem-solving

Multidisciplinary management

- To provide a regular and consistent information source for multidisciplinary treatment and management

Methods and theoretical basis

- The programme utilises an integrative approach to problems of anger and aggression. This includes

psycho-educational, cognitive-behavioural, psychodynamic and group counselling models
- The multidisciplinary team through ward rounds refers patients to the group. Suitability of referred members is finalised in shift handover on the day of the group
- The group is run with two assistant psychologist facilitators

The methods used in the group are:
- discussions
- role plays
- flip chart exercises
- picture exercises

Members are encouraged as much as possible to participate in all the different segments of the sessions. An effort is made to make the sessions as interactive and enjoyable as possible.

Group boundaries

The importance of group boundaries cannot be overestimated. Considering the patient population of the PICU, it is particularly important to have consistent group boundaries, which aid in the communication, containment and focus of the group (Nitsun 1996). The group boundaries are presented to the group members at the start of each session and members are reminded about them if at any point in time the boundary is in danger of being broken.

Difficulties

Running an inpatient group can be quite a challenging task due to the heterogeneity and mental state of these patients. On a PICU, due to a short length of stay, the composition of the group is constantly changing, adding to the difficulty. Some of the other difficulties that can occur in the Anger Management Group are as follows.
- The involuntary status of most PICU patients and the locked ward environment may produce feelings of frustration and resentment among the

members. This could lead to the formation of the 'anti-group' – which are the disruptive and destructive elements in the group (Nitsun 1996). The limited group cohesiveness can allow the space for such destructive anti-group processes to manifest themselves in a variety of ways ranging from deliberate disruption of the group to excessive dropout. The hostile angry feelings that can be evoked during group sessions can place a strain on the facilitators and threaten the integrity of the group. In short, managing anti-group processes is a potentially challenging task for the facilitators, who have to utilise alternative management strategies to strengthen the therapeutic process in the group.

- Facilitators need to be aware of their own emotional responses (countertransference) to negative and hostile acting-out in the group. Facilitators not addressing such countertransference responses can lead to their potentially acting-out and/or the emergence of feelings of burnout and amotivation.
- Often it is difficult for members to establish a therapeutic relationship in the group because of their short length of stay on the unit. As group members become more settled in the group and get to know other members and facilitators/staff better, they are transferred back to the ward from where they were referred. This adds to difficulties with group cohesiveness and group identity formation.
- For some members, behaving aggressively and violently may be an intrinsic part of their culture and identity (Robin and Novaco 1999); for example, some members may have learned that aggression seems to be the only way to prevent violence being directed towards them. Furthermore, some members may feel that to show destructive aggression is a part of their being and they may consider anger management a direct threat to their sense of self, or may simply consider that the group is not suitable for them.
- Gender issues may need to be considered in anger management. For example, many traditional views of masculinity assert that aggression (fights, verbal abuse/threats) is an acceptable and necessary part of daily life (Bem 1981). Members may feel that to show anger and aggression is to show their power

and if an attempt is made to shift this behaviour, they may feel disempowered and less dominant. This feeling may be more prevalent among the male members. As a result, resistance to attend the group may be evident in such a situation. However, the reason for this resistance may need to be untangled. Other social and personal reasons for resistance to group attendance and change should also be considered, such as social class, cultural ethnicity issues as well as intrapsychic and other personal reasons.

In summary, the Anger Management Group provides a psycho-educational and interactive experience for the members with an emphasis on understanding and dealing with anger and aggression in an appropriate way. The difficulties inherent in running such a group within a PICU setting need to be borne in mind. Particularly important is that facilitators recognise and work with patient resistance as well as their own emotional responses to the group.

- 'The group was very educative and constructive'
- 'The group was useful to me'
- 'I explained stuff, interesting chat'
- 'I enjoyed the handout'
- 'Interesting and constructive'

REFERENCES

Beck AT, Steer RA, Kovacs M, Garrison B. 1985 Hopelessness and eventual suicide: a 10-year prospective study of patients hospitalized with suicidal ideation. Am J Psychiatry 142: 559–563

Beck AT, Brown G, Steer RA. 1989 Prediction of eventual suicide in psychiatric inpatients by clinical ratings of hopelessness. J Consult Clin Psychol 57: 309–310

Beck AT, Brown G, Berchick RJ *et al.* 1990 Relationship between hopelessness and ultimate suicide: a replication with psychiatric outpatients. Am J Psychiatry 147: 190–195

Bem SL. 1981 Gender schema theory: a cognitive account of sex typing. Psycholo Rev 88: 354–364

Bradshaw J. 1991 Homecoming. New York: Piatkus

Chaudhry K, Kingsley M, Ghafur S. 2006 The Anger Management Group at Pathways PICU. National Association of Psychiatric Intensive Care Units Bulletin 4: 19–21

Clinton C. 2000 Pathways PICU. [Unpublished survey] Goodmayes Hospital, Essex

Dawson P, Galis A, Hughes L, O'Shaughnessy. 2003 Development of an Anger Management Group Programme in PICU [Unpublished manuscript]. Pathways PICU. Goodmayes Hospital, Essex

Dawson P, Kingsley M, Pereira S. 2005 Violent patients within psychiatric intensive care units: treatment approaches, resistance and the impact upon staff. J Psychiatr Intensive Care 1: 45–53

Department of Health. 2002 The National Suicide Prevention Strategy for England. London: Department of Health Publications

Dewar S. 1999 Clinical Governance Under Construction. London: Kings Fund

Docker-Drysdale B. 1991 The Provision of Primary Experience: Winnicottian Work with Children and Adolescents. New Jersey: Jason Aronson

Evans M, Morgan HG, Hayward A, Gunnell, DJ. 1999 Crisis telephone consultation for deliberate self-harm patients: effects on repetition. Br J Psychiatry 175: 23–27

Faddon G, Bebbington P, Kuipers L. 1987 The burden of care: the impact of functional psychiatric illness on the patient's family. Br J Psychiatry 150: 285–292

Flett GL, Hewitt PL. eds. 1994 Perfectionism: Theory, Research and Treatment. Washington DC: American Psychological Association

Gabbard GO. 1994 Psychodynamic Psychiatry in Clinical Practice. Washington, DC: American Psychiatric Press

Goldstein MJ. 1999 Psychological Approaches to Management of Violence. Paper delivered at King George Hospital, Goodmayes, Essex

Harriss L, Hawton K. 2005 Suicidal intent in deliberate self-harm and the risk of suicide: the predictive power of the Suicide Intent Scale. J Affect Disord 86: 225–233

Hawton K, Fagg J. 1988 Suicide, and other causes of death, following attempted suicide. Br J Psychiatry 152: 359–366

Hawton K, Townsend E, Arensman E et al. 2003 Psychosocial and pharmacological treatments for deliberate self-harm (Cochrane Review). In: The Cochrane Library, Issue 3, 2003. Oxford: Update Software

Heisel MJ, Marnin J. 2004 Suicide ideation in the elderly. Psychiatr Times XXI (3)

Heisel MJ, Flett GL, Hewitt PL. 2003 Social hopelessness and college student suicide ideation. Arch Suicide Res 7(3): 221–235

Hewitt PL, Norton GR, Flett GL, Callander L, Cowan T. 1998 Dimensions of perfectionism, hopelessness, and

attempted suicide in a sample of alcoholics. Suicide Life Threatening Behav 28: 395–406

Hinshelwood RD. 1999 The difficult patient. Br J Psychiatry 174: 187–190

Kaplan HI, Sadock B, Grebb J. 1994 Synopsis of Psychiatry, 7th edn. Baltimore, MD: Williams and Wilkins

Kernberg OF. 1975 Borderline Conditions and Pathological Narcissism. New Jersey: Jason Aronson

Linehan MM, Goodstein JL, Nielsen SL et al. 1983 Reasons for staying alive when you are thinking of killing yourself: the reasons for living inventory. J Consult Clin Psychol 51: 276–286

MacLeod AK, Tata P, Tyrer P, Schmidt U, Davidson K, Thompson S. 2005 Hopelessness and positive and negative future thinking in parasuicide. Br J Clin Psychol 44 (4): 495–504

Malone KM, Oquendo MA, Haas GL, Ellis SP, Li S, Mann JJ. 2000 Protective factors against suicidal acts in major depression: reasons for living. Am J Psychiatry 157: 1084–1088

Mann JJ, Waternaux C, Haas GL, Malone KM. 1999 Toward a clinical model of suicidal behaviour in psychiatric patients. Am J Psychiatry 156(2): 181–189

Mervis J. 1999 Workshop on loss and grief. Presented to Mental Health Professionals at Tara Hospital, Gauteng, South Africa

Miller A. 1987 For Your Own Good. London: Virago

Miller A. 1995 The Drama of Being a Child: The Search for the True Self. London: Virago

Milnes D, Owens D, Blenkiron P. 2002 Problems reported by self-harm patients: perception, hopelessness, and suicidal intent. J Psychosom Res 53 (3): 819M

Nitsun M. 1996 The Anti-Group: Destructive Forces in the Group and their Creative Potential. London: Routledge

Ostman T, Wallsten, Kjellin L. 2005 Family burden and relatives' participation in psychiatric care: are the patient's diagnosis and the relation to the patient of importance? Int J Soc Psychiatry 51(4): 291–301

Owens D, Dennis M, Read S et al. 1994 Outcome of deliberate self-poisoning. An examination of risk factors for repetition. Br J Psychiatry 165: 797–801

Owens D, Horrocks J, House A. 2002 Fatal and non-fatal repetition of self-harm: systematic review. Br J Psychiatry 181: 193–199

Petrie K, Chamberlain K, Clarke D. 1988 Psychological predictors of future suicidal behaviour in hospitalized suicide attempters. Br J Clin Psychol 27: 247–258

Robin S, Novaco RW. 1999 Systems conceptualisation and treatment of anger. J Clin Psychol 55: 325–337

Salter D, Platt S. 1990 Suicidal intent, hopelessness and depression in a parasuicide population: the influence of social desirability and elapsed time. Br J Clin Psychol 29: 361–371

Seager M. 2006 The concept of 'psychological safety' – a psychoanalytically informed contribution towards 'Safe, Sound & Suppotive' Mental Health Services. Psychoanal Psychother 20(4): 266–280

Sidley GL, Callam R, Wells A, Hughes T, Whitaker K. 1999 The prediction of parasuicide repetition in a high risk group. Br J Clin Psychol 38: 375–386

Sinclair J, Hawton K. 2004 Suicide and deliberate self-harm. In: Guthrie E (ed) Handbook of Liaison Psychiatry. Cambridge: Cambridge University Press

Sutherby K, Szmukler GI, Halpern A et al. 1999 A study of 'crisis cards' in a community psychiatric service. Acta Psychiatr Scand 100: 56–61

Szanto K, Reynolds CF 3rd, Conwell Y et al. 1998 High levels of hopelessness persist in geriatric patients with remitted depression and a history of suicide attempt. J Am Geriatr Soc 46(11): 1401–1406

Szasz T. 1998 The involuntary patient. Br J Psychiatry 15: 216–225

Townsend E, Hawton K, Altman DG et al. 2001 The efficacy of problem-solving treatments after deliberate self-harm: meta-analysis of randomised controlled trials with respect to depression, hopelessness and improvement in problems. Psychol Med 31: 979–988

Wallace ER IV. 1983 Dynamic Psychiatry in Theory and Practice. Philadelphia: Lea & Febiger

Watts D, Morgan G. 1994 Malignant alienation: dangers for patients who are hard to like. Br J Psychiatry 164: 11–15

Wetzel RD, Margulies T, Davis R, Karam EI. 1980 Hopelessness, depression, and suicidal intent. J Clin Psychiatry 41: 159–160

Winnicott DW. 1971 Playing and Reality. New York: Basic Books

Winnicott DW. 1975 Through Paediatrics to Psycho-Analysis. New York: Basic Books

Zahl D, Hawton K. 2004 Repetition of deliberate self-harm and subsequent suicide risk: long-term follow-up study of 11583 patients. Br J Psychiatry 185: 70–75

7

Psychological approaches to longer-term patients presenting with challenging behaviours

Brian Malcolm McKenzie

Introduction

Severely disturbed behaviour posing a risk to the patient, the treating team or other patients can co-exist with or arise out of acute and chronic forms of psychosis, although a direct relationship is often obscure. These behaviours may settle as soon as the florid aspects of a psychosis dissipate; at other times they may come more sharply into focus as the psychosis improves. On many occasions the intensive care aspect is, de facto, more about the management of challenging behaviours than any psychotic condition. A wide range of behaviours may be construed as challenging. Effectively any behaviour sufficiently persistently disruptive or dangerous to the treatment setting might be defined as challenging. Common examples in psychiatric settings are:

- non-compliance with medication
- extreme withdrawal on the ward
- physical violence to staff, other patients or property
- sexual aggression
- self-harm and suicide attempts
- firesetting
- persistent verbal abuse

Before considering psychological interventions it is important to note that the task of treating patients with a combination of psychotic and behavioural disorder is very frequently made more difficult by the fact that other dimensions of the patient's life may equally show impairment. Shepherd (1999) defines the 'challenging behaviour group' as having a combination of severe and intractable clinical symptoms, a range of behavioural problems and profound social dislocation. One might add problems of family conflict, degradation of living skills and perhaps disorders of personality.

Challenging behaviour within this conception is not a new phenomenon. Individuals with these characteristics were described in a survey of repeated admissions to psychiatric facilities 25 years ago as the 'new long stay' (Mann and Cree 1976). A more recent national audit has indicated that, if anything, this group had increased in size within UK National Health Service psychiatric facilities (Lelliott and Wing 1994). They pose both short- and long-term problems but invariably their treatment requires intensive resources over the longer term. The difficulty in treating this group is perhaps seen in the fact that many patients having this combination become revolving door patients (Lelliott and Wing 1994).

Whatever the ultimate conception of this group, the combination of psychosis, hostility, social alienation, poor living skills and not being able to manage their emotions or behaviours will be a common experience to practitioners working in this field.

This chapter concentrates on psychological approaches to conceptualising and managing the *behavioural problems* this group brings. The other aspects of their need, especially the psychotic

Psychiatric Intensive Care, 2nd edn., eds. M. Dominic Beer, Stephen M. Pereira and Carol Paton.
Published by Cambridge University Press. © Cambridge University Press 2008

dimension, are not directly touched upon. However, it should be stressed from the outset that the problems overlap greatly and psychological treatment responses *must interconnect with medical, nursing and social interventions* if any success is to be hoped for. Furthermore the negatively reinforcing nature of the multilayered needs of this group demand that psychological treatment occurs *simultaneously at individual and systemic levels.*

Instead of focusing on a specific form of challenging behaviour, such as sexual aggression, this chapter attempts to draw out general principles of understanding and approach to treatment. Specifically as a starting point patients exhibiting challenging behaviours are conceptualised as bringing three clinical problems to the treating team, i.e.:

- they present highly complex processes of thought, emotion and behaviours which are difficult to understand
- they pose profound difficulties of engagement
- they bring pressures to bear on the treatment teams

The chapter divides into two sections: understanding challenging behaviours, and treatment approaches

Understanding the complex patterns of thoughts, emotions and behaviours that make up challenging behaviours

Many of the patients in this group act in such a way as to tax the understanding of the team. Their behaviour often seems beyond the comprehension of ordinary insight. There is a resulting temptation to place the behaviour in the realm of psychotic disturbance and thereafter disregard any need for any functional or psychological analyses of the behaviour. It is true that there might be very deeply held disturbed beliefs underlying the behaviour, seemingly profoundly at odds with reality. An example might be the belief that a member of staff is attempting to poison that patient.

However, many disturbed behaviours seem to reflect psychological or emotional processes that are not directly part of a psychotic process or are

disinhibited by the psychosis. Consider the following example.

Case history

A's diagnosis was unclear. She appeared mildly thought-disordered at times and had made a serious suicide attempt. She had also been violent to staff and generally presented angrily and assertively. The staff would attend and use de-escalation techniques that would calm her. She would apologise and a genuinely positive interaction would ensue. Any difficulties and concerns she had would be resolved to the best of the parties' abilities. She would return to her room feeling exhausted and saying that she wished to sleep. Some hours later she would emerge in a furious and abusive state, forcing intervention from the nursing team, often leading to restraint which would damage relationships. When calm enough to be interviewed she could only say that she had felt suicidal while lying down. She could not elaborate any further.

The intense violence of her presentation after a positive exchange seemed puzzling. However, simply from the short description above a number of hypothesis could be proposed for her seeking conflict as shown below.

Some possible reasons for challenging behaviour

- She was seeking more positive attention
- A more paranoid view of staff had set in
- Her anger had not been properly resolved
- She could not tolerate being alone
- She did not like having a good relationship with staff
- She could not tolerate her suicidal feelings

This list is far from exhaustive. However, it makes the point that there are at least a number of areas that might provide a lead for a functional analysis of the behaviour. Recent developments in a number of psychological theories might provide a basis for these hypothesis: *understandings of personality disorder put forward in the cognitive–behavioural theory, attachment theory*, and *developments in therapeutic communities*. These are set out directly below.

Before turning to these developments it should be stressed that at the basis of the psychological approaches is the understanding that *all behaviour is fundamentally interpersonal*. Challenging behaviour is therefore to be understood within its interpersonal context.

Concepts from modern psychoanalysis

Modernity is only a relative concept here but the most vivid, and seemingly accurate, account of emotional functioning in psychotic conditions is to be found in Melanie Klein's outline of the 'Paranoid – Schizoid position'. This is hypothesised to be the earliest stage of emotional development. At this level interpersonal relating is dominated by fear of loss of those seen as 'good' and threat from those seen as 'bad' (Segal 1964). Staff will be percieved in a very black and white fashion with litle chance of the client's seeing realistic shades of grey. This holds dangers of significant distortion in perception of staff. Those staff perceived as good will be wished to be 'possessed' and their absence may trigger a traumatic sense of having nothing good and being alone with persecutors. Withdrawal, self-harm or suicide may follow. For staff perceived as threat, hatred and a wish for their destruction are reserved. These wishes provoke a sense of guilt and fear of retaliation which worsen the situation. Staff may be subject to verbal or physical attack. The task of the staff is not to retaliate and respond in a benign way, hopefully ameliorating the cycle of paranoia. A good example of this is the case of a psychotic patient who had been on 4 months of 2:1 observations at a previous hospital because of her risk of assaulting staff and was transferred to the ward. No assaults followed and she was soon off observation. Staff were puzzled. She continued however to voice a description of clearly fantastic tortures at the previous unit. It seems mentally she had located her persecutors outside the unit allowing her to have a reasonably good relationship with staff who, in reality, were not all that much different from those on the previous unit.

Concepts from modern cognitive therapy

Cognitive therapists have traditionally put forward the view that situations, thoughts, emotions and feelings are closely connected. Thoughts are seen to play a primary role in interpreting events and regulating emotional responses. Disturbances in thought are thereby seen as critical in maintaining disturbances of emotion. A prime example is an 'automatic thought'. An example might be the thought 'I'm useless' which occurs whenever something goes wrong in the individual's life. Such negative automatic thoughts displace the possibility of more positive thoughts; for example, 'everyone has failures, let me try again'.

Furthermore thought patterns play a fundamental role in interpreting events, often skewing our perception. Beck (1996) lists a number of faulty thought processes.

Case history

B was referred with a problem of repeatedly getting into fights in social situations. He had a history of ridicule and rejection at the hand of his father and being bullied and teased at school. Ultimately he had fought back and developed a reputation for violence. Now when he walked into a social situation he felt tense and aroused with the expectation of confrontation. Any glance from other men he interpreted as being a challenge and a threat. He would brood on this matter, believing he could not let this challenge pass as it would mean he was less than a man, in fact he was worthless. This thought would lead to his feeling bad about himself. Ultimately he would react angrily and challenge his perceived rival. If a fight ensued all negative thoughts and feelings would be lost.

Faulty cognitive styles

- All or nothing thinking
- Catastrophising
- Personalising
- Negative focus

Case history

C had made a number of serious attempts on her life and severe acts of self-injury. She stated she did this to get rid of persecuting memories of serious sexual, physical and emotional abuse she had suffered as a child. These thoughts brought on 'black feelings' of which she could identify self-hatred. They made her feel terrible. Harming herself brought relief.

Case history

D would glance over at the nursing station and try to catch the eye of a nurse busy at work. The nurse would look away and return to her paperwork. This would arouse feelings in D of rejection and exclusion. D would then knock on the door of the nursing station, some-times angrily, and demand something in the nurse's ambit, for example an escorted trip to the patients' bank. The nursing staff, often under pressure, would indicate that nothing could be done that shift. An angry alterca-tion would follow and D would storm off to D's room where D would brood about the injustice of the mat-ter. Later in the afternoon D would explode violently at a seemingly trivial incident with a ferocity which took staff aback.

Faulty cognitive styles

• Living by fixed rules
• Jumping to conclusions

Sets of automatic thoughts, self-statements, percep-tual distortions and faulty cognitions may become organised into cohesive wholes. These are called schemas. Schemas provide an organising focus for experience, rules and beliefs. They therefore act in an executive manner. Maladaptive schemas are seen as the self-reinforcing basis of disturbances in behaviour. An example of a maladaptive schema and the connection to disturbed behaviour might be seen below.

One can see a reinforcing relationship between expectation and perception of the situation, beliefs about self, emotions and behaviour. B would mis-takenly read perceptual cues and would reach faulty

Table 7.1. Cognitive analysis of personality disorders.

Personality disorder	Automatic thoughts	Strategy
Dependent	I am helpless	Attachment
Avoidant	I may get hurt	Avoidance
Passive–aggressive	I could be stepped upon	Resistance
Paranoid	People are adversaries	Wariness
Narcissistic	I am special	Self aggrandisement
Histrionic	I need to impress	Dramatics
Obsessive–compulsive	I cannot make mistakes	Perfectionism
Antisocial	People are there to be taken	Attack
Schizoid	I can't allow myself to be close	Isolation

conclusions about himself. Further his aggression resolved his bad feelings about himself.

'It is the consistent failure of schemas to manage feelings relating to interpersonal functioning that cognitive theorists believe define personality disor-der' (Beck and Freeman 1990; Beck 1996). They put forward the view that certain maladaptive schemas correspond to the various personality disorders. This is outlined in Table 7.1.

Problems of internal control

Beck and Freeman (1990) go on to further develop the concept. Patients with personality disorder have a maladaptive schema that attempts to control inter-nal feelings and external interpersonal events. *When the maladaptive schema fails the result is profound levels of anxiety.* The individual then attempts to rec-tify the situation with further disturbances in affect, behaviour and cognition in a desperate attempt to re-establish control. The authors refer to this *as prob-lems of internal control* (Beck and Freeman 1990). In cases of severe disturbance of personality or of behaviour these authors argue that the maladaptive schemas are coupled to disorders of internal con-trol. *In doing so it would appear that they have put forward a conceptual framework capable of understanding the basis of challenging behaviour.*

Case history

E had a long-standing pattern of repeated absconding, angry outbursts in which verbal abuse and damage to property occurred, as well as times occasioning minor physical violence. Although deemed to be chronically psychotic, this side appeared not to trouble E unduly. Many behavioural programmes had been put into place without much success. E's keyworker unflaggingly tried to keep a rapport going but was little rewarded, as E would rarely stay any length in conversation. E could be loquacious, although this could end unpredictably. E seemed an impulsive law unto himself.

A behavioural contract was suggested and presented, leading to E'storming out of the room in anger. E returned an hour later and said he would sign it. The contract set clear goals but tolerated a level of failure. It also required regular update and brief feedback sessions that emphasised positive reinforcement. Much to the surprise of the team E began to use this contract to relate to all staff members. It appeared that E had found a useful and safe way to relate. E became far less verbally abusive.

Concepts from modern behavioural therapy

Emotional dysregulation and affect intolerance

A very similar concept is put forward by Linehan in her study of self-harm in borderline personality disorder conditions. She argues that the core problem is *affect intolerance* (Linehan 1993). Certain feelings are unacceptable to the borderline patient and the patient embarks on a disturbed process of behaviour, *or substitution of different affects*, to minimise the effect of these feelings. Such behaviours are frequently seen in self-harm. Linehan (1993) refers to this process as *affect intolerance or emotional dysregulation*. Such processes might be seen in the following examples.

C appears to substitute physical pain, which she was in control of, for psychic pain.

Here we can see an entrenched schema which appears to organise D's perception and cognition

to cue into any behaviour which may be taken as rejection. Such feelings could not be tolerated and could only be worked out through the explosion of anger and the taking of revenge. The above example perhaps opens up an understanding of a distorted schema that might coincide with a dependent personality disorder. Although the behaviour on initial glance seems simply violent, an analysis based on emotional dysregulation and problems in internal control now suggests itself. Furthermore if one accepts a concept of *affect substitution* the treatment team has the beginning of powerful tools to understand the seemingly paradoxical behaviour of challenging behaviour patients.

Concepts from mentalisation approaches

Mentalisation refers to the developmental achievement of being able to reflect on the behaviours of oneself and others (Fonagy *et al.* 2004). This provides a 'buffering' process between emotionally charged behaviours of others and the patient's emotional reaction (Schore 2003) allowing for control of behaviour and reattribution of the motives of others. It is found to be deficient in those with borderline and psychotic conditions (Bateman and Fonagy 2004).

The process can be broken down into constituent parts and addressed within a therapuetic relationship. These are set out by Leiper (2005) as:
- establish a secure framework
- bear in mind the deficits
- focus on mentalisation
- bridge the gaps
- work with current mental states
- use the therapeutic relationship
- retain psychological closeness

Concepts from attachment theory

Ainsworth (1969) indicates that around 4% of infants show a pattern of attachment that might be defined as insecure or disorganised. These infants are profoundly affected by separation from the primary caretaker and cannot sustain any purposeful or organised pattern of behaviour during their absence. Furthermore following separation these children show disturbed patterns of re-establishing and showing attachment. It is postulated that they become the future generation of borderline patients. It has also been shown that these children tend to have been subjected to major parental failure (Fonagy *et al.* 1997).

The same authors make the point that the disturbed bonds and the behaviour that marks that which become set between child and caretaker transfer or are carried as a model of interaction to adulthood. Relationships with members of caring staff of social institutions would therefore become characterised by disturbed patterns of attachment. Furthermore the absence of a containing relationship or attachment on the ward might lead to disturbed and disorientated behaviour.

Ainsworth *et al.* (1978) identified the following insecure attachment patterns in infants:
- *avoidant*, in which attachment figures are avoided
- *ambivalent*, where there is distress on separation and failure to settle on reunion
- *disorganised*, where there is extremely disorganised and disturbed behaviour in the context of having no attachment strategy

George *et al.* (1996) identify three corresponding adult states of mind:
- *dismissing*: attachment-related behaviour or the need for attachment is dismissed
- *preoccupied*: there is a preoccupation with attachment failures
- *unresolved*: this group shows a striking lack of ability to think about attachment

These styles will dictate how patients relate to staff and explain difficulties in establishing a normal process of relating, frequently even when the psychosis is absent.

Case history

F had a long history of intimidation and property damage. His aggressive behaviour continued with frequency on the ward. The team decided on a plan to impose strict boundaries with respect to his verbal and physical aggression. Alongside this was a programme of positive reinforcement. F was known to enjoy socialising at a hospital social centre. The shift was divided into short time periods. For every period he achieved free of aggression he would be rewarded with time to visit the social club. This was to act as the primary reinforcer. Help on adopting different strategies to the verbal and physical aggression he had employed in the past was taken up in regular keyworker sessions.

When the plan was presented to F by the team his reply was, 'I know what you are up to. You can F off. There is no way I am going to work for my ground leave. You and your behavioural programme can get stuffed.'

Faulty cognitive styles

- Avoidant/dismissing
- Ambivalent/preoccupied
- Disorganised/unresolved

Disturbances in attachment might underlie what appears to be very disturbed behaviour on the ward. The overly isolated and schizoid patient may be acting out an avoidant/dismissing attachment pattern. Similarly the ambivalent or preoccupied patient may show disturbance when left unsupported.

The following example may make the unresolved or disorganised pattern clear.

Case history

G had been on an acute ward for a number of months. Several attempts had been made to re-establish him in the community but all had failed through his verbal and sometimes physical aggression. On the ward he remained a difficult to manage patient, being frequently verbally aggressive and physically destructive. He also wished to dominate the patient group, often demanding to watch his television programme despite others wishing to watch another. One evening in a conflict about who had the right to choose which channel to watch, he became so aroused that he broke the television set. This was nothing new to the staff group which was inured to him by this point. However, at a ward meeting the rest of the patient group was so angry and voiced such complaints about G that the staff group then decided to refer him to a challenging behaviour unit.

Concepts from therapeutic communities

Problems in dependency

Experiences in therapeutic communities have led to useful understandings in disturbed ward behaviour. Green (1986) makes the observation that often violence on the ward is preceded by a period in which relationships between staff and patients appear to be getting better. He explains this as a period in which there is an opening up in the emotional relationships towards each other. However, this openness upsets the psychological equilibrium of the patient and exposes the individual to intolerable feelings of both intrusion and exclusion. The good relationship must then be damaged.

This is closely related to the 'core complex' described by Glasser (1979). He emphasises that the severe anxieties associated with separation and with suffocation or disregard for the individuated self can rapidly alternate, leaving the carer with seemingly contradictory disturbances in behaviour.

Case history

H's admission had come about after violence to staff on an open ward. On the ward H kept up a steady barrage of hostility for many weeks, flouting a number of ward rules and agreements made by her. H demanded that a date be set for discharge. On the other hand a reading of H's history indicated that it was just such setting of dates that precipitated the worst violence on staff members.

Case history

J had started to see the ward psychologist. She had a prolonged but not severe psychosis. The psychologist (perhaps incorrectly) had begun to challenge some of her avoidance of her own emotions, leading to some anger in J. Later that day she made loud allegations

that he and other members of staff had made sexual advances towards her. She was clearly sexually vulnerable and slightly disinhibited. Although retracted, these allegations led staff members to feeling anxious and unable to engage in treatment.

Problems in interpersonal functioning

Campling (1999) identifies a number of related problematic dynamics that work against a positive therapeutic relationship. The first is hostile dependency. This occurs when the patient, experiencing dependency needs, feels them to become overwhelming and has to relieve them by attacking the carer. This in turn leaves the patient anxious, more vulnerable and more dependent.

The second dynamic she identifies is one of envy. This is a strong hostile wish to destroy any good qualities in the person trying to care for them. A third related concept outlined by Campling is the negative therapeutic reaction; an attempt to sabotage everything that points to success. Another quality that she feels requires urgent attention in therapeutic communities is deceitfulness; this, she states, often covers up more profound feelings of emptiness and shame and neglect.

Summary

The concepts of affect intolerance, affect substitution, disorders of attachment behaviour and disorders of dependency give strong tools to the practitioner in understanding the development of disturbed behaviour on mental health wards. These concepts again become very relevant in the two following sections.

Problems in engagement

It is extremely rare with patients exhibiting challenging behaviours for the patient to sit down with a member of the treating team, agree that he or she has a problem behaviour, and ask for help and guidance from the therapist. However, the collaborative nature of goal setting is one of the most important features of any therapy (Beck *et al.* 1979).

Understanding the marked resistances of this group is therefore important. In discussing the cognitive-behavioural treatment of personality-disordered patients, Beck and Freeman (1990) have commented that the course of cognitive therapy is far more complicated when there is a combination of behavioural disturbance with mental illness or personality disorder.

One of the most important treatment considerations in working with personality disordered patients is to be aware that therapy will evoke anxiety because individuals are being asked to go far beyond changing a particular behaviour or reframing a perception. They are being asked to give up who they are and how they have defined themselves for many years. (Beck and Freeman 1990, p. 9)

Furthermore not only is the patient's behaviour inextricably bound up in defending their self-concept, but it is also defined in opposition to the treating team from whom they have long been alienated. This alienation may have little to do with the treating team. Campling (1999), working in therapeutic communities, indicates that patients with severe personality disorders, presumably because of grossly inadequate parenting, have no basis for trusting that people in caring positions have their welfare at heart. Key figures, Campling says, may have neglected and abandoned the patients in the past. These relationships become prototypes for future relationships with authority figures, undermining the treating team.

While the above observations are findings in respect of personality disorders, the situation appears, if anything, more pronounced in challenging behaviour. It might be a trite observation but unless these factors are understood the most technically sound interventions might fail. Case history F (p. 94) might illuminate this. Here the team attempted to use behavioural principles to positively reinforce the desired behaviour of non-aggressive behaviour.

It should be noted that staff had been careful not to mention the phrase 'behavioural programme' but clearly he knew exactly where the team was coming from. Hence the proposal and rejection of the behavioural programme became part of the problematic interaction and not part of the solution.

Understanding the genesis of the resistance or breakdown in the therapeutic relationship is extremely complex. However, again, the approaches adopted by attachment theory and issues of problems of dependency are highly pertinent here. One need only think of the avoidant/dismissing style of attachment and the problem in forming a working relationship. The central point to be taken is that all insecure forms of relating are fragile and riven by anxiety. In cases where there is an accompanying psychosis these anxieties must be profoundly magnified. Furthermore if patients are able to form relationships these will be, in part, marked by destructive acting out. All the above factors undermine the collaborative therapeutic relationship.

Pressures on the treating teams

The treating team is in a complex relationship with the patient. In this interaction perceptions of patient behaviour and the thresholds of acceptance vary. A judgement of whether a patient is presenting with challenging behaviour will in part depend on how much the team is put under stress or pressure by that patient, or by other parts of the system.

Consider this example.

As can be seen in the case history of G above, the threshold and impetus for referring to G as a 'challenging behaviour patient' emerged with the pressure applied by another part of the system, i.e. the patient group. This process reflects a very central aspect to understanding challenging behaviour: challenging behaviour patients place pressure on staff teams, directly or indirectly. Understanding the nature of these pressures and the anxieties held by treatment teams often identifies the necessary focus of treatment. However, pressure on teams often leads to the team becoming polarised and unable to pursue clear therapeutic strategies.

Subjective pressures and their responses

The behaviour of certain patients impacts emotionally on individual members of the treating staff, thereby communicating itself to the treating group. The following examples, though not exhaustive, are commonplace in challenging behaviour wards.

- *Attack on the relationship with the staff.* One may start with the psychoanalytic view expressed by Jeammet (1999) who, working with disturbed adolescents in an inpatient setting, sees challenging behaviour invariably as representing an attack on the therapeutic setting and ultimately on the people who are caring for the patient. An act of destructive behaviour often seems to undo the hard work put in by the team and breaks trust and confidence in the patient–carer relationship. Staff may feel angry and want to reject the patient in turn.

- *Undermining of team therapeutic confidence.* These patients often create a situation where, whatever the staff does, they 'fail'. Patients often vacillate between opposite demands, criticising staff for not meeting their needs at the particular point they are at. Attempts to rectify the immediate demands result in criticism that the other side of the continuum is ignored. One such potential impasse is seen in unresolved dependence–autonomy needs (Green 1986). An example of this might be seen in case history J: staff felt bewildered and at odds with each other; their ability to manage and therapeutically help the patient felt undermined.

- **Raising staff levels of anxiety.** 'Challenging behaviour' patients can easily raise levels of personal anxiety in staff, either through direct threat or by acting in such a way that their behaviour exposes staff to censure. The following example illuminates the point.

Intrinsic structural pressures

The pressures described above have their origin in the patients' behaviours. However, it is a very important principle to keep in mind that, from the patients' subjective perspective, these behaviours are often entirely with reason. In part this may have to do with their history and this was discussed particularly in the previous section. However, it is also important to remember that the context of being on a ward, particularly a locked ward, is a ready source of tension and may go some way to explaining the above difficulties in staff and patient interaction.

These conditions are clearly outlined by Cahn (1998).

- The ward is most often part of an infrastructure for medical treatment. Accordingly the institution is expected to operate with the objectivity and rationality that characterise medicine. Tensions therefore inevitably arise with the subjective aspects or needs of the patient. These are characterised by emotionality, irrationality and ambivalence, all of which fail to follow the expected orderly course of treatment.

- Admissions are seldom made voluntarily. The ward therefore takes on a law-and-order function that is only partly explicit and this is in tension with the subjectively perceived needs of the patient.

- Patients who have exhibited a great deal of violence are often admitted into a Psychiatric Intensive Care Unit (PICU) / challenging behaviour ward. The ward is therefore required to contain and control this violence, which becomes a policing function. Again this produces a tension with the subjective needs of the patient.

- The ward must often accept all patients referred. Hence patients are very different in terms of age, outlook and social interactions. The equilibrium of group life is often under enormous stress.

- Often there is no mutual agreement on treatment. Staff have no choice of whether to work with someone or not and vice versa. Interpersonal tensions might therefore be generated.

It is clear that if the team does not guard against these structural tensions the subjective aspect of the patient can be devalued. If this occurs, Cahn argues, the experience of staff is very much drawn into the problem of devaluation. If the patients feel devalued it would be easy to identify the staff as the devaluers and in reprisal devalue any work done by staff.

Unless these tensions and pressures are taken into account and managed at a systemic level they will lead to an elevation in the disturbance of behaviour at ward level and impede therapeutic engagement, with medical, psychological and social treatments.

Treating challenging behaviours in ward settings

If the above analysis is correct, then psychological approaches should, as a starting point, focus on the goals summarised below:

- Contribute interventions that aim at understanding the complex thought, emotion and behavioural processes that underlie the difficult cycles of interaction that exist between treating staff and the 'challenging behaviour' patient. This would include both understanding the patient and contributing to the engagement of the patient
- To express empathy
- To develop discrepancy, i.e. for the patient to look at both sides of the problem – positive and negative features
- To avoid arguments
- To 'roll with' resistance
- To support self-efficacy

Box 7.1. Principles of motivational interviewing

- Help develop the integrated treatments
- Help develop structures and processes of communications that go some way to ameliorating problems in team cohesion and ward tensions and pressures
- Contribute to the general understanding of the impact of patients on staff members and act supportively towards treating staff members

---

The following sections of the chapter attempt to address practically the above goals by looking at current practices in associated areas.

Cognitive-behavioural approaches to challenging behaviour

Identification of problematic schemata

Beck (1996) suggests therapists should collect information from various sources indicating the automatic thoughts, beliefs and self-concept by which the patient lives. Beck suggests that the first cognitive approach should recover automatic thoughts, the almost instantaneous sense the patient makes of a situation. An example of it might be, 'staff don't care for me'. Generally from there the therapist must elicit the distorted cognitions built into or making up the automatic thought. An example may be a number of 'conditional assumptions' or distorted beliefs about interpersonal functioning, such as 'If I'm not liked I am worthless'.

Distorted cognitions that make up a schema

The following cognitions may be elicited, which could be organised into a coherent schema

- 'If they don't pay attention to me they don't like me'
- 'I cannot bear not to be liked'
- 'If I'm not liked I am worthless'

The therapist then has the task of translating these underlying interpersonal beliefs as they form the basic motivations of maladaptive interpersonal strategies. This, as discussed above, is in itself a difficult process. Beck (1996) recommends the use of cognitive probes. This is a method in which the therapist and patient identify incidents that illuminate the problems and clearly focus on a particular actual incident. Beck and Freeman (1990) suggests the use of imagery to re-imagine the experience and recover the automatic thoughts.

Identifying problematic thinking styles

In addition to maladaptive beliefs and thoughts, cognitive therapists, as discussed above, focus on distortion in thought. Linehan (1993), working with borderline personality disordered patients, identifies a number of problematic thinking patterns. These include: arbitrary inferences, (conclusions based on insufficient evidence), exaggeration, inappropriate attribution of all blame and responsibility for negative events to oneself, inappropriate attribution of all blame and responsibility for events to others. Catastrophising (unrealistic expectation or pessimistic predication based on selective attention to negative events in the past) predominates in this group.

Countering problematic beliefs and patterns of behaviour

The beliefs underlying disturbed behaviour then need to be challenged. A variety of techniques can be identified: discussion, re-attribution, use of homework and adducing empirical evidence for such judgements. Linehan (1993) has developed what she believes are core skills needed for the borderline patients. These seem equally appropriate with challenging behaviour patients.

Mindfulness skills
These essentially are based on teaching the patient to take a non-judgmental stance and to observe their own behaviour; that is, what are the events, emotions and behavioural responses?

Distress tolerance skills
Emphasis here is on learning to bear pain and the ability to tolerate and accept distress. Distress tolerance can lower impulsive and reactive destructive behaviour. Many cognitive skills are put into place, such as not catastrophising or being over-judgmental.

Emotional regulation skills
Linehan indicates that many borderline individuals are affectively intense and labile and argues that they would benefit from learning to regulate affective levels. She suggests that the emotions are initially validated, then that they are identified and labelled, again from the patient's perspective. Thirdly

the patient is taught to understand the function and the connection between the emotion and destructive behaviours.

Interpersonal skills
These are similar to those taught in assertiveness or interpersonal problem-solving classes.

Self-management skills
Behavioural targets are set with realistic goals, self-monitoring and carrying out contingency management skills.

Case history

K was an extremely angry woman who could be physically violent and physically destructive to property. A psychiatric report identified a long psychiatric history, the presence of personality disorder and was equivocal as to the presence of psychotic features.

She was admitted to the challenging behaviour ward. After an initial assessment the psychiatric team identified mood instability and she was treated accordingly. The psychologist attempted to take up her intense feelings of rage and work in anger management or appropriate expression of anger. The nursing team, however, experienced the full force of her daily anger, deviancy and non-engagement. They rapidly adopted a defensive position in which the best option was to avoid confrontation with K during the shift. The phenomenal task became one of increasingly avoiding her altogether. Soon very powerful arguments began to develop between various elements of the team as to the purpose behind her continuing stay on the ward. Little understanding of each other's position could occur. The normative and existential tasks had become increasingly shunned.

Approaches to the problem of engagement

Therapeutic contracting

Campling (1999) makes the point that one of the main differences between working psychotherapeutically with more disturbed patients in comparison to less disturbed patients is that one cannot take the therapeutic alliance for granted. The relationship cannot be left to develop, and mistrust needs to be analysed as it arises. Trust is to be created and the therapeutic alliance built up in a way that is tangible and understood by the patient. She (Campling 1999) suggests the following preparation for engagement on the ward:

- Staff should not focus on disruptive behaviour and its consequences.
- Staff should be ready to reinforce the next appearance of appropriate behaviour even if it comes very soon after disruptive states. Even on wards containing the most difficult or disruptive patients they will be behaving appropriately for 85% of the time. The temptation for staff, of course, is to focus on the remaining 15% of time during which the patients cause trouble, thereby unconsciously reinforcing this mode of personal interaction. The task of the staff is to positively reinforce every time the patient behaves appropriately.
- Identify and target appropriate behaviours – situations such as talking to others, watching TV, smiling, cooking, playing, doing repairs, eating appropriately, using the bathroom appropriately and sleeping.
- Take time in the assessment phase to look at the patients' fears about therapy.
- Make it clear that progress will be slow and sometimes matters will become worse.
- A therapeutic contract should be established that spells out the staff responsibilities, the patient's responsibility and the need to work in partnership.

Case history

L was constantly wrapped up in concerns about other patients, often approaching staff with these worries and asking for advice. However, she could rarely think of her own emotions and needs. Staff formulated the response of asking her what her feelings were in relation to the problem, and encouraged her to try to develop her own plan of action.

Case history

M had a long history of emotional instability and self-injurious behaviours, some quite severe and life-threatening. After a number of ups and downs she appeared to make a concerted effort to re-establish a more normal pattern of life. Things improved and she went for a number of visits to her sister, who was married. One evening her sister and husband had an intense and lengthy argument. Nothing negative was expressed to or about M.

She returned to the ward saying all was well. She went to her room and took an overdose of antidepressants. She reported their argument at the weekend had upset her. On closer questioning she indicated that at the time of the argument she had felt very alone and had decided to take the tablets. Clearly she had been storing tablets for some time. One knew from past treatment that she self-harmed when feelings became unbearable and often these had to do with feelings of anger and rejection.

An interesting experiment in partnership occurred in the 1980s at the Littlemore Hospital in Oxford. The Eric Burden Community and Young Adult Unit was set up. Its admission criteria were very similar to those which might be established for a challenging behaviour unit today, i.e.:

- Diagnosis of a functional psychosis or borderline personality disorder
- Normal intelligence
- No or partial response to conventional medical treatment
- Breakdown of social network

Anyone on a young adult unit case register had the right to request admission. The patients had the right to set the level of medication and manage the thresholds of symptoms to those that they felt were acceptable. It was not the staff's role to eliminate delusions or hallucinations. Clear emphasis was placed on communalism as a strong cultural value on the ward. It was found that psychotic patients used the therapeutic community in much the same way as personality-disordered contemporaries elsewhere (Pullen 1999).

Therapeutic forbearance

Holmes (1993) describes secure attachment as that when an individual is in proximity to his or her attachment figure, he or she feels safe and can engage in exploratory behaviour. This is important for the therapeutic relationship between patient and therapist. The attitude of the therapist may contribute to the patient's progress from insecure to secure attachment to the treating team. The team, like a good mother, picks up cues from the patient's affect or behaviour, and feeds them back to him or her in an appropriate way.

Motivational interviewing

Motivational interviewing is an approach to developing a therapeutic alliance, originally developed in the addiction services, particularly with problem drinkers (Miller and Rolnick 1991). The approach evolved out of Rogerian principles in that the critical conditions for change are accurate empathy, non-possessive warmth and genuineness. The therapist's role in this view was not a directive one providing solutions. Confrontation is seen as counterproductive.

Miller and Rolnick (1991) argue that the fundamental goal is to let the patient consider both advantages and disadvantages to change. The patient should therefore experience ambivalence.

Alongside this they outline a number of traps to avoid: avoiding confrontation and denial, avoiding what they call the 'expert trap', avoiding the labelling trap and avoiding a premature focus trap. The motivational interviewing techniques are entirely appropriate for this highly resistant group and should inform any approach to working with challenging behaviour patients.

Approaches from dialectical behaviour therapy

Linehan (1993), working with borderline patients, articulates a view she calls 'dialectical behaviour therapy'. The 'dialectic' can be described as trying to hold in mind a balance of both where the patient is struggling and the reasons for his or her difficult behaviour, as well as the goals of less destructive behaviour. In defining what is distinctive about this approach she states

the most fundamental . . . is the necessity of accepting patients just as they are within a context of trying to teach them to change. The tension between patients' alternating excessively high and lower aspirations and expectations relative to their own capabilities offers a formidable challenge to therapists. It requires moment to moment changes in the use of supportiveness and acceptance versus confrontational and change strategy. (Linehan 1993, p. 10)

In addition to the focus on acceptance, Linehan emphasises treating 'therapy-interfering behaviours' as legitimate aims of treatment. Linehan identifies three groupings of behaviour that interfere with therapy:
* *Inattentive behaviour.* This includes not attending, attending late, taking substances before coming to the session, having feelings or behaviours which preclude therapy
* *Non-collaborative behaviour.* Being oppositional, distracting and digressing
* *Non-compliant behaviours.* These include failure to carry out agreed tasks

These, she says, should be taken up and treated cognitively and dialectically. This serves to provide a useful approach to challenging behaviours.

Constructive institutional responses

Defining tasks and boundaries

Roberts (1994) has explored failing organisations within the National Health Service (NHS). She establishes a number of common problems including vague task definition, defining methods instead of aims, avoiding conflict over priority, confusing tasks with aims and failing to manage boundaries. It might be argued therefore that central to the successful running of a challenging behaviour ward is for the management team to define the primary task, the subordinate tasks and the systems to manage them.

The primary task

The concept of a primary task can seem to be an oversimplification, given the complexities that challenging behaviour patients bring. However, as a starting point it is invaluable. In this respect Miller and Wright (1967) describe establishing the primary task as a useful concept which allows the team to explore ordering of multiple activities. If one conceptualises challenging behaviour as the breakdown of the ordinary treatment relationship, then the primary task is to re-establish a working patient–carer relationship. The tasks of addressing specifically the disruptive behaviours and underlying psychological problems that disrupt the relationship then become clear. This conceptualisation has become much more prevalent in the treatment of personality-disordered patients where 'therapy disruptive behaviours' form legitimate and initial focuses for treatment, rather than reasons for exclusion from treatment (Campling 1999; Linehan 1993; Beck 1996; Beck and Freeman 1990).

Tasks understood by the organisation

Lawrence (1977) described how in any institution there can be task confusion. He distinguishes between them as follows:

- *Normative primary task*, which is the formal operationalisation of the organisation
- *Existential primary task*, which is the task which people from the enterprise believe they are carrying out
- *Phenomenal primary task*, which can be inferred from people's behaviour and of which they may not be consciously aware

If there is task confusion the treating team can be split with arguments. Case history K hopefully shows how severe challenging behaviour patients can stress the organisation's definition of itself.

In this example a clear definition of the ward tasks as restoring the treatment relationship and dealing with the behaviours that prevent the formation of such a relationship would help prevent splits in the team and enable treatment to start.

Therapeutic structures at ward level

Systematically Cahn (1998) considers that intervention or organisation should occur at three levels. The entire institution is regarded as a therapeutic system or environment with each level needing to contribute to the primary task.

The managing group

Here the task must be to endeavour to create and keep open an environment in which therapeutic processes can take place. This should be in part to define tasks and structures and to support the subgroups.

Ward structures and treatment teams

The ward constitutes a boundaried environment in which the patient should be given concrete, tightly drawn and firm rules. This provides security.

Staff–patient ward groups

Most therapeutic communities stress the need for regular meeting of staff and patients (Byrt 1999). The principle seems important for all ward groups, in particular in the light of the structural pressures outlined above. Cahn (1998) says that ward meetings should represent the entire ward with all its subgroups. Patients should be free to bring up subjects of their own. The group leaders must often provide structural help. As far as possible collaboration needs to occur and agreements drawn up that staff and patients can become partners. In practice there need to be agreed minute-takers, chairpersons and a formal process for decisions to be taken to the appropriate hospital manager/clinician if the matter cannot be dealt with at the ward meeting.

There clearly needs to be communication between each level.

Integrative treatment approaches

The task of the ward should be discussed and integrated. There is a constant stress on this and the focus for the psychological practitioner is to suggest means of integrating and communicating the primary task of the ward and to explain how that translates in respect of the patient. Some useful therapeutic approaches can be adopted that strengthen this goal and the tasks outlined above.

The RAID programme for challenging behaviour

One method for maintaining a positive style by all treating staff in the face of difficult behaviours is the adoption of the RAID programme. This is a programme developed by Davies (1993).

RAID is an acronym standing for 'Reinforce Appropriate (behaviour), Ignore Difficult or disruptive (behaviour)'. Focus is placed on the positive aspects of the patient's behaviour while de-emphasising the more disruptive. This creates an environment in which more positive interaction occurs and helps the staff think positively of the patients despite the difficult behaviours exhibited by them. Reinforcing positive behaviours makes future positive action more probable and builds on the patients' sense of competence. Ultimately therefore success on the ward should strengthen the relationship between the staff and the patient.

Davies (1993) identifies an essential stance to be maintained by the treating team.

Psychosocial nursing

A particularly appropriate means of establishing the basis of positive interaction with patients is the development of psychosocial nursing. The aim of this approach is to strengthen social functioning. Essentially the stance taken by nurses is to maintain in mind a view of the patient's potential capabilities and encourage and foster responsibility for putting these abilities into action, rather than assuming the patient to be ill. The following example might make this process clear.

Integrating treatment

Functional analysis

This is based upon an understanding of challenging behaviour as disorders of attachment, dependency and emotional dysregulation. To do effective work at this level it is necessary to perform a clear functional analysis of the behaviour. Once the problem is established intervention needs simultaneously to be integrated at the level of individual and ward approaches, and to make sure there is the least possible contradiction. Consider case history M.

The first step is to gain a very clear and detailed understanding of the whole chain of the behaviour, its antecedents and consequences. Linehan (1993) calls this 'chaining'. She argues that a clear analysis of a whole chain of an episode of disturbed behaviour must be made; understanding the trigger, the underlying cognitive, affective and behavioural schemata. Similarly Beck and Freeman (1990) suggest an analysis of the view of self, the view of others, one's own negative beliefs and basic strategies. The latter authors call these flow charts.

If one couples this with the understanding brought by the concepts of affect intolerance, disturbances of internal control, problems in dependency and disturbances of patterns of attachment, then the approach of functional analysis provides an extremely powerful method of understanding the behaviour.

Using this as a basis one can postulate that the argument between M's sister and brother-in-law is the trigger for the behaviour. M's perception is that she is ignored and excluded. This re-awakens powerful feelings of rejection which are not tolerable. M then takes the overdose. This paradoxically is a matter of psychological or emotional survival. The focus of treatment is needing to tolerate pain and anxiety associated with feelings of rejection. This can be addressed in individual treatment. Furthermore the patient needs to be taught more appropriate means of expression. This is most probably done best at ward level on a daily level, perhaps using the RAID approach. The ward can also do supportive work at community group level, countering the strong cognitions of rejection. Intensive work needs to be done on maintaining relationships both at ward and individual levels.

The following flow chart (Fig. 7.1) provides an example of an integrated approach to treatment.

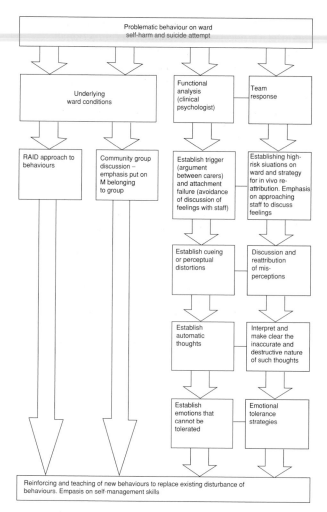

Figure 7.1. An example of treatment of challenging behaviours at ward level

Conclusion

Figure 7.1 shows how chronically disturbed behaviour could be managed on a ward. The approach also hopefully allows for an integration of thoughts from different theoretical standpoints. The ultimate emphasis of this chapter is how to understand the powerful processes that undermine the working patient–carer relationship and adopt treatment approaches aimed specifically at re-establishing the relationship. Once established many of the problems this group faces can then be effectively treated.

REFERENCES

Ainsworth M. 1969 Object relations and dependency and attachment: theoretical review of mother infant relationship. Child Dev 40: 969–1025

Ainsworth M, Blehar RM, Waters E *et al.* 1978 Patterns of Attachment: A Psychological Study of the Strange Situation. Hillsdale N.J.: Lawrence, Erlbaum Associates

Bateman A, Fonagy P. 2004 Psychotherapy for Borderline Personality Disorder: A Mentalisation-Based Approach. Oxford: Oxford University Press

Beck AT, Freeman A. 1990 Cognitve Therapy of Personality Disorders. New York: Guilford Press

Beck AT, Rush J, Shaw B, Emery G. 1979 Cognitive Therapy of Depression. New York: Guilford Press

Beck JS. 1996 Cognitive therapy of personality disorders. In: Salkovskis PM (ed) Frontiers of Cognitive Therapy. New York: Guilford Press

Byrt R. 1999 Nursing: the importance of the psychosocial enviroment. In: Campling P, Haig R (eds) Therapeutic Communities Past, Present and Future. London: Jessica Kingsley

Cahn T. 1998 Beyond the treatment contract: psychoanalytical work in the public mental hospital. In: Pestalozzi J *et al.* (eds) Psychoanalytic Psychotherapy in Institutional Settings. London: Karnac

Campling P. 1999 Chaotic personalities: maintaining the therapeutic alliance. In: Campling P, Haig R (eds) Therapeutic Communities Past, Present and Future. London: Jessica Kingsley

Davies W. 1993 The RAID Programme for Challenging Behaviour. Leicester: Association for Psychological Therapies

Fonagy P, Target M, Steele M, Steele H. 1997 The development of violence and crime as it relates to security of attachment. In: Osofsky JD (ed) Children in a Violent Society. New York: Guilford Press, pp. 150–177

Fonagy P, Gergely G, Jurist E, Target M. 2004 Affect regulation, mentalisation and the development of the self. London: Karnac

George C, Kaplan N, Main M. 1996 Adult Attachment Interview, 3rd edn. Unpublished Manuscript. University of California, Berkeley: Department of Psychology

Glasser M. 1979 Some aspects of the role of aggression in the peversions. In: Rosen I (ed) Sexual Deviation. Oxford: Oxford University Press

Green A. 1986 On Private Madness. London: Karnac

Holmes J. 1993 Attachment theory: a biological basis for psychotherapy. Br J Psychiatry 163: 430–438

Jeammet P. 1999 Links between internal and external reality in devising a therapeutic setting for adolescents who present with serious conduct disorders. In: Amastasopoulous D, Laylou-Lignos E, Wadder M (eds) Psychoanalytic Psychotherapy of the Severely Disturbed Adolescent. London: Karnac

Lawrence G. 1977 Management Development. Some ideals, images and realities In: Coleman AD, Geller MH (eds) Group Relations Reader No. 2. Washington, DC: Rice Institute

Leiper R. 2005 Mentalisation and beyond. Presented at Salomons continuing professional development training December 2005

Lelliott P, Wing JK. 1994 A national audit of new long stay psychiatric patients. II: Impact on services. Br J Psychiatry 165: 170–178

Linehan M. 1993 Cognitive Behavioural Treatment of Borderline Personality Disorder. New York: Guilford Press

Mann S, Cree W. 1976 New long stay psychiatric patients: a national sample survey of fifteen mental hospitals in England and Wales 1972/1973. Psychol Med 6: 603–616

Miller EJ, Wright AK. 1967 Systems of Organisation: The Control of Task and Central Boundaries. London: Tavistock

Milner WR, Rolnick S. 1991 Motivational Interviewing: Preparing People to Change Addictive Behaviour. New York: Guilford Press

Pullen G. 1999 Schizophrenia: hospital communities for the severely disturbed. In: Campling P, Haigh R (eds) Therapeutic Communities: Past, Present and Future. London: Jessica Kingsley Publisher

Roberts VZ. 1994 The organisation of work: contributions from open system theory. In: Obholzer A, Roberts VZ (eds) The Unconscious at Work. London: Routledge, pp. 28–38

Segal H. 1964 Introduction to the work of Melanie Klein. London: Heineman

Schore A. 2003 Affect Regulation and the Repair of the Self. New Jersey: Lawrence Erlbaum

Shepherd G. 1999 Social functioning and challenging behaviour. In: Meuser KT, Terrier N (eds) Handbook of Social Functioning and Schizophrenia. Massachusetts: Allyn and Bacon

8

Seclusion – past, present and future

Roland Dix, Christian Betteridge and Mathew J. Page

Introduction

Whether seclusion has a place within the treatment of the mentally disordered is one of the longest running debates in the history of mental health care and it is likely to continue. Controversial deaths in mental health facilities and their subsequent inquiries will further fuel speculation as how best to manage challenging behaviour. The Independent Inquiry into the Death of David Bennett (Norfolk, Suffolk and Cambridgeshire Strategic Health Authority 2003) questioned whether the use of seclusion may have been preferable to prolonged restraint.

The use of seclusion is at least 2000 years old and many of the related questions have remained consistent, surviving to the modern day. It is not the intention of this chapter to re-describe the moral, ethical and legal paradigms that have punctuated much of seclusion's history. The focus here will be to provide an overview of the history of seclusion, its value or otherwise, its alternatives and the necessary supporting policies for its use. Finally, we will offer a practical framework within which seclusion may be considered in the context of Psychiatric Intensive Care Units (PICUs) and Low Secure Units (LSUs).

For the purpose of this chapter seclusion is defined as 'the forcible confinement of a patient alone in a room for the protection of others from serious harm' (Mental Health Act 1983: Code of Practice; Department of Health 1999).

Seclusion is widely used throughout the world (Mason 1994). Not surprisingly, different cultures have different attitudes and, as a result, different variations on the use of seclusion. While it would be unwise to ignore the experiences of other countries, the theme of this chapter will be the use of seclusion in the United Kingdom.

No attempt to deal with the use of seclusion can be completely divorced from the simple question of whether seclusion should be used or not. To do so would deny the emotive nature of the issues innate to the subject. Having recognised this, the authors will not offer a definitive view as to whether PICUs and LSUs should have seclusion, but will rather provide a balanced guide to thinking, informing the decision-making process for anyone planning such a service. The arguments for and against the use of seclusion will be apparent throughout the chapter.

History of seclusion

It is difficult to define an era that marks the birth of seclusion in the management of mental disorder. The Greeks had rooms designed to entice the mentally ill patient to sleep so that they would dream their way back to sanity (Wells 1972).

Even in Ancient times, physicians of the Roman Empire such as Soranus advocated a compassionate attitude towards the insane. He suggested that

Psychiatric Intensive Care, 2nd edn., eds. M. Dominic Beer, Stephen M. Pereira and Carol Paton.
Published by Cambridge University Press. © Cambridge University Press 2008

sufferers should be, as far as possible, protected from fear, anger and, most interestingly, blame (Nolan 1993). This epoch in history may not only mark the first recorded use of seclusion, but also the beginning of one of the longest debates in mental health care.

During the Middle Ages and Renaissance, different religions attached their own meanings to the disordered mind. Therefore, the extent to which severe methods of management featured, including the use of seclusion, varied considerably (Mora 1967). The eighteenth and nineteenth centuries saw a shift towards the institutional model for the housing of the insane, and with it brought the use of seclusion that more closely resembles modern-day methods, i.e. for management of the most disturbed behaviour. During the 1790s Philippe Pinel demonstrated that his asylum, the Bicêtre in Paris, could operate without a profound reliance on the use of seclusion and restraint (Renvoize 1991). Pinel was confident that with the correct method of communication, paying attention to the in-mates' individuality and self-respect, *few* restraints were necessary (Hunter and Macalpine 1963). While it is apparent that Pinel had stumbled on the value of de-escalation, it is difficult to overlook the use of the term '*few*', which clearly signals that physical confinement was still deemed unavoidable in some circumstances. In Britain, William Tuke, a layman superintendent of the Retreat asylum in York, also advocated a more humane approach based on his Quaker 'moral therapy' philosophy. In 1892 an interesting debate about the use of seclusion between Tuke and another British pioneer, John Conolly, quoted Tuke as arguing:

If Conolly attached too much importance to this mode of treatment [*seclusion*], the other extreme, of regarding the padded room as never useful, is a very questionable position to take. (cited by Angold 1989)

It is difficult to avoid the feeling that in the twenty-first century this debate is no nearer to a conclusion. The latter half of the nineteenth century marked increased attempts to more clearly legislate for the legal and conceptual underpinnings of mental health care. There emerged several consistent themes, often in conflict with each other, attempting to improve the experience of the patient while at the same time addressing the fears of society. A number of attempts were made to balance the determined efforts by the medical profession to claim the scientific high ground with law makers, who argued that mental health care was a legal rather than medical concern (Rogers and Pilgrim 1996). While this situation produced various degrees of focus on the humane treatment of the patient, by and large the experience of the patient remained unchanged with the continued and unregulated use of mechanical restraint and seclusion.

During the 1920s there was growing concern about the conditions in many psychiatric hospitals for staff and patients alike. Staff were expected to work 14 h a day with only half a day off per month. In September of 1922 tensions reached such a pitch that staff and patients of the Nottinghamshire County mental hospital joined forces in fighting against police who were sent there to restore order (Nolan 1993). In 1923 an inquiry at Hull Asylum reported on the lack of privacy, dirty conditions, patients having to bath in the same water and most worryingly 'patients being confined in dungeons for long periods of time'. Conditions for all within many of the institutions during the early 1920s left little time or interest for singling out the use of seclusion for debate, amongst what appeared to be far more important concerns. In 1922 Dr Montagu Lomax published his book entitled *The Experiences of an Asylum Doctor*. This book was highly critical of the conditions in many institutions, the appalling arrogance and behaviour of many medical superintendents and also the barbaric methods of treatment including the use of seclusion. A storm of debate resulted from the book's publication. Even amidst aggressive attempts by medical superintendents to discredit Dr Lomax, the Royal Commission recommended wide-reaching improvements, which included limiting patient seclusion to certain clearly defined circumstances. Patients also had to be carefully monitored whilst in seclusion (Nolan 1993). This was possibly the first appearance of standard regulation on the use of seclusion.

The outbreak of war in 1939 preoccupied much of the 1940s. Mental hospitals, as far as it was possible, were emptied to accommodate the wounded. This also resulted in a renewed interest in the science of mental illness, in particular the use of electroconvulsive therapy for the treatment of shell shock and depression (Merskey 1991). Another addition included the introduction of psychotherapeutic techniques. Even with these innovations the widespread and unregulated use of seclusion continued. This is chillingly illustrated by the personal accounts of nurses working in hospitals during the 1940s, collected by Nolan (1993). One nurse recalls:

Patients were subjected to hours and hours of endless boredom in the airing courts . . . We counted patients in and out . . . In side rooms, there were patients locked up for weeks on end; the staff had become so used to the screaming of these patients that they totally ignored it.

The 1950s saw the introduction of chlorpromazine, hailed by many as a miracle cure for psychosis. Even though the true efficacy of chlorpromazine remained in debate, a new era had dawned with many hospitals opening their doors during the 1950s and 1960s. Many wards now had open-door policies with new freedoms given to many patients, although for a significant minority of patients locked wards and seclusion continued.

A new Mental Health Act in 1983 resulted in the publication of a Code of Practice in 1993, which made a determined attempt to finally regulate the use of seclusion. A revised Code of Practice was also published in 1999, although no advice has been added regarding seclusion. The Mental Health Act Commission (MHAC) was appointed to support the 1983 Act and to prevent the emergence of mental hospital brutality scandals that riddled the 1970s. In spite of this, the 1992 Cutting Edge television documentary again exposed appalling practice involving seclusion at Rampton special hospital, as they had done 12 years earlier. The vice chair of the MHAC was forced to concede the Commission has failed where investigative journalism had succeeded (Rogers and Pilgrim 1996).

The 1970s to the 1990s were characterised by a massive increase in debating the moral, practical and conceptual issues attached to the use of seclusion. A snap-shot survey of the professional press in 1999 showed 314 papers containing the word seclusion in three popular databases. In recent years a number of often polarised arguments have been advanced resulting, in some cases, in the abolition of seclusion altogether in many hospitals. As far as PICUs are concerned, Beer et al. (1997) in their survey found that of 110 PICUs in the UK 40% had no seclusion room. Of those that did have seclusion, 15 units admitted to having no written policy on its use. Department of Health figures for 2004 confirm that of PICUs and LSUs, 50% continue not to have seclusion.

Even today, apart from the academic debate, the press has also recorded deaths of secluded patients. In America, the use of mechanical restraint and seclusion remains a routine procedure in many modern psychiatric hospitals (Hamolia 1985). Appelbaum (1999) reports on 142 deaths in American seclusion rooms between 1988 and 1998. While allowing for the Americans' favouring of seclusion more than their European counterparts, it is interesting that the House of Representatives has introduced a bill entitled the 'Patients' freedom from restraint act 1999' (Tenth Congress, First Session, March 25 1999). It appears that unease surrounding the use of seclusion has even penetrated the long-held hard line of many states of America. In Britain the famous and disturbing case of the death in seclusion of Orville Blackwood left the panel of inquiry concluding that a 'macho culture' existed around the use of seclusion in Broadmoor special hospital, in addition to their lacking procedures (Prins 1994). The Independent Inquiry into the death of David Bennett (Norfolk, Suffolk and Cambridgeshire Strategic Health Authority 2003) also comments on seclusion, this time not as a situation to be avoided, but rather as a possible safer alternative to prolonged restraint. This point has also been raised by other authors such as Paterson et al. (2003) and these views will be more closely examined later in the chapter.

Amidst the often passionate and polarised arguments presented by supporters and opponents of seclusion, one thing is clear: seclusion continues to be used in many hospitals and when staff are in the position of having to manage serious aggression, one is often reduced to few options. This point was succinctly made by Mason (1994) who concluded his international review of seclusion with the following comments:

When the patient is no longer susceptible to the paradigms of treatment, when they are in the throes of assault, when they are combatant – there remain only four things one can do: seclude them, restrain them, medicate them, or pass the problem on to some one else (transfer them).

The remainder of this chapter aims to illuminate a path through the maze of argument surrounding the modern-day use of seclusion, which will guide the thinking of PICU/LSU staff.

Factors that affect the modern-day use of seclusion

Opponents of seclusion are rapidly growing in numbers and as we will see later in this chapter, arguments for its abolition are profound and diverse. Seclusion continues to hold a precarious position in modern psychiatric hospitals and its continued use is under close scrutiny. The survival or demise of seclusion depends upon clear and honest analysis of what factors affect its use. Furthermore, alternative interventions and their impact on seclusion rates need to be examined. Until recently there was an identified lack of available guidelines for making decisions regarding seclusion (Outlaw and Lowery 1992). This has been corrected with the publication of the National Institute for Clinical Excellence (NICE 2005) Guidelines for the short-term management of disturbed/violent behaviour in psychiatric inpatient settings and emergency departments. NICE does not presume that all services have access to seclusion but where it is available it should follow its recommendations. The National Institute for Mental Health in England's (2004) Mental Health Policy Implementation Guide for Developing Positive Practice to Support the Safe and Therapeutic Management of

Aggression and Violence in Mental Health Inpatient Settings recognises that seclusion may be used as a strategy for managing violence and refers to the MHA Code of Practice (Department of Health 1999).

Patient behaviour

Patients in psychiatric hospitals can display a wide diversity of challenging behaviours to various degrees. The decision to implement seclusion is a complicated process fraught with problems. Much of the empirical literature reveals alarming variations in the rationale offered for the use of seclusion. Angold (1989) noted violence, in particular interpersonal violence towards staff, to be the most common rationale for seclusion. Likewise Tooke and Brown (1992) found that both staff and patients viewed destructive, aggressive behaviour but also inappropriate sexual behaviour as the main reasons for seclusion. A review of ten studies undertaken by Soloff *et al.* (1985) concluded that seclusion was most frequently used to contain disruptive, agitated or excited behaviour. Also it was the clear belief of the staff that much of the behaviour represented a serious risk of escalation into actual violence. The conclusion of this extensive review was that early use of seclusion dramatically reduced the incidence of actual violence.

Morrison and Lehane (1996) concluded that physical assaults on staff were the single most common cause of seclusion, closely followed by: threats to staff, self-inflicted injury, damage to property, disturbed behaviour, physical assault on patients, threats to patients and self seclusion. Moreover, physical assaults on staff and patients only accounted for one-third of the total episodes of seclusion. Surprisingly, the majority of episodes were precipitated by non-violent behaviours (Morrison and Lehane 1996).

During a year-long study of the use of seclusion and restraint use in eighty-two medical centres in America, the primary reason given for its use was disruptive behaviour disturbing the ward environment, not necessarily violent behaviour itself. Closely following in descending order were patient agitation, physical and verbal aggression (Betemps *et al.* 1992).

Meehan *et al.* (2000) found that seclusion was, for most patients, a negative experience and one which was often felt to be unnecessary. Conversely some respondents recalled it as being an opportunity to regain control of their behaviour.

Ward characteristics

General ward characteristics and staffing levels have also proven to have had a significant impact on the use of seclusion. Staffing levels in particular have been the focus of many studies that have consistently found a strong correlation between increased staffing levels and reduced incidence of seclusion (Outlaw and Lowery 1992; Morrison 1995). Craig and Hix (1989) found that staffing levels, education and experience in dealing with disturbed behaviour made a significant impact on the use of seclusion. Jose de Cangas (1993) linked staffing levels to frequency of seclusion; however, factors rated more highly were unit layout, degree of crowding and conflicting personalities.

Attitudes and culture

There is also good evidence that the attitudes and general ethos of staff groups are significant in the use of seclusion. Indications that staff are reluctant to be self critical with regard to seclusion have been presented. Jose de Cangas' (1993) study found that staff viewed seclusion use to be more affected by unit factors than variations in their own attitude and performance. In contrast, De Cangas and Shopflocker (1989) recorded that nursing staff held a positive attitude towards seclusion, were open minded about its implementation and believed that it was an effective intervention. Steele (1993) surveyed staff attitudes in four hospitals and revealed that 80% of staff claimed to refuse to consider seclusion until verbal intervention had been attempted and had failed. The majority of staff viewed seclusion as a last resort which had some therapeutic benefit.

Further evidence of the importance of staff attitude was presented by Gerlock and Solomons (1983), who established a correlation between staff attitude, ward culture and the frequency of seclusion. Tolerance levels towards disturbed behaviours, anxiety levels, the need to control behaviour because of low staffing levels as well as perceptions of the therapeutic benefits of seclusion were all found to be highly significant. Considering the literature concerning attitudes, it is clear that some staff teams are more motivated towards proactive interventions that can de-escalate behaviours which would otherwise warrant seclusion. Reasons for failing to engage in proactive intervention are offered by Morrison (1990), who argues that nurses are too often engaged in non-clinical tasks, resulting in lost opportunities to prevent escalating behaviour which culminates in seclusion. It is reasonable to hypothesise that those units with a positive attitude towards seclusion as a therapeutic treatment and low motivation towards creative interventions will undoubtedly have higher rates of seclusion.

Forster *et al.* (1999) found that introducing an interdisciplinary quality improvement workgroup and associated training around issues of prevention of aggression and promotion of least restrictive methods of management significantly reduced the incidence of seclusion. Plaskey and Coakley (2001) also found a dramatic reduction in the reliance on seclusion after a package of education and procedural changes was made.

Patient characteristics

Correlations between seclusion and patient characteristics such as gender, age and race have been established. Soloff and Turner (1981) found an alarmingly disproportionate number of black patients were being secluded. Lack of communication and cultural understanding between predominantly white staff and black patients was one proposed explanation. However, in a follow-up study four years later Soloff *et al.* (1985) found that young patients are secluded more often than older patients and that race and gender bore no significance. More recent British studies have shown that black people were over-represented in seclusion rates, were given higher doses of medication and tended to spend longer in hospital than white patients (Browne 1997).

Swett (1994) found slightly higher seclusion rates for males than for females but again confirmed being younger (under 35 years) was much more likely to result in seclusion. In terms of general patient characteristics, it is difficult to make confident assertions about their relevance to seclusion. However, there appears to be more than enough evidence to think seriously about perceptions of age and race.

Summary of important factors that affect the use of seclusion

To conclude our analysis of factors that affect the use of seclusion, a number of clear themes emerge. The literature has identified a deficit of descriptive accounts of the nature and degree of verbal and physical violence that precede seclusion. The lack of empirical data that describe the intricacies of violent behaviour has serious implications for future practice. Indeed, Breakwell (1997) strongly supported careful monitoring of patterns of violent behaviour for the purposes of future clinical predictions and practice. Without better data on details of aggressive behaviour that are deemed to warrant seclusion, much of the decision-making process will be left to individual staff. Finally there are many other variables, for example staff attitudes and perceptions of age and race, that simply should not affect the decision to seclude or otherwise.

Box 8.1. Key points

- Justifying the use of seclusion purely on the grounds of managing violence is simply not supported by the evidence
- There is good indication that seclusion is used to supplement staffing levels
- Staff attitudes to seclusion are important
- Adequate staff training in seclusion is needed
- There is no satisfactory explanation for the over-representation of non-white patients in seclusion statistics

---

Does seclusion have a place in contemporary psychiatric practice?

The arguments for and against seclusion are complex. Many authors have advanced both evidence and argument to support their particular viewpoint. In order to promote clarity, and provide a context within which to consider the evidence, it is helpful to categorise the debate under three main headings: morality, consequentialism and treatment.

Morality: there are those who believe that the use of seclusion is morally wrong. Put simply, it is held that within modern practice the procedure of locking a patient alone in a room cannot in principle be justified (Hammill 1987).

Consequentialism: there are those that maintain a consequentialism approach to ethical reasoning; that the decision whether or not seclusion is used results from a direct appraisal of the potential consequences that arise for the patient and others (Morrison and Lehane 1995). In other words, when faced with extreme aggression the end justifies the means, and that, in some cases, seclusion may be the least damaging option for the patient as well as others.

Treatment: some commentators have maintained that seclusion is a useful treatment modality (Orr and Morgan 1995). They do not, in the first instance, overly concern themselves with moral or ethical debate, but rather maintain that the practice can produce positive effects in the mental and behavioural state of the patient.

The moral argument

Within the literature it is not difficult to find examples of powerful condemnation of seclusion. Some commentators have described the practice as an 'archaic, controversial form of tyranny' and 'an embarrassing reality' in the management of mental disorder (Pilette 1978; Rosen and DiGiacomo 1978; Soloff 1979). The Royal College of Nursing has been quoted to regard seclusion as an anti-therapeutic intervention that will ultimately become redundant

(Topping-Morris 1994). Topping-Morris goes on to suggest that 'as patient advocates, nurses should seek to expose the issue of seclusion as a lingering relic of the past'.

Although the comments listed above are generally representative of the views held by opponents of seclusion, they do not in themselves provide a solid foundation from which to debate. The consistent themes are that seclusion is a very distressing patient experience (Norris and Kennedy 1992; Tooke and Browne 1992; Meehan *et al.* 2000; Griffiths 2001), and that it is outdated and outmoded. These views are fuelled by evidence that patients can perceive seclusion as a form of torture (Chamberlin 1985; Jensen 1985). They illustrate the general unease associated with the notion of locking away disturbed behaviour as a simple method of management. Hammill (1987) asks 'Why has the practice continued? Is it because it is still easier to isolate an out of control patient behind a locked door, rather than deal with the underlying problem?' Many of these arguments are based on the overwhelming evidence that, when available, seclusion will be implemented with dubious rationale, be inconsistently used and that its frequency is related to many other variables not necessarily dependent on degrees of violence. These issues have been given appropriate attention previously in this chapter, and from our analysis of factors affecting the use of seclusion are undeniably valid. The basic core of the moral argument is that if one has seclusion as an available option, patients will be secluded inappropriately, suffer extreme distress and staff will not be motivated to develop superior methods of dealing with violence (Drinkwater and Gudjonsson 1989). It is reasonable therefore not to have seclusion at all.

The consequentialist argument and alternatives to seclusion

Beauchamp and Childress (1994) defined the application of consequentialism to an ethical debate as 'the right act in any circumstance is the one that produces the best overall result, as determined from an impersonal perspective that gives equal weight to the interests of each affected party'. It is not difficult to see the attraction of this theory for supporters of seclusion as a method for managing violence. Verbal de-escalation, restraint, medication and the use of increased observation in an extra care area have all been proposed as alternatives to seclusion (Kinsella and Brosnan 1993; Kingdon and Bakewell 1988; Donat 1998; Myers 1990; Department of Health 2002). We will examine evidence for their effectiveness and attempt to balance this with arguments advanced by those who maintain that they do not in every case provide a preferable alternative to seclusion.

Verbal de-escalation

The value of verbal de-escalation in preventing actual physical assault has long been accepted (Infantino and Mustingo 1985; Stevenson 1991; Turnbull *et al.* 1990). Shepherd and Lavender (1999) showed that of 127 violent incidents 50% could be managed with verbal interventions alone. They report seclusion being used in only two of the total incidents. A clinical trial demonstrated a drop in the use of seclusion by 50% after the introduction of a model of de-escalation (Morales 1995). Following a change in seclusion policy in a secure unit, Torpy and Hall (1994) found a highly significant reduction in seclusion rates. They suggested that the staff had become considerably more skilled at alternative interventions, in particular verbal de-escalation.

In line with the experience of many mental health nurses, most if not all advocates of de-escalation accept that at best the technique can only dramatically reduce, rather than eradicate, physical violence. Some authors point out that verbal de-escalation is a complex process and during interaction the dynamics can easily work in the opposite direction, escalating aggression (Blair 1991; Maier 1996). Soloff *et al.* (1985) found in their review of the literature that there was overwhelming empirical support for using seclusion to limit the progression of disruptive behaviour to actual violence. Although seclusion has been advocated as a quick and effective method of preventing progression towards physical assault, it must be accepted that a determined attempt at verbal de-escalation is an obvious first intervention.

Physical restraint

The introduction of control and restraint (C&R) training to a medium secure unit showed several benefits (Parks 1996). Seclusion was only used in 12% of the total number of violent incidents. It was suggested that staff were now in the position to hold a patient safely until either verbal de-escalation or medication could work. This was balanced however with an increase in injuries to staff in comparison to figures before the introduction of C&R. Increased staffing levels are highly significant in reducing seclusion use. One explanation for this could be that if more staff are available then restraint is more readily attempted. Evidence of this is provided by Palmstierna and Wistedt (1995) who showed that increased staff numbers reduce the severity of violent incidents, but not their frequency.

Physical restraint as an alternative to seclusion can in itself be a very problematic intervention. While it is permitted in many American states to use four-point mechanical restraint, in the UK restraint has been traditionally understood to involve the holding of a person by another (MHA Code of Practice; Department of Health 1999). Betempts and Buncher (1992) showed that some patients spent up to 72.2 h in a single episode of mechanical restraint in American hospitals. In the UK prolonged restraint has been known to result in sudden death from asphyxia (Paterson *et al.* 1998). Indeed, many of the deaths that actually occur while a patient is in the seclusion room have been correlated with a violent struggle immediately before the patient was secluded (Kumar 1997). The authors work in a PICU without seclusion and we have ourselves experienced situations where the patient continues to fight with staff, requiring continued restraint on some occasions for up to 40 min. Mindful of the potential problems associated with restraint, it is reasonable to suggest that, when compared, 40 min spent in a seclusion room may be preferable as well as safer for both the patient and staff to the same length of time spent in physical restraint. The evidence or otherwise supporting seclusion as a safer alternative to prolonged restraint is an extremely important issue. Restraint is being covered in Chapter 9, and readers are encouraged to read that chapter to complement their understanding of seclusion.

Rapid tranquillisation

Rapid tranquillisation (RT) is covered in depth in Chapter 4 so we shall only briefly touch on its relevance to seclusion. The appropriate use of medication has been proposed as a method of reducing or even eradicating the use of seclusion (Klinge 1994). Not surprisingly Pilowsky *et al.* (1992) showed that, when given intravenously, RT had eradicated the need for seclusion. Intramuscular RT has also proved highly effective with only a small minority of cases requiring restraint or seclusion following its use. It is beyond question that RT is largely effective in calming an agitated, angry and potentially assaultative patient. However, its use has been shown to produce distressing side-effects and is also correlated with sudden death (Laposata 1988; Paterson *et al.* 1998).

The extra care area (ECA)

The use of an extra care area (ECA) in which a single patient may receive intensive nursing intervention is advocated in the Mental Health Policy Implementation Guide: National Minimum Standards in Psychiatric Intensive Care Units and Low Secure Environments (Department of Health 2002) as an alternative to seclusion, and has become a popular method of managing acute disturbance (Kinsella and Brosnan 1993; Dix and Williams 1996). The principles of the ECA appear to fulfil much of the function of seclusion by removing a patient, who is liable to assault others, from the general ward population. It also has the advantage of keeping staff in contact with the patient through the aggressive episode so that they can develop the enhanced skills necessary for dealing with disturbed behaviour (Kinsella and Brosnan 1993). The use of graded observation in concert with the ECA was reported by Kingdon and Bakewell (1988) to have successfully completely replaced seclusion. They report no increase in violent incidents or any cases of refused admission as a result of a new non-seclusion policy.

Again this method is also not without its problems. Kinsella and Brosnan (1993) reported on the occurrence of patients receiving positive reinforcement towards disturbed behaviour as a result of the special attention they receive from prolonged use of the ECA. The ECA can also be difficult for staff. In terms of the numbers of staff needed, there is a danger of creating a ward within a ward (Dix and Williams 1996).

Summary of seclusion alternatives and their consequences

To summarise the seclusion debate within the context of consequentialism: alternatives to seclusion should be carefully appraised in relation to the problems they themselves may cause. It is very easy to maintain a no seclusion policy, while at the same time failing to recognise the possibility of equally undesirable, and sometimes dangerous, consequences of alternative interventions. The basic position of this philosophy is that while all possible action should be taken to avoid the need for seclusion, there are rare circumstances in which it remains the least damaging intervention. Of particular importance is the need for a detailed analysis of the cases of sudden death that occur during prolonged restraint (Paterson and Leadbetter 2004).

Box 8.2. Key points

- Verbal de-escalation is valuable in reducing and managing the incidence of assaults, although it cannot eradicate them.
- Physical restraint is effective for the immediate management of assault; when used for extended periods, it can be potentially dangerous for the patient and arguably is not preferable to seclusion.
- Rapid tranquillisation is effective in the immediate management of disturbed behaviour. There can be difficult delays (unless administered intravenously) in achieving

---

sedation. There is also the possibility of severe side-effects.
- The extra care area is effective in containing a patient liable to assault others. It can be very expensive in terms of time and resources. There is also a possibility of producing a secondary behavioural disturbance in order to maintain intensive contact with the staff.

The treatment argument

Several authors have produced evidence that seclusion can promote positive mental and behaviour change in the patient (Mason 1993; Orr and Morgan 1995). In short, they advance the argument that, more than just a method of emergency management, seclusion can be an effective treatment. Before we examine some of this evidence, we must clearly state that the concept of seclusion as a treatment is simply not acceptable within the English Mental Health Act Code of Practice (Department of Health 1999), where part 19.16 clearly states that:

Its [seclusion] sole aim is to contain severely disturbed behaviour which is likely to cause harm to others . . . Seclusion should not be used as part of a treatment plan.

Most of the support for seclusion as a treatment comes from the USA. Khan *et al.* (1987) concluded that patients who were exposed to low stimulation, mechanical restraint and seclusion experienced a significant reduction in psychotic symptoms. Hamolia (1985) again argues that seclusion can be therapeutic as a result of the patient's being contained, removed from the circumstances in which they responded aggressively, and by receiving reduced sensory input. She further suggests that 'Their [the patients] distortions create such psychic pain that seclusion may provide some relief and may be the only place they feel safe from their persecutors'. In addition seclusion is suggested to be a place where the patient can learn to exercise control over their impulses. In a survey by Steele (1993), 60% of the staff felt that seclusion had therapeutic as well as emergency management value. In a minority of the sample group, some studies of patients' perception of seclusion have recorded positive comments in relation to the experience of being secluded (Norris and Kennedy 1992). Feelings such as safety, reassurance from the regular observations, and the time to reflect in the quiet of the seclusion room were reported.

The major problem with demonstrating that seclusion has any treatment value is the overwhelming evidence that staff and patients perceive seclusion very differently (Plutchik *et al.* 1978; Soliday 1985; Heyman 1987; Richardson 1987; Nolan 1989). Staff tend to underestimate the negative experience of the patient while simultaneously overestimating the positive effects. In addition, it is very difficult to establish a control group of non-secluded patients who have similar mental and behavioural profiles to those who were secluded and against which therapeutic value may be measured.

To conclude the treatment argument, it is beyond question that the vast majority of patients perceive seclusion as a negative experience. Much of the evidence for positive effects can easily be questioned in terms of its scientific rigour (Whittington and Mason 1995). In any event in Britain at least, this modality of 'treatment' is as good as outlawed by the Mental Health Act Code of Practice (Department of Health 1999).

Policy for the use of seclusion

During this chapter it has become clear that the use of seclusion is by and large a personal affair dependent on the characteristic of wards and their team members. While it may have to be accepted that the very nature of aggression and the use of seclusion in its management will always produce variation in practice, it is inexcusable to maintain the seclusion option without a clear, agreed and well thought through policy.

Principles of a working seclusion policy

Wherever possible seclusion should be avoided (Mental Health Act Code of Practice; Department of Health 1999). All other avenues must be exhausted before resorting to this final measure. Professionals faced with the prospect of having to seclude need to be knowledgeable regarding the legal framework applicable. Furthermore the policy should be informed by evidence offered in the literature. This necessity may produce a degree of discomfort inasmuch as the policy will need to cater for some potentially sensitive issues. These include, for example, staff attitudes, staffing levels and perceptions of age and ethnicity.

Legal position: Common Law

In England and Wales according to Jones' (1999) analysis, two Common Law authorities are relevant. Firstly, Lord Griffiths viewed one authority as 'imposing temporary confinement on a lunatic who has run amok and is a manifest danger either to himself or others – a state of affairs as obvious to a layman as to a doctor.' Secondly, Lord Keith outlined the authority to detain where someone was mentally ill and likely to harm self or others. This judgement may also extend to the use of seclusion (Jones 1999). The importance of being able to justify detention was emphasised. Common Law appears to be at odds with the Mental Health Act Code of Practice as it appears to tolerate the seclusion of a patient who may present a risk to themselves. This should not however be used to supersede the Code.

Mental Health Act 1983

Seclusion is not covered by the 1983 Mental Health Act itself, although there is comprehensive guidance in the Mental Health Act Code of Practice. The Mental Health Act provides no statutory duty to adhere to the Mental Health Act Code of Practice (Department of Health 1999). However, as a statutory document, if the Code's principles are not adhered to, then this evidence could be used in legal proceedings. The Code of Practice clearly states that seclusion should be used for the shortest period of time possible, and that it must not be used as a punishment, a treatment, because of staff shortages, or because of self-harm or suicide risk.

The sole aim of seclusion is 'to contain severely disturbed behaviour which is likely to cause harm to others'.

Unit policies on seclusion should actively incorporate the Code's guidelines by ensuring the safety of the secluded patient in a designated room meeting the Mental Health Act Commission's standards for seclusion. NICE (2005) guidance should also be clearly represented in any seclusion policy. Professionals must offer care and support during and after seclusion. The difference between time out and seclusion must be emphasised clearly, the former being an agreed strategy with therapeutic aims and without a locked door.

The evidence and policy making

The published evidence sends clear messages in a number of areas that must be heard by policy makers. They include accounting for varying attitudes of staff, the need to monitor the effects of staffing levels and perceptions of age and ethnicity. In addition, accurate records of all patient behaviours and ward environmental factors that preceded seclusion must be kept and regularly reviewed. In terms of audit, the authors suggest the input of professionals divorced from the unit, for both an independent perspective and the credibility of the monitoring process.

The example policy shown in Figure 8.1 incorporates these important issues. It begins with a philosophy statement to which all the staff must contribute and agree. There is also a list of clear statements that must be considered by the decision maker implementing seclusion. These two components aim to minimise inconsistencies that result from personal attitudes. There are also instructions relating to procedure.

The example seclusion form offered in Figure 8.2 requires the decision maker to give a clear description of what actually happened, to consider an assault rating scale of the level of aggression that actually occurred, and in the opinion of the staff the level that was avoided by using seclusion. These

requirements aim to prevent vague rationale being used to implement seclusion. Moreover they help the staff to focus on what level of real threat they are dealing with, hopefully diminishing impulsive reactions while under stress. It is required for staff to describe what alternative interventions were attempted, again promoting the emphasis of avoiding seclusion. On the seclusion form, the numbers of staff on duty and the patient's age and ethnicity are also required. These data will provide a solid basis for audit, which will need to occur at least every 6 months. The policy also requires staff to comment on the length of time physical interpersonal restraint may have been required if seclusion was not implemented. The basic assumption here is that prolonged restraint is less safe than seclusion, assuming the option to seclude is available. In order to save space the example policy documents suggested here are not as comprehensive as they might be in reality, but they do contain most of the important issues.

Conclusion

The number of PICUs and LSUs are increasing (Reed Committee 1992; Dix 1995; Department of Health 2005). In line with the Reed Committee's (1992) recommendations and the Department of Health (2002) Policy Implementation Guide, most if not all local mental health services will have access to PICUs as part of their standard inpatient provision. By definition the PICU will often be the facility that has responsibility for the most disturbed patients (Pereira *et al.* 1999). Already many of these units house the only seclusion room in the hospital. There may be a danger of complacency amongst service managers resulting from the notion that seclusion has been hidden away in corners of PICUs, rather than in view of all patients and staff in every general adult ward. In the 50% of PICUs without seclusion rooms (Beer *et al.* 1997; Department of Health 2005), it is beyond question that it is possible to operate without them. We have seen throughout this chapter that seclusion continues to be an enormously complex issue. To date, the polarised positions held by

Jones Ward PICU policy for the use of seclusion

Philosophy statement

Seclusion is a serious infringement on a person's civil liberty. It should be avoided wherever possible. It can only be used as a last resort when all other interventions have been tried and failed and for the shortest possible time. Staff must be confident that they can justify the implementation of seclusion.

Seclusion may only be considered when the following conditions are met:

1. The patient is behaving in a way that is likely to injure others in the immediate future.
2. Staff have made a clinical assessment taking into account clinical and actuarial indicators that there is an immediate serious risk of harm to other people.
3. All other interventions have been considered or attempted especially verbal de-escalation including listening skills, negotiation skills aiming for a win/win situation, anger management techniques and diversional activities.
4. The decision maker has carefully considered their own stress levels and ensured that they are not adding bias to the decision to seclude.
5. Seclusion is not being used as a therapy or as a punishment.
6. Seclusion is not being used to manage self harm or suicidal behaviour.
7. Inadequate staff numbers are not influencing the decision to seclude.

Procedure for seclusion

1. Once a patient is in seclusion a designated member of staff must remain within sight and sound of the room at all times.
2. That a member of staff will make a written observation on the seclusion form (see Figure 8.2) of what the patient is doing, at least every 15 min.
3. As soon as the risk of serious assault has diminished seclusion should be discontinued. This will be indicated when the patient is verbally/non-verbally calm. It is not acceptable for the seclusion record to show that the patient is asleep, lying or sitting quietly on two consecutive entries without seclusion being discontinued.
4. Inform the duty doctor immediately that seclusion is commenced who must attend and make an entry in the health record.
5. The need for seclusion must be reviewed by:
   (a) two nurses every 2 h
   (b) a doctor every 4 h
   (c) a multidisciplinary team including the patient's RMO and ward manager, if seclusion continues for 8 h
6. If the need for seclusion is disputed by any member of the team then it should immediately be referred to a senior manager for review.

Figure 8.1. Suggested policy for the implementation of seclusion

---

Jones Ward PICU Seclusion Form

Reason for seclusion (terms such as aggression, disturbed in isolation are not acceptable)

_____

_____

_____

From the rating scale (Lanza and Campbell 1991) below record the level of aggression resulting from the patient's behaviour by entering the appropriate number in the boxes provided

Level actually demonstrated =   ARS Number ☐

Level that was assessed to be
likely if patient was not secluded =   ARS Number ☐

        Assaultive Rating Scale (ARS)
        1. Threat of assault but no physical contact
        2. Physical contact but no physical injury
        3. Mild soreness/surface abrasion/small bruises
        4. Major soreness/cuts/large bruises
        5. Severe lacerations/fractures/head injury
        6. Loss of limb/permanent physical injury
        7. Death

Describe the interventions attempted to avoid seclusion

Seclusion Details

Time In Seclusion ☐   Time Out ☐   Number of Staff on duty ☐

Name of person making the decision to seclude _____

Patient Name _____ Sex ____ Ethnicity _____ Age ____

Name of Staff Member observing _____

    Time   Observation

    _____   _____

    _____   _____

    _____   _____

    _____   _____

    _____   _____

    _____   _____

Please attach any continuation sheets

Figure 8.2. Suggested seclusion form

many commentators have not been helpful in progressing into the new millennium with any more clarity than the last. Furthermore, attitudes have started to change as a result of sudden death associated with prolonged restraint. Supporters and antagonists of seclusion often leave confusion in their wake.

Recently, seclusion has also become a central issue in the tragic deaths of two people in the UK, one patient, Mr David Bennett, and one member of staff, Mr Eshan Chattun. Mr David Bennett died whilst being restrained having knocked one nurse unconscious and continuing to struggle, only three yards from the seclusion room (Norfolk, Suffolk and Cambridgeshire Strategic Health Authority 2003). Mr Chattun entered a seclusion room located on the ground floor of a two-storey PICU. He was beaten to death before assistance could be called (Carvel 2005).

A number of important questions could be raised in relation to these tragic events:

- How does seclusion compare with restraint and medication in terms of safety, in particular for the patient?
- Once a person has been secluded, are serious risks being managed, or are we just delaying the risks until seclusion is discontinued?
- How does the experience of being secluded affect the patient–staff relationship?

Recent debate has focused on the tragic occurrence of sudden death during restraint (Parkes 2002; Paterson *et al.* 2003; Paterson and Leadbetter 2004). In recent years it has become increasingly difficult to discredit the use of seclusion purely on the basis of moral discomfort. There remains the need for detailed and objective analysis of the risk factors contained within prolonged restraint. The argument that a period in seclusion could be safer for the patient than prolonged restraint appears to be gaining ground.

Much of the published analysis is undertaken from an academic foundation which often leaves unanswered questions for staff who actually face violence on a daily basis. To break from this tradition, the authors will conclude with thoughts based on first-hand experience of dealing with aggression both with and without seclusion.

The authors have recently been involved in a situation where a patient had spent over a week within the ECA of a LSU. Many of the negative effects, as discussed during this chapter, of using the ECA for extended periods started to emerge during our recent experience. These effects may be simply summarised by the following paradox, 'the patient is in the ECA because they behave problematically; the patient behaves problematically because they are in the ECA'. As a result of an episode of prolonged restraint within the ECA, the seclusion room was used for the first time since the unit opened nearly three years ago. Having resorted to seclusion once, it has since been used with the same patient twice more.

The need for, or the desirability of, seclusion must be informed by systematic analysis of the evidence supporting least risk to the patient and staff comparing seclusion with all its alternatives. The debate does not rest here however. And the evidence is overwhelming: if you have seclusion, eventually you will use it, and not always for the most extreme situations.

REFERENCES

Angold A. 1989 Seclusion. Br J Psychiatry 154: 437–444

Appelbaum P. 1999 Seclusion and restraint: congress reacts to reports of abuse. Psychiatr Serv 50(7): 881–885

Beauchamp T, Childress J. 1994 Principles of Biomedical Ethics, 4th edn. Oxford: Oxford University Press

Beer D, Paton P, Pereira S. 1997 Hot Beds of general psychiatry: a national survey of psychiatric intensive care units. Psychiatr Bull 21: 142–144

Betemps E, Buncher M. 1992 Length of time spent in seclusion and restraint by patients at 82 VA Medical Centres. Hosp Community Psychiatry 43(9): 912–916

Betemps E, Somoza E, Buncher C. 1992 Hospital characteristics and staff reasons associated with use of seclusion and restraint. Hosp Community Psychiatry 44(4): 367–371

Blair DT. 1991 Assaultive behaviour: does provocation begin in the front office? J Psychosoc Nursing Mental Health Serv 39: 21–26

Breakwell G. 1997 Coping With Aggressive Behaviour. Leicester: BPS Books

Browne D. 1997 Black people and sectioning. London: Little Rock Publishing, p. 47

Carvel J. 2005 Hospital trust faces sentence for staff death. The Guardian, 18 April 2005

Chamberlin J. 1985 An ex-patients response to Soliday. J Nervous Mental Dis 173(5): 288–289

Craig C, Hix C. 1989 Seclusion and restraint: decreasing the discomfort. J Psychosoc Nurs Mental Health Serv 27(7): 16–19

De Cangas JP. 1993 Nursing staff and unit characteristics: do they affect the use of seclusion? Perspect Psychiatr Care 29(3): 15–22

De Cangas J, Shopflocher D. 1989 The practice of seclusion and factors affecting its use. In: Chi-Hui (Kao) Lo (ed) Proceedings of the Sigma Theta Tau International Research Congress. Advances in International Nursing Scholarship Taipei: Sigma Theta Tau, p. 83

Department of Health. 1983 Mental Health Act 1983: Code of Practice. London: Department of Health and Welsh Office

Department of Health. 1999 Mental Health Act 1983: Code of Practice. London: Department of Health

Department of Health. 2002 Mental Health Policy Implementation Guide: National Minimum Standards in Psychiatric Intensive Care Units (PICU) and Low Secure Environments. London: Department of Health

Department of Health. 2005 Survey of Physical Environments in PICU and LSUs in England and Wales. London: Department of Health

Dix R. 1995 A nurse led psychiatric intensive care unit. Psychiatr. Bull 19: 285–287

Dix R, Williams K. 1996 Psychiatric Intensive Care Units, a design for living. Psychiatr Bull 20: 527–529

Donat D. 1998 Impact of a mandatory behavioural consultation on seclusion/restraint utilisation in a psychiatric hospital. J Behav Ther Exp Psychiatry 29: 13–19

Drinkwater J, Gudjonsson G. 1989 The nature of violence in psychiatric hospitals. In: Howells K, Hollin C (eds) Clinical Approaches to Violence. Chichester: John Wiley and Sons Ltd, pp. 287–307

Forster PL, Cavness C, Phelps MA. 1999 Staff training decreases use of seclusion and restraint in an acute psychiatric hospital. Arch Psychiatr Nurs 13 (5): 269–271

Gerlock A, Solomons H. 1983 Factors associated with the seclusion of psychiatric patients. Perspect Psychiatr Care 21(2): 46–53

Griffiths L. 2001 Does seclusion have a role to play in modern mental health nursing? Br J Nurs 10(10): 656–661

Hammill K. 1987 Seclusion: inside looking out. Nurs Times, 4 February, pp. 38–39

Hamolia C. 1985 Managing aggressive behaviour. In: Stuart G, Sundeen S (eds) Principles and Practice of Psychiatric Nursing, 5th edn. St Louis, Mo.: Mosby, pp. 719–741

Heyman E. 1987 Seclusion. J Psychosoc Nurs Mental Health Serv 25(11): 8–12

Hunter R, Macalpine I. 1963 Three hundred years of psychiatry 1535–1860: a history presented in selected English texts. Oxford: Oxford University Press

Infantino J, Mustingo S. 1985 Assaults and injuries among staff with and without training in aggression control techniques. Hosp Community Psychiatry 36: 1312–1314

Jensen K. 1985 Comments on Dr Stanley M. Soliday's comparison of patient and staff attitudes towards seclusion. J Nervous Mental Dis 173(5): 290–291

Jones R. 1999 Mental Health Act Manual, 6th edn. London: Sweet and Maxwell

Khan A, Cohen S, Chiles J, Stowell M, Hyde T, Robbins M. 1987 Therapeutic role of a psychiatric intensive care unit in acute psychosis. Compr Psychiatry 28: 3, 264–269

Kingdon D, Bakewell E. 1988 Aggressive behaviour: evaluation of a non-seclusion policy of a district service. Br J Psychiatry 153: 631–634

Kinsella C, Brosnan C. 1993 An alternative to seclusion? Nurs Times 89(18): 62–64

Klinge A. 1994 Staff opinions about seclusion and restraint at a state forensic hospital. Hosp Community Psychiatry 45: 138–141

Kumar A. 1997 Sudden unexplained death in a psychiatric patient – a case report: the role of the phenothiazines and physical restraint. Med Sci Law 37: 170–175

Lanza M, Campbell R. 1991 Patient assault: a comparison of reporting measures. Qual Assurance 5: 60–68

Laposata A. 1988 Evaluation of sudden death in psychiatric patients with special reference to phenothiazine therapy: forensic pathology. J Forensic Sci 33: 432–440

Lomax M. 1922 The Experiences of an Asylum Doctor. London: George Allen & Unwin

Maier GJ. 1996 The role of talk down and talk up in managing threatening behaviour. J Psychosoc Nurs Mental Health Serv 34(6): 25–30

Mason T. 1993 Seclusion theory reviewed: a benevolent or malevolent intervention? J Med Sci Law 33: 1–8

Mason T. 1994 Seclusion: an international comparison. Med Sci Law 34: 54–60

Meehan T, Vermeer C, Windsor C. 2000 Patients' perceptions of seclusion: a qualitative investigation. J Adv Nurs 31: 370–377

Merskey H. 1991 Shell-shock. in: Berrios G, Freeman H (eds) 150 years of British Psychiatry, 1841–1991. London: Gaskell, pp. 245–267

Mora G. 1967 History of psychiatry. In: Freeman AM, Kaplan HI (eds) Comprehensive Text Book of Psychiatry. Baltimore, Md.: Williams and Wilkins

Morales T. 1995 Least restrictive measures. J Psychosoc Nurs Mental Health Serv 33(10): 42–43

Morrison P. 1990 A multi-dimensional scalogram analysis of the use of seclusion in acute psychiatric settings. J Adv Nurs 15: 59–66

Morrison P. 1995 Research in the effects of staffing levels on the use of seclusion. J Psychiatr Mental Health Nurs 2(6): 365–366

Morrison P, Lehane M. 1995 Saffing levels and seclusion use. J Adv Nurs 55: 1193–1202

Morrison P, Lehane M. 1996 A study of the official records of seclusion. Int J Nur Stud 33(2): 223–235

Myers S. 1990 Seclusion: a last resort measure. Perspect Psychiatr Care 26(3): 25–25

National Institute for Clinical Excellence. 2005 Violence: The Short-Term Management of Disturbed/Violent Behaviour in Psychiatric Inpatient Settings and Emergency Departments. London: NICE

National Institute for Mental Health in England. 2004 Mental Health Policy Implementation Guide: Developing Positive Practice to Support the Safe and Therapeutic Management of Aggression and Violence in Mental Health Inpatient Settings. London: NIMHE

Nolan P. 1989 Face value. Nursing Times 85(35): 62–65

Nolan P. 1993 A History of Mental Health Nursing. London: Chapman Hall

Norfolk, Suffolk and Cambridgeshire Strategic Health Authority. 2003 Independent Inquiry into the Death of David Bennett. Cambridge: Norfolk, Suffolk and Cambridgeshire Strategic Health Authority. Available online at www.irr.org.uk/pdf/bennett_inquiry.pdf

Norris M, Kennedy W. 1992 The view from within: how patients perceive the seclusion process. J Psychosoc Nurs 30(3): 7–13

Orr M, Morgan J. 1995 The medical management of violence In: Kidd B, Stark C (eds) Management of Violence and Aggression in Health Care. London: Gaskell

Outlaw FH, Lowery BJ. 1992 Seclusion: the nursing challenge. J Psychiatr Nurs Mental Health Serv 30(4): 13–17

Palmstierna T, Wistedt B. 1995 Changes in the pattern of aggressive behaviour among inpatients with changed ward organisation. Acta Psychiatr Scand 91: 32–35

Parks J. 1996 Control and restraint training: a study of its effectiveness in a medium secure psychiatric unit. J Forensic Psychiatry 7(3): 525–534

Parkes J. 2002 A review of the literature on positional asphyxia as a possible cause of sudden death during restraint. Br J Forensic Pract 4(1)

Paterson B, Leadbetter D. 2004 Learning the right lessons. J Mental Health Pract 7(7): 12–15

Paterson B, Leadbetter D, McComish A. 1998 Restraint and sudden death from asphyxia. Nurs Times 94(44): 62–64

Paterson B, Bradley P, Stark C, Saddler D, Leadbetter D, Allen D. 2003 Deaths associated with restraint use in health and social care in the UK. The results of a preliminary study. J Psychiatr Mental Health Nurs 10: 3–15

Pereira S, Beer D, Paton C. 1999 Good practice issues in psychiatric intensive care units. Psychiatr Bull 23: 397–404

Pilette PC. 1978 The tyranny of seclusion: a brief essay. J Psychosoc Nurs Mental Health Services 16(10): 19–21

Pilowsky LS, Ring H, Shine PJ, Battersby M, Lades M. 1992 Rapid tranquillisation. A survey of emergency prescribing in a general psychiatric hospital. Br J Psychiatry 160: 831–835

Plasky P, Coakley C. 2001 Reducing the incidence of restraint and seclusion. In: Dickey B, Sederer LI (eds) Improving mental health care: commitment to quality. Washington DC: American Psychiatric Publishing

Plutchik R, Karasu T, Conte H, Siegel B, Jerrett I. 1978 Toward a rationale for the seclusion process. J Nervous Mental Disease 166(8): 571–579

Prins H. 1994 Report of the Committee of Inquiry into the Death of Orville Blackwood and a Review of the Deaths of Two Other Afro-Caribbean Patients. London: Special Hospital Service Authority

Reed Committee. 1992 Review of Health and Social Services for Mentally Disordered Offenders and Others Requiring Similar Services. London: Department of Health/Social Services Office

Renvoize E. 1991 The Association of Medical Officers of Asylums and Hospitals for the Insane, the Medico-Psychological Association, and their Presidents. In: Berrios G, Freeman H (eds) 150 Years of British Psychiatry, 1841–1991. London: Gaskell

Richardson B. 1987 Psychiatric inpatients: perceptions of the seclusion room experience. Nurs Res 36: 234–238

Rogers A, Pilgrim D. 1996 Mental Health Policy in Britain: A Critical Introduction. London: Macmillan Press Ltd

Rosen H, DiGiacomo JN. 1978 The role of physical restraint in the treatment of mental illness. J Clin Psychiatry 39: 228–232

Shepherd M, Lavender T. 1999 Putting aggression into context: an investigation into contextual factors influencing the rate of aggressive incidents in a psychiatric hospital. J Mental Health 82(2): 159–170

Soliday SM. 1985 A comparison of patient and staff attitudes towards seclusion. J Mental Nervous Dis 173: 282–286

Soloff PH. 1979 Physical restraining and the non psychotic patient: Clinical and legal perspectives. J Clin Psychiatry 40: 302–305

Soloff P, Turner M. 1981 Patterns of seclusion. J Nervous Mental Disease 169(1): 37–44

Soloff P, Gutheil T, Wexler J. 1985 Seclusion and restraint in 1985: A review and update. Hosp Community Psychiatry 36(6): 652–657

Steele R. 1993 Staff attitudes toward seclusion and restraint, anything new? Perspect Psychiatr Care 29: 23–28

Stevenson S. 1991 Heading of aggression with verbal de-escalation. J Psychosoc Nurs, 29: 6–10

Swett C. 1994 Inpatient seclusion. Bull Am Acad Psychiatry Law 22: 421–430

Tooke S, Brown J. 1992 Perceptions of seclusion: comparing patient and staff reactions. J Psychosoc Nurs 30(8): 23–26

Topping-Morris B. 1994 Seclusion examining the nurse's role. Nurs Stand 8(49): 35–37

Torpy D, Hall M. 1994 Violent incidents in a secure unit. J Forensic Psychiatry 4(3): 519–544

Turnbull J, Aitken J, Black L. 1990 Turn it around: short term management of aggression and anger. J Psychosoc Nurs 28: 6–12

Wells D. 1972 The use of seclusion on a university hospital floor. Arch Gen Psychiatry 26: 410–413

Whittington R, Mason T. 1995 A new look at seclusion: stress, coping and the perception of threat. J Forensic Psychiatry 6(2): 285–304

9

Restraint and physical intervention

Roland Dix

Introduction

Throughout the ages, virtually all complex societies have found the need for containment and control of behaviour by physical means. Indeed, it is difficult to imagine a world without prisons, police and the periodic need for society to impose its collective standard of behaviour on individuals.

While most people share a degree of comfort with the notion of physical intervention to maintain law and order, its use under the justification of mental health 'care' is deeply troubling to many, with some arguing it has no place at all (Davis 2004). The first words in any discussion about restraint must include the methods of avoiding the need for its use wherever possible. De-escalation, negotiation and the development of trusting relationships have been covered in detail elsewhere in this volume and the reader is advised to consider these issues as an essential first step. The focus here will be confined to the activity of restraint, assuming that due attention has already been paid to the methods of avoiding the need for its use.

Restraint and physical intervention: the questions

In mental health care, the use of restraint, both mechanical and inter-personal, has a long and chequered history. In recent years, the use of restraint has come under increasing scrutiny. In the UK and the USA, death during restraint has been increasingly reported (Appelbaum 1999; Paterson et al. 2003). The death of David Bennett during restraint in a Medium Secure Unit (Paterson and Leadbetter 2004) has intensified the debate to the extent that the coming years are likely to see major changes in the nature and practice of restraint in the UK. The beginning of these changes may be illustrated by the renaming of 'restraint' to the more sophisticated phrase of 'physical intervention' (NICE 2005; NIMHE 2004). At the same time, violence toward health care staff has become a major health and safety concern. Out of a total figure of 65 000 assaults per year, Beech and Bowyer (2004) reported three times as many assaults against staff in UK mental health and learning disability units as compared to general health care.

This point in the history of restraint in mental health care marks no better time for a detailed examination of the issues. Providers of inpatient mental health care in general, and leaders of Psychiatric Intensive Care Units (PICU)/Low Secure Units (LSUs) in particular, will be concerned with the following questions;

- What is the history and theoretical underpinning for systematised restraint?
- What are the legal and ethical issues related to restraint?
- What is the evidence for the efficacy of some of the methods commonly in use?

Psychiatric Intensive Care, 2nd edn., eds. M. Dominic Beer, Stephen M. Pereira and Carol Paton.
Published by Cambridge University Press. © Cambridge University Press 2008

- What principles underpin best practice?
- How do patients and front-line practitioners ensure that their experiences inform future developments?

In terms of the theory and practice of physical intervention, the remainder of this chapter aims to offer practical advice as well as a guide to the thinking for service leaders and practitioners within inpatient environments.

History of mechanical restraint

Throughout history, the use of physical restraint has been a consistent feature within the provision of mental health care. Before the advent of antipsychotic medication in the 1950s, forcible confinement of patients often represented the first-line approach to the management of disturbed behaviour (Dix 2004). The institutions of the nineteenth century record the use of a vast array of mechanical restraint equipment. Disturbing examples of their use include the story of James Norris, a former American Marine, who during the early 1800s spent 20 years shackled to a bed (Porter 1991). Industrialisation also brought ever more elaborate pieces of equipment designed to restrict movement and at the same time were being justified as treatment. Examples of these include machines capable of dropping a bound patient into hot and cold baths and spinning a patient around at high speed (Porter 1991). Some of these 'therapy' sessions were many hours in duration and were sanitised with the label of necessary treatment.

In the UK, increasing disquiet about practice in mental institutions fuelled momentum to abolish mechanical restraint. Reforms initiated by Gardiner Hill and Charlesworth at the Lincoln Asylum in 1837 managed to reduce the number of patients kept under permanent mechanical restraint from thirty-nine to only two (Henderson 1954). Subsequent decades saw increasing determination by reformist pioneers to eradiate the use of hobbles, chains and handcuffs.

The non-mechanical restraint philosophy of the British nineteenth century reformists penetrated well into the 1960s and 1970s and led to the almost total abolition of mechanical restraint in the UK for the management of disturbed behaviour.

As we advance into the twenty-first century, the developed world contains considerable variation in attitude and philosophy regarding the use of mechanical restraint in mental health care. In the UK, the use of mechanical restraint is generally considered as extremely rare and applied only with special independent scrutiny from the Mental Health Act Commission. In contrast, however, it could be argued that UK attitudes towards enforced psychoactive drugs with the aim of controlling behaviour may be more pronounced than many of the UK's counterparts. In the USA and many European countries, the practice of mechanical restraint continues, albeit with considerable regulation in clearly defined circumstances.

History and development of interpersonal systematised restraint in UK mental health services

History also records staff having to physically take hold of patients during episodes of disturbed behaviour and aggression. For decades, this often involved individual members of staff applying restraint in any way they could, often relying on superiority of numbers applying restraint in an uncoordinated fashion.

Many systems of interpersonal restraint have ancient roots arising from the practice of martial arts. In 1882, the Japanese philosopher Jigoro Kano developed judo, a system of self-defence that modified the combat orientated techniques of Ju-Jitsu to include methods of non-injury inflicting systematised holds (Hoar 1997). These techniques allowed for one person to hold another person securely without inflicting injury to either. The principle and practice of other non-injury-inflicting methods of self-defence such as Aikido, developed by Morihei Ueshiba in 1942, also can be said to represent the technical underpinning for many of the interpersonal restraint techniques taught in modern training programmes.

Recent decades have seen the introduction of systemised methods of physical restraint to mental health inpatient units (Lee *et al.* 2001). The UK prison service developed a systemised method of restraint in 1981 based on techniques borrowed from the martial arts and building on the experience of other organisations such as the police. Termed 'control and restraint' (C&R), this method aimed for the organised and safe restraint of prisoners relying on standard training, regulation and team working.

During the 1970s there was growing concern in UK mental health services regarding the ability and training of staff to safely deal with violence in psychiatric hospitals (Brailsford and Stevenson 1973; Bridges *et al.* 1981). The death in 1984 of Mr Michael Martin, a patient in Broadmoor high secure hospital, resulted in the publication of the Ritchie Report (1985). One of the report's main recommendations was that nursing staff should be properly trained in the use of C&R. Ironically, only two days before the death of Mr Martin, a management team from Broadmoor hospital had seen a demonstration of the prison service's new C&R method and immediately decided that it should be introduced to the hospital (Wright 1999).

By the mid 1980s, training in C&R had also been introduced to Medium Secure Units (MSUs). During the last decade, a number of surveys confirm that the term C&R, with variations on its methodology, has become firmly ingrained in the spectrum of inpatient mental health settings (Gournay *et al.* 1998; Lee *et al.* 2001; UKCC 2001). Training in the use of organised systems of restraint has become an accepted necessity within modern mental health practice (Department of Health and Welsh Office 1999; Pereira and Clinton 2002; NICE 2005; UKCC 1999).

Recent years have seen many different methods of systemised restraint introduced to mental health services within the UK (UKCC 2001). Hitherto, it is not clear how many varieties of restraint training are actually in use. Lee *et al.* (2001) uncovered training in a 'wide variety of techniques' in their survey of staff working in PICUs and MSUs in England and Wales. Some unpublished surveys have suggested that as many as twenty-nine different methods of restraint are currently being taught to staff. With such variation in practice the overarching principles of lawful and safe practice must provide the starting point for the development of any restraint policy.

Law and ethics related to restraint

Mental Health Act

Within the context of the UK inpatient mental health settings, one would expect the Mental Health Act (MHA) 1983 to be the starting point for the legality of restraint. However, the MHA does not specifically deal with the legal authority to restrain, and detailed guidance is only offered in the MHA Code of Practice (Department of Health and Welsh Office 1999). While the Code is not a statutory document, the case of Munjaz (MHAC 2005) – concerned with the use of seclusion – initially concluded that the code must be followed. Although this ruling was later challenged and modified by the Court of Appeal, the status of the Code was strengthened to more than mere guidance (Seligman and Feery 2006). In effect, practitioners need to demonstrate good reason to deviate from the Code and thus it must be considered in all episodes of restraint. The Code defines the circumstances in which restraint may be justified. These are summarised in Table 9.1.

Table 9.1. Code of practice guidance on justification and reasons for restraint

- To take control of a dangerous situation
- To contain or limit the patient's freedom for no longer than necessary and to end or significantly reduce the danger to the patient or others

Five most common reasons in the Code for restraint
- Physical assault
- Dangerous, threatening or destructive behaviour
- Non-compliance with treatment
- Self-harm or risk of physical injury by accident
- Extreme and prolonged overactivity likely to lead to physical exhaustion

The use of restraint in the prevention of absconding or returning a detained patient to hospital is also not an uncommon activity for mental health staff. Andoh (1995) debates whether the MHA imposes a duty for staff to retake absconders and concludes:

The MHA1983 does not expressly impose a duty on the police, hospitals or approved social workers to retake absconders from hospitals; but, does confer a power to do so.

Only brief mention is made of the use of restraint in relation to absconding in the MHA Code, which advises that the guidance offered for other reasons for restraint should apply.

Criminal law

The Criminal Law Act 1967 also allows for such force 'as is reasonable' in the prevention of a person committing a crime. This has been interpreted by the MHA to mean that restraint is appropriate when someone with mental health problems is thought likely to harm themselves, someone else or property. This Act provides a legal framework for the restraint of those who may or may not be subject to the MHA. When considering the concept of 'reasonableness' the Central Police Training and Development Authority (2003) advises that the question will need to be decided in each individual case. Further guidance offered to police officers includes that force should only be used when:

- Considered an absolute necessity
- The minimum amount necessary is used
- It is proportionate to the perceived threat

Legality for the common uses of restraint in mental health

To summarise the law in relation to restraint in mental health, it may be helpful to consider the issues in terms of two general themes: firstly, specific mental health practice guidance and case law; secondly, more general relevant issues contained within criminal and common law.

The Mental Health Act Code of Practice offers detailed guidance which, following the case of Munjaz (2005), must be considered as extremely important to the legality of restraint. In addition, the use of restraint for the enforcement of treatment for those subject to the Mental Health Act (1983) must first ensure that the Code's advice in relation to informed consent has been paid close attention. If challenged in the civil courts, failure to do so may result in practitioners finding difficulty in accounting for their actions when justifying the use of restraint for the enforcement of treatment. The application of the relevant sections of the Mental Health Act does not in itself afford the right to use restraint in the delivery of treatment. The Mental Health Act contains the legal authority in specific circumstances to enforce treatment having first properly considered the consent guidance contained in the Code of Practice.

The second consideration can be said to arise from the application of criminal and common law. The common law doctrine of necessity provides authority to take steps that are reasonable and proportionate to protect a patient or others from harm. The Criminal Law Act 1967 provides a legal basis for physical intervention in the prevention of the committing of a crime. This is also relevant in issues of self-defence (Jones 2004). The key here is the concept of 'reasonableness' meaning that actions should be proportional in intensity and duration to the level of threat for which physical intervention is being applied.

Evidence and efficacy for methods of interpersonal restraint

The lack of consistency in the methods of restraint presents major obstacles to an empirical evaluation of current practice. However, there are far bigger problems for researchers aiming to produce quality evidence in the use of restraint. The randomised controlled trial (RCT) is the widely accepted gold standard of evidence for interventions used in health care. It is not difficult to advance the argument that the use of restraint simply cannot be tested using an RCT study design. One cannot imagine, or expect, ethical approval for a study using techniques that may inflict serious injury in order to compare them with techniques that may not. The UKCC (2001) comprehensive review on managing inpatient violence commented:

We could find no high quality studies that evaluate either the use of restraint or seclusion in those with mental illness.

Much of the theoretical underpinning for the use of systematised restraint can be said to arise from common sense. Put simply, it must be preferable for staff to act in a consistent, coordinated fashion in relation to restraint than the alternative of an improvised spontaneous approach. Parkes' (1996) evaluation of the introduction of C&R to an MSU showed a reduction in the need for seclusion. This may suggest that staff felt more confident in their ability to effectively deal with aggression as a result of their C&R training. Interestingly, Parkes' (1996) evaluation also noted an increase in injuries to staff as compared to before the introduction of C&R. To date, it appears that there simply is not sufficient systematic evaluation of restraint practice to draw any reliable conclusions about efficacy. In the UK, the Department of Health (DoH) has commissioned an extensive review of physical interventions used in the management of violence with the aim of introducing standardised accreditation for training and practice. The National Institute for Clinical Excellence (NICE) (2005) has also produced guidance which must be central to any consideration of how restraint should be practised. While accepting the lack of high-quality empirical evaluation of restraint, the literature contains sound advice and directs practitioners towards the major issues.

Safety

The very nature of aggression and restraint will always contain an element of unpredictability. It can reasonably be said that it may be impossible to account for all potential hazards in attempting to bring an often highly charged and frightening episode of physical aggression or disturbance under safe control. In order to maximise the safety of the person being restrained, a number of considerations have been proposed (Parkes 2002; Paterson and Leadbetter 2004; MacPherson et al. 2005; Metherall et al. 2006). It is helpful to consider these factors under two broad headings – factors that are innate to the person being restrained and factors that may emerge as a product of the restraint process.

Safety factors innate to the person being restrained

Wherever possible it is important that staff have a detailed knowledge of the person who may be subject to restraint. This is essential not only for maximising the potential to avoid the need for physical intervention in the first place, but also to diminish the likelihood of injury or collapse. Table 9.2. contains a list of issues reported as significant to maintaining the safety of a person being restrained.

In many circumstances (arguably in the majority) it should be possible for staff to complete an assessment of the factors in Table 9.2 before restraint is applied. PICU/LSU patients will often be known to staff, and where acute disturbance is possible, an early multidisciplinary review of the risk factors can be undertaken. Furthermore, this can also provide an opportunity to include the patient in a discussion

Table 9.2. Factors increasing the risk of injury and cardiac/respiratory failure during restraint

Pre-existing medical conditions especially cardiac or
   respiratory, e.g. heart disease, asthma
Pre-existing skeletal or muscular injury or disease
Pregnancy
Extreme fear as a function of delusional beliefs
Obesity
Substance misuse
High doses of medication

of how best to help them through an episode of acute disturbance including the notion of advanced directives in the methods of management.

Beyond the factors that the patient brings to the episode of restraint, the restraint process itself also requires close scrutiny to identify safety concerns that may emerge. It requires no great extension of common sense to recognise that even for an otherwise fit and healthy person, the spectacle of a violent struggle also poses serious risks. In order to manage these risks, constant awareness is required from staff involved in the restraint – often no easy task when their attention will inevitably be focused on bringing the situation under control.

Factors that affect safety during the restraint process

Authors such as Parkes (2002), Paterson and Leadbetter (2004), Metherall *et al.* (2006) and MacPherson *et al.* (2005) and the report into the death of David Bennett (Norfolk, Suffolk and Cambridgeshire Strategic Health Authority 2003) offer guidance on how to recognise higher risk situations that may arise during the restraint process. Metherall *et al.* (2006) described the creation of medical emergency response teams (MERT) available to respond quickly to episodes of restraint over the 24-h period. The MERT includes an assessor trained to intermediate life support standards, whose sole role is to monitor the physical condition of the patient being restrained. Table 9.3 outlines the considerations important to maintaining safety during the restraint process.

It is extremely important that a person independent to the restraint process is present with the sole purpose of monitoring the physical condition of the patient. In the event of prolonged restraint, a careful balance needs to be drawn between the risk to the patient of continuing restraint and the risk of further assault if restraint is discontinued. In some circumstances this may need to be weighted towards early discontinuation of restraint while accepting some

Table 9.3. Increased risk factors that may emerge from the process of restraint

Prolonged restraint – the longer restraint is applied the more risk of collapse or injury

The prone position – restraint in the face-down position is more dangerous to health

Increased body temperature – resulting from prolonged struggling and close proximity to shared body heat

Pressure applied to the thorax – body weight directly restricting breathing to the back or front of a patient being restrained

Table 9.4. Functions of the medical emergency response team (MERT) assessor during a restraint episode

- The MERT assessor's function is independent of the restraint process and is carried out in conjunction with the staff member responsible for holding the head of the patient during the restraint episode
- Monitor the airway, respiration and circulation of the patient and whenever possible utilise pulse oximetry
- The MERT assessor will ensure that the patient's well-being is monitored and physical observations are recorded
- Physical observations are assessed against a pre-arrest call set of criteria

risk of further assault. The role of the MERT assessor is to be aware of all the physical risk factors associated with restraint and implement the functions listed in Table 9.4 (Metherall *et al.* 2006).

While accepting the lack of high-quality evidence about the efficacy of restraint methods, there can be little excuse for not paying close attention to the known factors that impact on the safety of the patient during the restraint process. Metherall *et al.*'s (2006) concept of provision for close physical monitoring of the patient under restraint must be considered as a core principle underpinning best practice. Moreover, such provision is also recommended in NICE (2005) practice guidance. It also provides a solid foundation on which to build audit aimed at improving standards. This philosophy can be easily extended to the safety of staff, which also needs a robust system of monitoring and audit, probably best described within existing health and safety and human resource procedures.

Dignity

No matter how robust the justification, the experience of being physically restrained will be perceived by the patient as a significant assault on their dignity. In many cases where restraint is necessary, there will be opportunity to take meaningful and practical steps towards promoting the dignity of the person. In some cases the need for restraint may arise spontaneously, leaving little time for planning. Often however, there will be time to consider how best to minimise the distress that will likely result. Simple steps include careful consideration of the location for restraint, minimising the likelihood that the process will be observed by onlookers. The gender of the staff applying restraint should also ideally be the same as the person being restrained. In the case of giving rapid tranquillisation while under restraint, it will often be necessary to expose embarrassing parts of the body, in particular the upper outer quadrant of the buttock. The combination of being restrained while clothing is removed has the obvious potential to be perceived as sexual assault. Every effort should be made, in particular in the case of female patients, to ensure a gender match between staff and patient.

The practice of safer restraint must be considered in multifactorial terms, one component of which is the holding technique. Of equal importance is the close physical monitoring of the patient's condition. Also of great importance is making every effort to preserve as much dignity for the person as possible. Possibly the most important and difficult variable arising from the process of restraint is the staff's ability to remain closely in touch with the changing levels of risk, both to and from the patient, and ceasing restraint at the earliest possible moment.

Leadership and restraint

Episodes of acute disturbance and aggression are amongst the most challenging situations that mental health staff will encounter. Fear and anxiety are often close companions to highly charged situations that may culminate in restraint. If left unchecked, these emotions will often result in either lost opportunities for early de-escalation or increased potential for over-reaction with the application of restraint.

Within a ward community, the fear that arises from aggression is often highly infectious – although the confidence needed to engage it can be similarly 'caught' by the team. Without skilled leadership in taking forward crisis resolution strategies, situations will often become much worse than they may have needed to be. Leadership is an essential part of both avoiding the need for restraint and, where absolutely necessary, its minimum and safe application. It is extremely difficult to set out a list of definitive measures that can be applied to produce effective clinical leaders, in particular in dealing with crises. The following may be a reasonable starting point however:

- Highly developed communication skills
- Ability to empathise with the patient and the wider staff team
- Creative thinking towards options for resolving crises
- A willingness to take the initiative and lead from the front
- Effective training
- Role modelling a calm and receptive attitude
- Flexibility in overcoming potential conflict
- Willingness to take risks in allowing the discharge of frustration by the patient without quick resort to physical intervention
- Facilitating the patient and other staff in crisis resolution skills
- Effective post-incident debriefing with honest reflection on learning points
- Experience

The PICU/LSU may be an ideal learning environment in which much of the above can be cultivated toward producing effective leaders. Very important also is the atmosphere and ward culture that encourage insight and reflection amongst staff, thus allowing for the development of creative methods of dealing with acute crises.

Conclusion

Throughout this chapter, we have seen that the practical and conceptual issues associated with restraint of patients with mental health problems remain complex. Possibly the biggest challenge to advancing practice is trying to achieve a clear understanding of the basic human issues that arise when a staff group has the authority to lay hands upon a person within the context of health care. Liberty is generally considered as amongst humanity's most valued possessions. Indeed in most of the developed world, its removal can only be considered following careful and consistent application of a detailed process. The physical removal of an individual's free body movement must be considered as amongst the most severe infringement of civil liberty. It is not difficult for each of us to imagine the fear, loss of dignity and helplessness which we would inevitably experience when our very basic human instinct of free movement is taken from us. When patients are the subjects of systematised restraint, they must feel – and indeed are for that time – at the mercy of others. It is no wonder anger is also a very familiar companion to the process of restraint.

Many mental health nurses will have witnessed the distressing effects of systematised restraint on the recipient. In a majority of cases the efficiency of restraint applied by well trained staff must often leave the patient feeling without a chance of resisting its application. It can be all the more distressing when applied to enforce treatment on a person who is already experiencing mental torment.

The tragic death of Mr David Bennett during restraint offers a stark reminder of how badly wrong an episode of difficult restraint can go. It must also be remembered that a member of staff was knocked unconscious prior to Mr Bennett's restraint. No doubt extreme fear was present in all the staff involved in that tragic incident. The distress and consequences of acute disturbance and the need for restraint have many victims often including the staff and others who may happen to bear witness to its occurrence.

Given the incredibly high human cost of episodes of restraint, what can be done to improve practice? First and foremost, it is required for front line staff and patients who have first-hand experience of situations involving restraint to join together and define the future practice development agenda. In some organisations senior service managers and other policy-makers can be so divorced from the reality of aggression and restraint that the enormously complicated issues can be reduced to little more than intellectual interest. Policy and practice must be informed by detailed understanding of the nature of situations and process of restraint. The advent of the MERT assessor in monitoring patient safety is a direct example of developing practice within a detailed understanding of the issues.

Finally, even with major advances in de-escalation and understanding of many of the ways in which institutions can diminish confrontation, circumstances where restraint is unavoidable can still be considered as inevitable. Such are the potential human, risk and safety issues for all the people involved, restraint in all of its complexity must remain at the top of a service leader's agenda.

Acknowledgements

I would like to thank Mr Mathew Page for his help in preparing this chapter; Danni Kemmett for her feedback on earlier drafts and Andy Haywood for his insights as a restraint trainer.

REFERENCES

Andoh B. 1995 Jurisprudential aspects of the 'right' to retake absconders from mental hospitals in England and Wales. J Sci Med Law 35(3): 255–230

Appelbaum P. 1999 Seclusion and restraint: congress reacts to reports of abuse. Psychiatr Serv 50(7): 881–885

Beech B, Bowyer D. 2004 Management of aggression and violence in mental health settings. Mental Health Pract 7(7): 31–37

Brailsford D, Stevenson J. 1973 Factors related to violent and unpredictable behaviour in psychiatric hospitals. Nurs Times 69(3) Suppl 9–11

Bridges W, Dunane P, Speight I. 1981 The provision of post basic education in psychiatric nursing. Nurs Times, 23 December, pp. 141–144

Central Police Training and Development Authority. 2003 Personal Safety Manual. Harrogate: Centrex

Davis P. 2004 Critical thoughts on restraint in hospital. Mental Health Nurs 24 May, pp. 20–21

Department of Health and Welsh Office. 1999 Mental Health Act Code of Practice. London: The Stationery Office

Dix R. 2004 Advances in the management of acute schizophrenia and bipolar disorder: impact of the new rapid-acting atypical intramuscular formulations of treatment choice. Therapeutic Focus, 5–10

Gournay K, Ward M, Thornicroft G, Wright S. 1998 Crisis in the capital: inpatient care in inner London. Mental Health Practice 1: 10–18

Henderson D. 1954 A Text Book of Psychiatry. Oxford: Oxford University Press

Hoar S. 1997 The A–Z of Judo. Bristol: Ippon Books

Jones R. 2004 Mental Health Act Manual, 9th edn. London: Sweet and Maxwell

Lee S, Wright S, Sayer J, Parr AM, Gray R, Gournay K. 2001 Physical restraint for nurses in English and Welsh psychiatric intensive care and regional secure units. J Mental Health 10(2): 151–162

MacPherson R, Dix R, Morgan S. 2005 Revisiting guidelines for the management of acutely disturbed psychiatric patients. Adv Psychiatr Treat 11: 404–415

Mental Health Act Commission (MHAC). 2005 The House of Lords Munjaz Ruling. MHAC Policy Briefing for Commissioners, Issue 12, October 2005

Metherall A, Worthington R, Keyte A. 2006 Twenty four hour medical emergency response teams in a mental health in-patient facility – new approaches for safer restraint. J Psychiatr Intensive Care 1: 21–29

National Institute of Clinical Excellence (NICE) 2005 Violence – The Short-term Management of Disturbed/Violent Behaviour in Inpatient Psychiatric Settings and Emergency Departments. Clinical Guideline 25. London: National Institute for Clinical Excel-

lence. Available online at http://www.nice.org.uk/pdf/cg025niceguideline.pdf

National Institute for Mental Health in England (NIMHE). 2004 Mental Health Policy Implementation Guide – Developing Positive Practice to Support the Safe and Therapeutic Management of Aggression and Violence in mental Health In-patient Settings. London: Department of Health

Norfolk, Suffolk and Cambridgeshire Strategic Health Authority (2003) Independent Inquiry into the care of David Bennett. Cambridge: Norfolk, Suffolk and Cambridgeshire Strategic Health Authority. Available online at www.irr.org.uk/pdf/bennett_inquiry.pdf

Parkes J. 1996 Control and restraint training: a study of its effectiveness in a medium secure unit. J Forensic Psychiatry 7(3): 525–534

Parkes J. 2002 A review of the literature on positional asphyxia as a possible cause of sudden death during restraint. Br J Forensic Pract 4: 24–27

Paterson B, Leadbetter D. 2004 Learning the right lessons. Mental Health Pract 7(7): 12–15

Paterson B, Stark C, Sadler D, Leadbetter D, Allen D. 2003 Restraint- related deaths in health and social care in the UK: learning the lessons. Mental Health Pract 6(9): 10–17

Pereira SM, Clinton C. 2002 Mental Health Policy Implementation Guide: National Minimum Standards in Psychiatric Intensive Care Units (PICU) and Low Secure Environments. London: Department of Health

Porter R. 1991 The Faber Book of Madness. London: Faber and Faber

Ritchie S. 1985 Report to the secretary of state for social services concerning the death of Michel Martin. London: SHSA

Seligman M, Feery D. 2006 Seclusion: Lord Steyn's lament. J Psychiatr Intensive Care 2(2): 111–117

United Kingdom Central Council (UKCC) for Nursing, Midwifery and Health Visiting. 1999 Nursing in Secure Environments. Preston: University of Central Lancashire

United Kingdom Central Council (UKCC) for Nursing, Midwifery and Health Visiting. 2001 The recognition prevention and therapeutic management of violence in mental health care. London: Health Services Research Department

Wright S. 1999 Physical restraint in the management of violence and aggression in in-patient settings: a review of the issues. J Mental Health 8(5): 459–472

10

The complex needs patient

Zerrin Atakan and Venugopal Duddu

Introduction

Mental health workers are increasingly faced with patients who not only suffer from a severe mental illness, but also have a number of additional problems, which further complicate their treatment and management. This is especially so in urban inner city areas. Very often, the treatment of the mental illness alone is not sufficient and resources focused specifically to their needs are scarce or non-existent.

Such patients are often admitted to psychiatric intensive care or acute inpatient units due to their disturbed behaviour. Their management often tends to be problematic and incomplete, and unless attention is paid to meet their specific needs, a 'revolving door' phenomenon is a likely outcome. In Psychiatric Intensive Care Units (PICU), patients with complex needs are often those who cannot be transferred out or discharged within 8 weeks, either because their symptoms are resistant to treatment, or there are other needs that have not been adequately addressed. They display frequent verbal or physical violence and often find ingenious methods of abusing drugs, even in very carefully controlled ward environments.

We will attempt, in this chapter, to define the 'complex needs patient' and examine the commonly encountered diagnoses and additional problems (with reference to their possible aetiological factors) in such a patient. Finally, we will examine how such patients can be treated and managed.

> **Box 10.1.** Characteristics of complex needs patients in PICUs
>
> - Symptoms resistant to treatment
> - Frequent violent episodes
> - Substance misuse
> - Cannot be transferred/discharged within 8 weeks

Definition of 'complex needs patient'

Over recent decades, with the development of Community Care philosophy and policies, the recognition of a 'new' group of mentally ill patients has emerged: the 'new long-stay patient'. Other terms followed such as: 'young chronics', 'hard to treat', 'hard to place', 'treatment resistant', 'dual diagnosis' and 'challenging behaviour'. Most of these terms have overlapping meanings and are, to some extent, interchangeable.

Here we suggest the use of the term 'complex needs patient' to emphasise a needs-based approach to their management and to steer away from negative and pessimistic terminology. The complex needs patient suffers from a severe mental illness, mainly in the form of schizophrenia or bipolar disorder and, in addition, has one or more additional problems such as another mental illness, substance abuse, medical problems, homelessness, history of abuse or lack of social support. More often than not, the same patient

Psychiatric Intensive Care, 2nd edn., eds. M. Dominic Beer, Stephen M. Pereira and Carol Paton.
Published by Cambridge University Press. © Cambridge University Press 2008

has a number of these problems at once as one problem tends to lead to another.

> **Box 10.2.** Other terms used to describe complex needs patients
>
> - New long-stay patient
> - Young chronics
> - Difficult to treat
> - Treatment resistant
> - Dual or multiple diagnosis
> - Challenging behaviour

Background and characteristics of the complex needs patient

Mann and Cree (1976) first developed the 'new long-stay patient' concept. They defined this group as patients who had been in hospital continuously for more than 1, but less than 5 years. Their national survey revealed this group to have multiple disabilities and problems. This group, apart from being resistant to treatment, were socially isolated, unskilled, had little family support and suffered from poor physical health. In addition, they presented with behavioural problems such as violence towards others, self-harm and extreme antisocial behaviour. Of these patients, 60% suffered from a psychotic disorder and 40% of these had been diagnosed as suffering from schizophrenia.

> **Box 10.3.** Characteristics of complex needs patients
>
> Severe mental illness *plus* one or more of the following:
> - Another mental health problem
> - Substance abuse
> - Mild learning difficulty
> - History of abuse
> - History of brain injury
> - Medical problems
> - Homelessness
> - Lack of social support
> - Problems related to ethnicity

A similar national audit carried out in the UK in more recent times (Lelliott *et al.* 1994) examined a group of patients who had been in hospital continuously for more than 6 months but less than 3 years. This revealed similar findings to those found by Mann and Cree (1976). Compared with earlier findings, the new long-stay patients of the 1990s were more likely to have more pronounced positive symptoms, exhibit more violence and abuse substances. In addition, they were more likely to be detained under the Mental Health Act.

> **Box 10.4.** Characteristics of new long-stay patient (Mann and Cree 1976)
>
> - Psychotic illness
> - Treatment resistant
> - Poor physical health
> - In hospital for more than 1 but less than 5 years
> - Behavioural problems
> - Socially isolated
> - Unskilled

The terminology of 'treatment resistance', although more often conveying difficulties in response to medication, when studied closely may reveal similar characteristics to the term 'new long-stay'. Kane (1996) describes four main factors that can make patients difficult to treat; the first factor, refractoriness to treatment, appears to have changed over time. In the 1960s about 70% of patients got better with antipsychotic treatments, whereas in the 1990s only about 50% of patients responded to conventional treatments.

> **Box 10.5.** Characteristics of new long-stay patients (Lelliott *et al.* 1994) (in addition to Mann and Cree's findings)
>
> - More positive symptoms
> - Substance abuse
> - In hospital for more than 6 months, but less than 3 years
> - More violence
> - Detained under the Mental Health Act

Kane lists other factors as:

- Problems of adverse side-effects
- Non-compliance with treatment (as approximately 30% of patients become non-compliant within 1 year)
- The problem of co-morbid conditions

Antisocial and violent behaviours can also make patients difficult to treat. When we examine typical non-compliant patients, very often we see that they do not perceive benefits in taking medication, have little or no daily supervision to ensure their medication intake, they experience side-effects, have little or no awareness of their illness, and their symptoms make them suspicious, grandiose and anxious. These characteristics, coupled with substance abuse, further complicate the issue. Psychoactive substances can impair perception and interfere with judgement. Some drugs, especially alcohol, may act as chemical disinhibitors of aggressive impulses (Collins and Schlenger 1988). Behavioural disturbances and violence are further characteristics of the complex needs patient.

Box 10.6. Factors leading to treatment resistance (Kane 1996)

- Adverse side-effects
- Non-compliance
- Refractoriness to treatment (worse in 1990s compared with 1960s)
- Violence
- Co-morbidity

It is frequently observed that substances combined with a psychotic state can increase the risk of patients wanting to act on their delusions and display violence. It is known that persons experiencing especially persecutory-type delusions tend to act on them (Wessely *et al.* 1993). Symptoms such as hostility, paranoid ideation and substance abuse are the most significant short-term predictors of violent behaviour. Link and Stueve (1994) studied the principle of 'rationality within irrationality' when mentally ill patients feel threatened due to persecutory ideas and their internal control mechanisms are compromised. They argue that in these circumstances violence is more likely to occur. According to a detailed study they carried out, they have found that symptoms such as 'mind dominated by forces beyond your control', 'thoughts put into your head that were not your own' and 'there were people who wished to do you harm' were significantly correlated with acts of violence.

It would be useful to examine some commonly seen subtypes of complex needs patients in more detail. These subtypes are categorised for purposes of examining each in more detail.

As mentioned previously, in reality a patient will have more than two problems and the nature of these problems are such that one problem can easily lead to another. For instance, patients with a history of sexual abuse develop severe mental illness and, with the loss of daily living skills, lack social support and become homeless. They starts abusing substances to relieve their anxiety and, entering the subculture of the drug-dealing world, they develop serious physical problems and begin offending.

Severe mental illness and another mental health problem

Severe mental illness can lead to various disabilities, rendering the person suffering from it unable to function fully in society. Negative symptoms alone contribute enormously to psychosocial disability. As a result, the person can develop further mental health problems such as depression, anxiety and hypochondriacal and obsessive symptomatology. With reduced self-esteem and hope, it is not uncommon for a patient to become suicidal, make repeated suicidal gestures or become involved in self-destructive behaviour.

Another commonly seen diagnostic category, especially found at the PICU, is personality disorders. Antisocial, borderline and histrionic personality disorders or traits are among the most frequently encountered. In a study investigating the relationship between psychopathy and violence among patients with schizophrenia, it was found that co-morbidity of schizophrenia and psychopathy was higher in patients who displayed violence, compared with those who did not (Nolan *et al.* 1999).

Patients with co-morbid borderline or antisocial personalities, by their tendency to violent acting out, poor impulse control, general insensitivity to others' feelings and demand for immediate satisfaction of their needs, may cause severe management problems within their environments. In certain instances, this may even lead to divisions among staff. Very often this may be at the expense of their severe mental illness where staff, overwhelmed by the negative feelings emanated by the patient, may review their beliefs about the sincerity of the patient's underlying psychosis.

Severe mental illness and substance abuse (dual diagnosis)

Due to the significance of this co-morbidity, it is dealt with separately in Chapter 18.

Severe mental illness, mild learning difficulty and challenging behaviour

A commonly encountered group of patients in generic mental health services are those with co-morbid mental illnesses and varying degrees of learning disabilities (LD). The majority of these patients tend to fall through the gaps between the adult and the LD services, and end up being treated only by generic adult services. The co-existence of LD and mental illnesses poses a number of challenges to patient management. Symptoms in these patients are often coloured by the extent of the LD, and consequentially, are difficult to recognise and interpret. This causes difficulties in recognizing and diagnosing mental illness in these subjects.

Patients with LD often present with behavioural disturbances, which can be a result of a large number of non-mental-illness causes. Some behavioural disturbances, such as aggression, destructiveness, self-injurious, non-aggressive problematic behaviours and stereotypies, are described as 'challenging behaviours'. Challenging behaviour is defined by Emerson (1995) as 'culturally abnormal behaviour(s) of such intensity, frequency or duration that the physical safety of the person or others is likely to be placed in serious jeopardy, or behaviour which is likely to seriously limit use of, or result in the person being denied access to, ordinary community facilities'.

The management of disturbed behaviour depends on the cause, meaning and purpose of such behaviours. The inability to express oneself clearly can lead to frustration and formation of challenging behaviour. The patient learns to communicate with others in a dysfunctional way and staff, inadvertently, may further maintain this. However, there can be a neurological basis to such behaviours (Reeves 1997). Treating the underlying cause, and finding safe alternative strategies to achieve the same goals can be a way to change these unacceptable behaviours.

Further information about this patient group can be found in Chapter 15.

Severe mental illness and medical morbidity

Physical illnesses are known to occur in a large proportion of patients with mental illnesses. However, they are poorly recognised and undertreated in most psychiatric settings. The life expectancy of schizophrenic patients is 9–12 years shorter than that of the general population. While suicide accounts for a third of these deaths, the remaining are due to medical illnesses (Allebeck 1989; Lambert *et al.* 2003) Patients with schizophrenia are reported to be 2.9 times more likely to die of natural causes, especially cardiovascular disease, than people from the general population (Ruschena *et al.* 1998).

Several studies have shown poor detection rates for physical illness among people with mental illness. Koran *et al.* (1989) estimated that 45% of patients in California's public mental health system had physical disease and, of these, 47% were undetected by the treating doctor. A substantial proportion of these illnesses were judged to be either causing or exacerbating the patient's mental illness. A study by Koranyi (1979) of psychiatric clinic patients revealed similar findings. Hall *et al.* (1981) found that 46% of patients admitted to a ward had an unrecognised physical illness that either caused or exacerbated their psychiatric illness; 80% had physical illnesses requiring treatment; and 4% had precancerous conditions or illnesses.

The high rates of physical morbidity and mortality among mentally ill patients could be related to lifestyle, illness and medication-related factors. Negative symptoms, social disability and cognitive deficits render schizophrenic patients more liable to unhealthy diet (fast foods rich in saturated fats), sedentary lifestyles and obesity. High rates of co-morbid substance abuse (due to smoking, alcohol and illicit drug abuse) also increase the risk of a number of physical illnesses. Finally, side-effects of antipsychotic medications such as obesity, impaired glucose tolerance and hyperlipidemia further contribute to the high risk of physical illnesses in this population (Regier *et al.* 1990; Brown *et al.* 1999; Jablensky *et al.* 1999).

These risk factors notwithstanding, there are a number of barriers to the recognition and treatment of physical illnesses, which have an important influence on the high physical morbidity in this population (Anath, 1984; Jeste *et al.* 1996; Goldman 1999; Brown *et al.* 2000). Mentally ill patients tend to be reluctant to see their general practitioner and discuss their problems (physical and psychological). They are more likely to be non-compliant with suggestions made, treatments given and follow-up appointments arranged. They often also have difficulties in communicating their problems due to their mental state. Cognitive deficits can further affect their awareness of physical problems, and also their ability to understand and follow the advice given. Finally, physical symptoms could be masked because of high pain tolerance in some patients, and reduction in pain sensitivity associated with the use of antipsychotic drugs.

There are also a number of physician-related factors that impede the recognition of physical illnesses. While non-psychiatrists tend to be reticent in treating patients with mental illnesses, specialist psychiatrists often do not focus on medical illnesses, and assume them to be managed by their medical counterparts. As a result medical illnesses tend to be poorly managed by both psychiatrists and medical physicians. This situation is compounded by the patients' poor motivation and a tendency to avoid seeing general practitioners for their symptoms.

The issue of physical morbidity in the mentally ill has been reviewed comprehensively by a number of authors (Lambert *et al.* 2003; Dombrovski and Rosenstock 2004).

Obesity, diabetes and hyperlipidemia

Kraepelin noted (Diefendorf 1915) that an initial loss of weight among schizophrenic patients was followed sometimes by a marked (and rapid) increase. Some 40%–62% of people with schizophrenia are obese or overweight. However, concerns about weight gain became prominent only with the advent of atypical antipsychotics in the last few decades. Although both typical and atypical antipsychotics can induce weight gain, some atypicals have a greater propensity to cause this. Allison *et al.* (1999), in their meta-analysis, reported the following mean increases in body weight with atypical antipsychotics: clozapine, 4.45 kg; olanzapine, 4.15 kg; sertindole, 2.92 kg; risperidone, 2.10 kg; and ziprasidone, 0.04 kg. The data for quetiapine were insufficient. In a more recent review, Nasrallah (2003) reported that the most significant weight gain was with clozapine and olanzapine, while risperidone was associated with modest dose-independent weight gain, and quetiapine with modest dose-independent short-term weight gain. The risk of hyperlipidemia seems to parallel that of weight gain (Meyer 2002). The significance of weight gain lies in its potential metabolic complications. However, it has been suggested that metabolic risks of weight gain are location dependent. Intra-abdominal fat deposition is associated with adverse consequences. In fact, researchers now suggest the use of abdominal girth as a parameter for defining the 'metabolic syndrome'. Research is conflicting as to whether it is the illness or its treatment that results in intra-abdominal accumulation of fat (Thakore 2005).

Impaired glucose tolerance and diabetes mellitus are also more common in patients suffering from schizophrenia than in the general population (Dixon *et al.* 2000). In fact studies have identified the risk of diabetes to be two- to fourfold higher amongst schizophrenic patients, compared to the general population (Bushe and Holt 2004). However, a number of drawbacks have been identified in existing prevalence studies: differential exposure to antipsychotic medications, and active screening for diabetes itself could have confounding influences. In a recent study, Subramaniam *et al.* (2003) reported that 16% of a cohort of long-term facility residents with schizophrenia in Singapore had diabetes (after participants with a known diagnosis of diabetes were excluded). None of the patients had been exposed to second-generation antipsychotics.

Additionally, treatment with the second-generation antipsychotics clozapine and olanzapine is related to an increased risk of developing diabetes mellitus type 2 (Gianfresco *et al.* 2002; Newcomer *et al.* 2002; Marder *et al.* 2004). The Consensus Development Conference on Antipsychotic Drugs and Obesity and Diabetes (American Diabetes Association 2004) stated that the risk of diabetes is consistently increased in patients receiving clozapine or olanzapine. The risk was 'less clear' with risperidone and quetiapine. Data are limited with respect to aripiprazole, although there was no evidence of an increased risk of diabetes from available clinical trials. In a randomised controlled trial of 157 patients with schizophrenia and schizoaffective disorder, Lindenmayer *et al.* (2003) showed a significant increase in glucose levels with clozapine, olanzapine and haloperidol, but not with risperidone. These observations have prompted the US Food and Drug Administration (FDA) to issue a diabetes warning concerning the risk of diabetes associated with the administration of clozapine, olanzapine, risperidone, quetiapine, ziprasidone and aripiprazole (FDA Patient Safety News 2004).

Ryan *et al.* (2003) studied whether schizophrenia is inherently associated with abnormalities in glucose metabolism. They found that 15% of drug-naive patients with first-episode schizophrenia had impaired fasting glucose levels, compared with none in the control group. They were also more insulin resistant, and had higher levels of insulin and cortisol than controls. A previous study by the same group found an increase in visceral obesity in drug-naive first-episode patients (Thakore *et al.* 2002; Thakore 2004). It has been hypothesised that the findings may be related to a subtle disturbance of the hypothalamic–pituitary–adrenal axis. Other factors may include poor diet and sedentary lifestyle.

The occurrence of diabetes mellitus and hyperlipidemia in schizophrenic patients after treatment with second-generation antipsychotics has mostly been attributed to weight gain. However, weight gain does not entirely account for these metabolic abnormalities, and it is postulated that other factors may also be involved. Some authors have suggested that direct receptor-mediated effects of atypical antipsychotic medications may also induce impairment of insulin sensitivity (Dwyer *et al.* 2001). The role of central nervous 5-HT_{2A} regulation in metabolic syndrome and physical activity is increasingly recognised (Muldoon *et al.* 2004). There is some preliminary evidence to suggest that 5HT_2 antagonism itself might be related to impaired glucose tolerance (Gilles *et al.* 2005).

Overall, the evidence suggests a high prevalence of obesity, lipid abnormalities, glucose intolerance and insulin resistance among schizophrenic patients. This constellation of metabolic abnormalities has been called the 'metabolic syndrome'. The World Health Organization has suggested the following criteria to identify this syndrome (Thakore 2005):

Insulin resistance and/or impaired fasting glucose and/or impaired glucose tolerance and two or more of the following:

1. Waist: hip ratio >0.90 (men)/ >0.85 (women) or body mass index $\geq 30\,\text{kg/m}^2$.
2. Triglyceride ≥ 1.7 mmol/l, or high-density lipoprotein (HDL) <0.9 mmol/l (men) and <1.0 mmol/l (women).
3. Blood pressure $\geq 140/90$ mm Hg (or treated hypertension).
4. Microalbuminuria.

Cardiovascular disease (hypertension, cardiac arrhythmias)

Cardiovascular illnesses are recognised as the most common natural cause of death among patients with schizophrenia. These include most cardiac risk factors (mentioned previously) as well as specific conditions such as hypertension, arrhythmias, syncope, heart failure, stroke, transient cerebral ischemia, and diabetes (Curkendall *et al.* 2004). A Canadian study found mortality rates from cardiovascular (and all other) causes were reported to be high in this population (Curkendall *et al.* 2004). It is likely that lifestyle factors (smoking, alcoholism, poor diet, lack of exercise) contribute to this increased risk of cardiac problems.

Sudden death and QTc prolongation

Patients with schizophrenia appear to be prone to a higher risk of sudden death (Davidson 2002). This is thought to be related to prolongation of the QTc interval and ventricular arrhythmias (torsade de pointes). A number of risk factors have been identified and include co-morbid heart disease, electrolyte imbalance, female sex, advanced age, polypharmacy and antipsychotic drugs (Hennessy *et al.* 2002; Haddad and Anderson 2002). Antipsychotic medications are thought to bring about this effect on the QTc through their effects on the potassium channels. However, it is not entirely clear whether this effect is dose dependent or an idiosyncratic response, and also whether antipsychotic drugs independently cause ventricular tachyarrhythmias. However, the Cardiac Safety in Schizophrenia Group (Ames *et al.* 2002) cited the QTc prolongation by antipsychotics as a risk factor for sudden death in its 2002 report. There is evidence of higher risk with thioridazine, mesoridazine, pimozide, sertindole and droperidol. A modest risk of QTc prolongation is associated with parenteral haloperidol, trifluoperazine, chlorpromazine, sulpiride and ziprasidone.

Cancer and schizophrenia

Studies have yielded conflicting results on the relationship between schizophrenia and cancer. Some suggest that schizophrenics have a higher risk of developing cancer, while others suggest a lower or the same risk as the general population (Dombrovski and Rosenstock 2004). There is some evidence to suggest that although people with schizophrenia are no more likely to develop cancer overall, in the event of their developing cancer they have a 50% lower chance of survival. Some gender differences have been reported in the risk for individual cancers; for example, an increased risk of breast cancer for women, and a reduced risk of lung cancer for men (Lambert *et al.* 2003).

Other physical illnesses

Patients with schizophrenia have accelerated rates of osteoporosis, which is attributed to antipsychotic-medication-related decrease in oestrogen and testosterone, reduced calcium due to smoking and alcoholism, and polydipsia. Antipsychotics (typicals, risperidone and amisulpiride) raise prolactin levels, causing galactorrhoea, amenorrhoea, oligomenorrhoea, sexual dysfunction, reduced bone mineral density, and also contribute to cardiovascular disease. The incidence of irritable bowel syndrome in people with schizophrenia is 19% (versus 2.5% in the general population). The prevalence of *Helicobacter pylori* infection is significantly higher in people with schizophrenia (odds ratio, 3.0; Lambert *et al.* 2003).

Severe mental illness and positive HIV status

With the growing concern of human immunodeficiency virus (HIV) infection and acquired immunodeficiency syndrome (AIDS), there have been efforts to target certain at-risk groups to prevent further spread of the infection. Unfortunately, psychiatric populations do not appear to have been targeted, despite the evidence that they represent a vulnerable and disadvantaged segment of the population with a high risk of developing HIV infection. Large numbers of patients with severe mental illness may be living in the main drug-abusing neighbourhoods of inner-city areas and also have unprotected sex. According to a review article by Grassi (1996), several recent studies have shown that high-risk behaviour, especially intravenous drug abuse and non-protected sexual intercourse, is reported by 20%–50% of psychiatric patients, particularly those affected by bipolar disorders and schizophrenia. Carey *et al.* (1997) studied the risk behaviours of sixty severely mentally ill patients and found that 48% of men and 37% of women reported either having unprotected sex or sharing needles. Many participants were misinformed about HIV transmission and risk reduction. They tended to rate themselves at only slight risk for infection, undermining their motivation for condom use.

The prevalence of positive-HIV status in severely mentally ill patients is higher compared to the general population and nearly half of them are found to be unaware of their HIV status (Grassi 1996). About 50% of all patients with schizophrenia are also known to be abusing drugs and some of them may prefer substances such as cocaine due to its short 'high'. This creates a need for more frequent injections which in turn leads to an increasing likelihood of sharing syringes and HIV transmission (Davis 1998). In another study, the likelihood of injecting drugs was four times greater among psychiatric patients with a history of intranasal substance use compared with those without such use, three-and-a-half times greater among black patients than others, and five times greater among patients aged thirty-six or older (Horwath *et al.* 1996). In addition, a 3-year longitudinal study shows a considerably higher risk of having more frequent future relapses for patients with manic depressive illness who are also intravenous drug users with HIV infection (Johnson *et al.* 1999).

Although patients with a primary diagnosis of a severe mental illness are in the high-risk group of developing the infection, the prevalence of a first-onset psychotic illness among HIV-positive patients is rare. According to a study where 1046 HIV-positive patients were screened, only 9 (0.9%) suffered from a psychotic illness; 7 of them were in late stages of the infection (Niederecker *et al.* 1995). These data do not indicate a markedly elevated prevalence of psychosis in HIV-positive or AIDS patients.

The HIV status of a severely mentally ill patient should be of concern to the clinicians, especially when the patient has a history of drug abuse

and unprotected sex. Establishing informed consent when carrying out an HIV test is crucial.

Severe mental illness and homelessness

Homelessness is one of the major problems a severely mentally ill patient is likely to have. Surveys of homeless persons carried out in different parts of the world show that a significant proportion of them suffer from serious mental and physical health problems. The reasons why a severely ill person becomes homeless may be varied and complex. However, according to a survey carried out in Munich, Germany, two-thirds of the mentally ill homeless had become homeless after the onset of mental illness (Fichter *et al.* 1996). In the same survey, amongst 146 homeless males, the lifetime prevalence rates were 12.4% for schizophrenia and 41.8% for affective disorders.

The presence of a dual diagnosis such as schizophrenia and substance abuse constitutes a major risk to remaining homeless or to becoming homeless again (Koegel *et al.* 1988). According to a study carried out in New York, the combination of abusing drugs, persistent symptoms and impaired global functioning at the time of discharge increased the risk of being homeless again within 3 months of hospital discharge (Olfson *et al.* 1999).

Furthermore, homelessness increases the risk of victimisation for the severely mentally ill. In one study, it was found that living in the city, abusing substances, having a secondary diagnosis of personality disorder and homelessness increased the risk of being a victim of a violent crime, at a rate two-and-a-half times greater than that of the general population (Hiday *et al.* 1999). In another study, 44% of the subjects had been the victim of at least one crime during the previous 2 months and the effect of the incident had had a significant impact on their outcomes in terms of increased homelessness and decreased quality of life (Lam and Rosenheck 1998).

Severe mental illness and sexual or severe physical abuse

It is known that there is an established link between early sexual abuse and the development of mental health problems in adulthood. In a longitudinal prospective study, childhood sexual abuse and the development of major depressive illness, conduct disorder, suicidal behaviours and substance abuse at age 18 were significantly correlated (Fergusson *et al.* 1996a). In the same study, it was found that most of the sexually abused children came from families with high levels of marital conflict, impaired parenting and parents who reported problems with alcohol. There appears to be a link especially between severe sexual abuse and an earlier onset of affective illness and personality disorder (Fergusson *et al.* 1996b; Giese *et al.* 1998; Cheasty *et al.* 1998).

When assessing a patient with severe mental illness, special attention should be given to earlier traumatic experiences. Very often the patient may not volunteer information on emotionally sensitive issues such as sexual or severe physical abuse, and yet such traumatic events may have a severe impact on their later behaviour and conduct.

Severe physical abuse in early years may also lead to later mental health problems and it is not uncommon for physical and sexual abuse to go together. Growing up in an environment where physical violence is part of life, a child will develop various strategies to cope. Some may seek solace in abusing drugs or alcohol from very young ages while others may accept physical or verbal violence as a way to 'resolve' problems, thus repeating the dysfunctional interaction patterns which they have 'learnt' within their family settings. In fact, both physical and sexual abuses are associated with an increased likelihood of the use of alcohol, cannabis and almost all other drugs for both males and females. Early onset of multiple drug abuse is especially common among those who have been both sexually and physically abused (Harrison *et al.* 1997).

Severe mental illness and ethnicity

Modern British society has become increasingly multicultural and multi-ethnic over the past few decades. The relationship between ethnicity and mental health has been the focus of much debate for several years now. Earlier preoccupations with *racial differences* and ethnic *predispositions* to mental illness have been replaced by *ethnic inequalities* in service experience and outcome. Ethnicity and culture are important variables that can complicate the care of patients within any mental health setting, but especially so within PICUs/Low Secure Units (LSUs). In fact, culture/ethnicity can have a pathoplastic (illness-shaping) effect on the problems involved in the management of many complex needs patients. Despite this, there is hardly any research on the mental health care experience of minority ethnic groups and on the outcome of mental health care in minority ethnic groups. Available research has been conducted either on treatment rates or on community-based national samples. The former have potential drawbacks as they mainly represent an aspect of illness behaviour, rather than a measure of illness prevalence itself.

Studies in Britain have consistently reported elevated rates of schizophrenia (and higher rates of first contact and of admission) among black African and Caribbean people compared with the white population (Bagley 1971; McGovern and Cope 1987; Harrison *et al.* 1988; Littlewood and Lipsedge 1988; Cochrane and Bal 1989; King *et al.* 1994; Van Os *et al.* 1996). These patients typically tend to be young men. Some studies (Harrison *et al.* 1988) have suggested that the rates are very high among young black Caribbean people who were born in Britain (although these data, like most work in this area, are dependent on a very small number of identified cases).

In contrast to findings from studies based on treatment contact, the EMPIRIC study and the Fourth National Survey of Ethnic Minorities (FNS) (both community based) found that Caribbean populations did have a raised prevalence of psychotic symptoms in comparison with the white British group, but not to the level reported elsewhere. And when differences were considered across gender, age and migration status, it was found that the prevalence of psychotic symptoms was not particularly high among young Caribbean men or those born in Britain. In fact, the difference between Caribbean and white people in estimated prevalence of psychotic illness in the FNS was largely accounted for by the relatively high prevalence among Caribbean women (Nazroo 1997; King *et al.* 2005).

Research findings on ethnic differences between South Asian and white populations are even more conflicting. Treatment-contact-based studies by Cochrane and Bal (1989) and Bhugra *et al.* (1997) suggested that rates of first contact with treatment services (and also admission rates) for psychotic illness among South Asian people are similar to those among white people. However, King *et al.* (1994), in another study using the same methods in a different part of London, suggested that rates of psychotic illness were raised to similar levels among South Asian people to those found among black Caribbean people. The study also found that the majority of white people identified as having a first onset of psychotic illness were not of British origin (they were mostly of Irish origin).

In contrast to the findings for contact with treatment services, the community-based EMPIRIC and FNS studies suggested that Indian and Pakistani subjects had higher rates of psychosis than the white group, although none of these differences was statistically significant. In contrast, the Bangladeshi group had a lower rate than the white group for both of these items, but not significantly so (Nazroo 1997; King *et al.* 2005). However, when these findings were examined by migration status, it seemed that the lower rates only applied to those South Asian people who had migrated to Britain, with non-migrants having rates that were identical to the white British rates. In support of the conclusions drawn by King *et al.* (1994), the FNS also reported a high rate of psychosis among white people who were not of British origin (they were predominantly, though not exclusively, of Irish origin), for whom the rate was 75% higher than for the white British group.

These ethnic variations in treatment contact rates and illness prevalence rates notwithstanding, there are a number of barriers to effective treatment of patients from ethnic minorities. These include such factors as cultural differences in illness experience and expression, cultural influences on help-seeking behaviours, stigma and ethnicity-based stereotyping

of psychotically ill patients. Black African-Caribbean patients are often stereotyped as being more hostile, violent and dangerous than their white counterparts. As a result, black service-users and carers in contact with statutory services feel undervalued and misunderstood, and tend to withdraw from active participation. Those remaining engaged with mainstream services often find themselves amidst a patronising environment shaped by stereotypical attitudes. They often express dissatisfaction with mainstream mental health services, and argue that services misrepresent, misunderstand and seek to control their experiences and methods of expression. A number of similar myths exist about South Asian patients which impede their ability to access care for their illnesses.

In one study that looked at the satisfaction with the mental health services, Parkman *et al.* (1997) found that second-generation patients of Caribbean origin were significantly less satisfied with almost all aspects of the services that they received than either older patients born in the West Indies or white patients (Parkman *et al.* 1997). It was also found in the same study that their dissatisfaction was highly associated with the number of previous admissions. Some of the ethno-cultural aspects caring for patients from black and ethnic minorities have been highlighted in the David Bennett Inquiry (Norfolk, Suffolk and Cambridgeshire Strategic Health Authority 2003). The Inquiry recommended that all staff who work in mental health services should receive training in cultural awareness, sensitivity and competency. This should include training to tackle overt and covert racism and institutional racism. It also recommended that the Care Programme Approach (CPA) care plans should have a mandatory requirement to include appropriate details of each patient's ethnic origin and cultural needs. Finally, the workforce in mental health services should be ethnically diverse. Where appropriate, active steps should be taken to recruit, retain and promote black and minority ethnic staff.

Effective treatment of all acutely ill patients needs to be based upon the development of a therapeutic alliance between the treating team and patients and carers. This alliance is essential for adequate information sharing and collaborative decision making, which are both essential for engagement with patients in the longer term. Communication difficulties (due to language incompatibilities), and insensitivity to cultural and ethnic values and practices can create an atmosphere of mistrust and hostility, and contributes to the perpetuation of unhelpful cultural/ethnic myths and stereotypes. These in turn often lead to prejudicial attitudes and cause major impediments to the development of a therapeutic alliance. In many ways these could contribute to lower rates of engagement and poorer outcomes.

In order that the needs of ethnic minority patients are appropriately assessed and met, it is essential that PICU/LSU mental health staff members are sensitive to the ethnic and cultural needs of individual patients, and incorporate the same in individualised care plans. Flexibility is necessary to develop an ethnically sensitive service. For example, the timing of medications may need to be scheduled around religious services or other obligations such as religious education lessons. Single-sex sections or activities may be required to take into account some cultural or religious obligations – these are especially for Asian patients/carers. Dietary restrictions may need to be taken into account for some patients who eat specific kinds of foods. Finally, effective communication between all parties involved is very important. Problems can arise if there is poor communication between the patients, carers and staff. This is particularly relevant for non-English-speaking patients (usually from South Asian backgrounds, and more recently from Eastern European cultures). Being able to communicate is essential so as to discuss treatment plans and medication changes. This is particularly relevant in a PICU/LSU setting where verbal de-escalation techniques are entirely based on verbal communication skills. Communication is also vital in gaining the support of carers in formulating care plans for the patients.

These basic principles of *sensitivity, flexibility* and *communication* need to be founded upon a reasonable *knowledge* base of the cultural values and practices of different ethnic minorities.

Mental health staff need to be trained so as to improve their awareness, understanding and knowledge of different communities. Cultural differences should not be viewed as cultural problems. Instead showing that they are beneficial will add a whole new dimension to an existing service. Staff training should also include aspects of the following:

- Providing accurate information about mental illness, correcting misconceptions
- De-stigmatising mental illness
- Developing trust in the community – local contacts
- Overcoming language barriers, facilitating decision making
- Sensitivity to cultural and religious values and practices, and incorporating these in the ward schedules
- Listening and understanding issues and experience of those from different cultures and faiths
- Providing a service patients can identify and communicate with
- Offering consistent support

Management

The treatment and management of severely mentally ill patients with additional serious problems pose significant challenges for both inpatient and community psychiatric services. This complexity is well recognised and acknowledged in the Mental Health Policy Implementation Guide: National Minimum Standards for General Adult Services in Psychiatric Intensive Care Units and Low Secure Environments (Department of Health 2002). This guide emphasises the need for a multidisciplinary approach in assessing the multiple needs of PICU/LSU patients, and also the importance of a broad bio-psychosocial approach in their management. Specifically, it recommends the need for biological, psychological, social and environmental interventions in order to meet the complex needs of many patients in this setting.

Complex needs patients are usually 'well known' within the service and their repeated admissions often cause a sense of 'failure' among staff members.

It is always disheartening to see previous good therapeutic work quickly being dissolved by the adversities a patient may encounter in the community. When patients are re-admitted, they will very often deny the severity of their problems and the existence of mental illness or substance abuse, despite the clear previous evidence for both. There may be some minimal cooperation whilst in hospital, especially in a locked environment such as a PICU/LSU. Problems are often compounded by ethnic/cultural disparities between the patient and the team members. Whilst on the ward, patients often make 'promises' to abstain from substances and other problem behaviours, but more often than not these 'promises' are forgotten soon after discharge with resultant relapses and 'revolving door' experiences. This (and resource constraints) seems to be the most common cause for prolonged (more than 8 weeks) admissions to PICUs. In places where there is no intensive care provision, such patients may be nursed on acute psychiatric wards where, due to low staff: patient ratios and at times lack of specialised training, patients may not receive the attention and care they require. Even in intensive care units, the management of such patients is often difficult due to inadequate recognition of additional problems, lack of specialised training for staff members or an inappropriate/inadequate treatment plan.

It is the experience of some psychiatric services in the UK that specialised units have been an essential addition to form a part of the comprehensive local mental health service. In the North West Region of England, a network of seven 'High Dependency Units' has been set up as a regional initiative. In South East London, there are two 'Challenging Behaviour Units' at the Bethlem Royal Hospital and at Oxleas NHS Trust. These units offer a low secure service to the patients with complex needs who may require admissions of 3–24 months in order to address complex psychiatric, psychological, social and organic factors. A full multidisciplinary team is therefore essential when attempting to treat these patients. The types of therapeutic and psychological interventions are specified in the chapters on these subjects in Part I.

The experience of staff members in such units suggests that some complex needs patients require a further period of highly staffed care following discharge. This may be in a hospital setting such as an open rehabilitation ward or in the community in a registered hospital hostel, possibly subject to the Mental Health Act, or in a highly staffed community hostel. A small minority of patients may even require longer-term low secure care in a hospital setting if their needs and behaviour cannot be managed in a less secure setting.

Although there is a clear need to have more specialised services and treatment programmes tailored to the needs of patients with complex problems across the UK, employing certain strategies listed below may be beneficial when dealing with patients within existing services.

Assessing the complex need areas

It is not always the patients themselves but the clinicians that need to acknowledge the existence of additional problems. The likelihood of failure of treatment in the long term increases if these additional problems have not been adequately recognised and assessed. The emphasis can no longer be on the treatment of the mental illness alone. A needs-based approach will see the patient as an individual with individual needs and focus on all the problem areas.

The personality traits and additional mental health problems of a patient need to be elicited whilst assessing the mental state, bearing in mind that they are likely to be present in a 'difficult to treat' patient. It is crucial to recognise an underlying depression for instance, as the patient with a severe mental illness carries a higher than normal risk of suicide. A detailed needs assessment will also reveal other problem areas such as homelessness, lack of social support and purposeful activities. A thorough medical examination and regular tests may also reveal unrecognised physical health problems in a patient who does not readily complain of poor health and is prone to develop serious illnesses.

At times some patients with mild learning difficulty may go unrecognised, especially if they have not been previously assessed for this. Atypical presentation of a psychotic illness should alert the assessor that there may be a mild learning difficulty. Furthermore, some repetitive problem behaviours can also be explained once this additional problem is acknowledged.

Again, it is well known that individuals who have been abused physically or sexually do not feel comfortable in disclosing their abuse. However, with thoughtful and tactful interviewing techniques, painful, traumatic experiences may be brought to the fore. In some cases, the abuse might still be going on, especially as patients with a severe mental illness can be open to exploitation.

Psycho-education

Patient empowerment plays an important part in the management of patients who have complex needs who may also feel that all control is being taken out of their hands, especially when they are receiving care at the intensive care units. Involving patients in decision making and taking responsibility for their actions require ongoing psycho-education. In addition to patients, carers also require information on aspects of mental illness and the impact of the additional problems and needs. This can be a daunting task, as very frequently it is seen that most patients cannot easily retain information. There is some evidence, however, that well-structured educational sessions can have some impact on the patient's insight into their mental health problems, although not on their medication compliance (Macpherson *et al.* 1996).

Patients with complex problems require information on a vast range of subjects. They will need to know about mental health issues, symptoms, the effects of substances, medications, their side-effects, employment guidance, the likely outcomes of unprotected sex, HIV infection and social skills training, to name only a few of the topics. Therefore, the timing and structure of the educational sessions are important. The language chosen has to be accessible. The information provided by the multidisciplinary team has to be consistent and well structured. Overwhelming the patient or the carer with too much information may lead to feelings of further alienation.

Box 10.7. Suggested topics for psycho-education:

- Mental health issues
- Medications and their side-effects
- Outcomes of unprotected sex
- Effects of substances
- Symptoms
- HIV infection
- Social skills
- Employment guidance

Staff-related issues and staff burnout

One of the most important aspects of good practice within the PICU/LSU setting involves cohesive multidisciplinary teamwork. A humane approach to all kinds of adversity as the adopted philosophy, a good mix of various complementary skills among the members of the team, availability of training and further staff empowerment, a well-structured ward programme and decent physical surroundings are among the essential elements needed to create a harmonious and cohesive PICU/LSU. However, it is also very easy for things to go terribly wrong in an emotionally charged environment.

One of the main problems in dealing with complex needs patients in PICU/LSUs is staff 'burnout'. Being exposed to violence on a daily basis can change an individual's reaction to patients over time. It is known that some may become emotionally exhausted and lose patience and tolerance, whilst others may feel demoralised and alienated from their patients and begin avoiding contact with them. Emotions experienced can vary, even within the same day, from anger and resentment to sadness, fear and anxiety. Staff may feel exhausted with such a strongly felt range of emotions experienced within a short period. Such emotions, if they are left unexplored and not briefed on an ongoing basis, may even lead to psychological disturbances. In a study carried out to measure and compare 'burnout' between staff who worked with patients displaying challenging behaviour in hospital-based bungalows and a community unit, it was found that hospital-based staff were less satisfied with their salaries, enjoyed their contact with their patients less, were more emotionally exhausted and found their training to be less adequate, compared with community-based staff (Chung and Corbett 1998).

It is important that staff understand the causes of challenging behaviours. If they do not, staff may inadvertently ensure the long-term maintenance of unwanted behaviour. In a study examining staff's beliefs about the causes of challenging behaviour and their responses to it, the belief systems of experienced and inexperienced staff were compared (Hastings et al. 1995). Experienced staff held beliefs that were consistent with present knowledge on challenging behaviours and distinguished between the behaviours in terms of their causes, whilst the inexperienced staff did not. These data are interpreted as emphasising the importance of a 'needs-based' approach and staff training, when managing challenging behaviour.

There are numerous ways of avoiding staff 'burnout'. It is crucial that the management team of PICU/LSUs take into account that 'burnout' is a strong possibility. Management should arrange regular staff support groups in addition to regular and relevant staff training to furnish staff with ways of coping and delivering appropriate and humane care to those most likely to have the most complex problems.

Summary

In this chapter, we have attempted to define the type of patient who has complex needs and examined them under several subheadings. Many of these patients are found in PICU/LSUs where they may require care for longer periods compared to patients with less complicated conditions. These patients not only suffer from a severe mental illness, but also have additional diagnoses or problems, which complicate and worsen their clinical outcome. Very often one problem can lead to another and there is an accumulation of adverse factors. Patients with schizophrenia appear especially prone to substance abuse and create serious management problems for the services. This chapter also includes information on management strategies for the complex needs patient and discusses the preferred choice of treatments.

REFERENCES

Allebeck P. 1989 Schizophrenia: a life-shortening disease. Schizophr Bull 15: 81–89

Allison DB, Mentore JL, Heo M et al. 1999 Antipsychotic-induced weight gain: a comprehensive research synthesis. Am J Psychiatry 156: 1686–1696

American Diabetes Association. American Psychiatric Association. American Association of Clinical Endocrinologists. North American Association for the Study of Obesity. 2004 Consensus development conference on antipsychotic drugs and obesity and diabetes. J Clin Psychiatry 65: 267–272

Ames D, Camm J, Cook P et al. 2002 Cardiac Safety in Schizophrenia Group. Minimizing the risks associated with significant QTc prolongation in people with schizophrenia: a consensus statement by the Cardiac Safety in Schizophrenia Group. Aust Psychiatry 10: 115–124

Anath J. 1984 Physical illness and psychiatric disorders. Compr Psychiatry 25: 586–593

Bagley C. 1971 The social aetiology of schizophrenia in immigrant groups. Int J Soc Psychiatry 17: 292–304

Bhugra D, Leff J, Mallett R, Der G, Corridan B, Rudge S. 1997 Incidence and outcome of schizophrenia in whites, African-Caribbeans and Asians in London. Psychol Med 27: 791–798

Brown S, Birtwistle J, Roe L, Thompson C. 1999 The unhealthy lifestyle of people with schizophrenia. Psychol Med 29: 697–701

Brown S, Inskip H, Barraclough B. 2000 Causes of the excess mortality of schizophrenia. Br J Psychiatry 177: 212–217

Bushe C, Holt R. 2004 Prevalence of diabetes and impaired glucose tolerance in patients with schizophrenia. Br J Psychiatry Suppl 47: S67–S71

Carey MP, Carey KB, Weinhardt LS, Gordon CM. 1997 Behavioural risk for HIV infection among adults with a severe and persistent mental illness: patterns and psychological antecedents. Community Ment Health J 33(2): 133–142

Cheasty M, Clare AW, Collins C. 1998 Relation between sexual abuse in childhood and adult depression: case-control study. Br Med J 316(7126): 198–201

Chung MC, Corbett J. 1998 The burnout of nursing staff working with challenging behaviour clients in hospital-based bungalows and a community unit. Int J Nurs Stud 35(1–2): 56–64

Cochrane R, Bal SS. 1989 Mental hospital admission rates of immigrants to England: a comparison of 1971 and 1981. Soc Psychiatry Psychiatr Epidemiol 24: 2–11

Collins J, Schlenger W. 1988 Acute and chronic effects of alcohol use on violence. J Stud Alcohol 4(6): 516–521

Curkendall SM, Mo J, Glasser DB *et al.* 2004 Cardiovascular disease in patients with schizophrenia in Saskatchewan, Canada. J Clin Psychiatry 65: 715–720

Davidson M. 2002 Risk of cardiovascular disease and sudden death in schizophrenia. J Clin Psychiatry 63 [Suppl. 9]: 5–11

Davis S. 1998 Injection drug use and HIV infection among the seriously mentally ill: a report from Vancouver. Can J Community Ment Health 17(1): 121–127

Department of Health. 2002 Mental Health Policy Implementation Guide. National Minimum Standards for General Adult Services in Psychiatric Intensive Care Units (PICU) and Low Secure Environments. London: Department of Health

Diefendorf R. 1915 Dementia Praecox. In: Clinical Psychiatry: A Text-book for Students and Physicians. Abstracted and adapted from the 7th German edition of Kraepelin's "Lehrbuch der psychiatrie" by A. Ross Diefendorf. London: The Macmillan Company, pp. 229–230

Dixon L, Weiden P, Delahanty J, Goldberg R, Postrado L, Lucksted A, Lehman A. 2000 Prevalence and correlates of diabetes in national schizophrenia samples. Schizophr Bull 26: 903–12

Dombrovski A, Rosenstock J. 2004 Bridging general medicine and psychiatry: providing general medical and preventive care for the severely mentally ill. Curr Opin Psychiatry 17: 523–529

Dwyer DS, Bradley RJ, Kablinger AS, Freeman AM. 2001 Glucose metabolism in relation to schizophrenia and antipsychotic drug treatment. Ann Clin Psychiatry 13: 103–113

Emerson C. 1995 In: Challenging behaviour. Analysis and intervention in people with learning difficulties. Cambridge: Cambridge University Press

FDA Patient Safety News; Show 28, June 2004. Warning about hyperglycemia and atypical antipsychotic drugs. URL address http://www.accessdata.fda.gov/scripts/cdrh/cfdocs/psn/printer.cfm?id_229

Fergusson DM, Lynskey MT, Horwood LJ. 1996a Childhood sexual abuse and psychiatric disorder in young adulthood: I. Prevalence of sexual abuse and factors associated with sexual abuse. J Am Acad Child Adolesc Psychiatry 35(10): 1355–1364

Fergusson DM, Horwood LJ, Lynskey MT. 1996b Childhood sexual abuse and psychiatric disorder in young adulthood: II. Psychiatric outcomes of childhood sexual abuse. J Am Acad Child Adolesc Psychiatry 35(10): 1365–1374

Fichter MM, Koniarczyk M, Greifenhagen A *et al.* 1996 Mental illness in a representative sample of homeless men in Munich, Germany. Eur Arch Psychiatry Clin Neurosci 246: 185–196

Gianfresco FD, Grogg AL, Mahmoud RA, Wang RH, Nasrallah HA. 2002 Differential effects of risperidone, olanzapin, clozapine, and conventional antipsychotics on type 2 diabetes: findings from a large health plan database. J Clin Psychiatry 63: 920–930

Giese AA, Thomas MR, Dubovsky SL, Hilty S. 1998 The impact of a history of childhood abuse on hospital outcome of affective episodes. Psychiatr Serv 49(1): 77–81

Gilles M, Wilke A, Kopf D, Nonell A, Lehnert H, Deuschle M. 2005 Antagonism of the serotonin (5-HT)-2 receptor and insulin sensitivity: implications for atypical antipsychotics. Psychosom Med 67: 748–751

Goldman LS. 1999 Medical illness in patients with schizophrenia. J Clin Psychiatry 60: 10–15

Grassi L. 1996 Risk of HIV infection in psychiatrically ill patients. AIDS Care 8(1): 103–116

Haddad PM, Anderson IM. 2002 Antipsychotic-related QTc prolongation, torsade de pointes and sudden death. Drugs 62: 1649–1671

Hall RC, Gardner ER, Popkin MK *et al.* 1981 Unrecognized physical illness prompting psychiatric admission: a prospective study. Am J Psychiatry 138: 629–635

Harrison G, Owens D, Holton A, Neilson D, Boot D. 1988 A prospective study of severe mental disorder in Afro-Caribbean patients. Psychol Med 18: 643–657

Harrison PA, Fulkerson JA, Beebe TJ. 1997 Multiple substance use among adolescent physical and sexual abuse victims. Child Abuse Negl 21(6): 529–539

Hastings RP, Remington B, Hopper GM. 1995 Experienced and inexperienced health care workers' beliefs about challenging behaviours. J Intellect Disabil Res 39(6): 474–483

Hennessy S, Bilker WB, Knauss JS, *et al.* 2002 Cardiac arrest and ventricular arrhythmia in patients taking antipsychotic drugs: cohort study using administrative data. Br Med J 325(7372): 1070–1074

Hiday VA, Swartz MS, Swanson JW, Borum R, Wagner HR. 1999 Criminal victimisation of persons with severe mental illness. Psychiatr Serv 50(1): 62–68

Horwath E, Cournas F, McKinnon K, Guido JR, Herman R. 1996 Illicit-drug injection among psychiatric patients without a primary substance use disorder. Psychiatr Serv 47(2): 181–185

Jablensky A, McGrath J, Herrman H *et al.* 1999 People living with psychotic illness: an Australian study 1997–98. Canberra: Commonwealth Department of Health and Aged Care, 1999. Available online at: http://www.health.gov.au/hsdd/mentalhe/resources/reports/pdf/psychot.pdf [accessed March 2003]

Jeste DV, Galdsjo JA, Lindamer LA, Lacro JP. 1996 Medical co-morbidity in schizophrenia. Schizophr Bull 22(3): 413–430

Johnson JG, Rabkin JG, Lipsitz JD, Williams JB, Remien RH. 1999 Recurrent major depressive disorder among human immunodeficiency virus (HIV)-positive and HIV-negative intravenous drug users: findings of a 3-year longitudinal study. Compr Psychiatry 40(1): 31–34

Kane JM. 1996 Factors which can make patients difficult to treat. Br J Psychiatry 169 [Suppl. 31]: 10–14

King M, Coker E, Leavey G, Hoare A, Johnson-Sabine E. 1994 Incidence of psychotic illness in London: comparison of ethnic groups. Br Med J 309: 1115–1119

King M, Nazroo J, Weich S *et al.* 2005 Psychotic symptoms in the general population of England–a comparison of ethnic groups (The EMPIRIC study). Soc Psychiatry Psychiatr Epidemiol. 40(5):375–81

Koegel P, Burnam MA, Farr RK. 1988 The prevalence of specific psychiatric disorders among homeless individuals in the inner city of Los Angeles. Arch Gen Psychiatry 45: 1085–1092

Koran LM, Sox HC, Marton KI *et al.* 1989 Medical evaluation of psychiatric patients. Arch Gen Psychiatry 46: 733–740

Koranyi EK. 1979 Morbidity and rate of undiagnosed physical illnesses in a psychiatric clinic population. Arch Gen Psychiatry 36: 414–419

Lam JA, Rosenheck R. 1998 The effect of victimisation on clinical outcomes of homeless persons with serious mental illness. Psychiatr Serv 49(5): 678–683

Lambert TJR, Velakoulis, D, Pantellis C. 2003 Medical comorbidity in schizophrenia in schizophrenia. Med J Aust 178 [Suppl. 5]: S67–S70

Lelliott P, Wing JK, Clifford P. 1994 A national audit of new long-stay psychiatric patients I: Method and description of the cohort. Br J Psychiatry 164: 160–169

Lindenmayer JP, Czobor P, Volavka J *et al.* 2003 Changes in glucose and cholesterol levels in patients with schizophrenia treated with typical or atypical antipsychotics. Am J Psychiatry 160: 290–296

Link B, Stueve C. 1994 Psychotic symptoms and the violent/illegal behaviour of mental patients compared to community controls. In: Monahan J, Steadman HJ (eds) Violence and Mental Disorder. Chicago, Ill.: University of Chicago Press, pp. 137–159

Littlewood R, Lipsedge M. 1988 Psychiatric illness among British Afro-Caribbeans. Br Med J 296: 950–951

Macpherson R, Jerrom B, Hughes A. 1996 A controlled study of education about drug treatment in schizophrenia. Br J Psychiatry 168: 709–717

Mann S, Cree W. 1976 'New' long stay psychiatric patients: a national sample survey of fifteen mental hospitals in England and Wales 1972/73. Psychol Med 6: 603–616

Marder SR, Essock SM, Miller AL *et al.* 2004 Physical health monitoring of patients with schizophrenia. Am J Psychiatry 161: 1334–1349

McGovern D, Cope R. 1987 First psychiatric admission rates of first and second generation Afro-Caribbeans. Soc Psychiatry 22: 139–149

Meyer JM. 2002 A retrospective comparison of weight, lipid, and glucose changes between risperidone- and olanzapine-treated inpatients: metabolic outcomes after 1 year. J Clin Psychiatry 63: 425–433

Muldoon MF, Kackey RH, Williams KV, Korytkowski MT, Flory JD, Manuck SB. 2004 Low central nervous system serotonergic responsivity is associated with the metabolic syndrome and physical inactivity. J Clin Endocrinol Metab 89: 266–271

Nasrallah H. 2003 A review of the effect of atypical antipsychotics on weight. Psychoneuroendocrinology 28 [Suppl. 1]: 83–96

Nazroo JY. 1997 Ethnicity and Mental Health: Findings from a National Community Survey. London: Policy Studies Institute

Newcomer JW, Haupt DW, Fucetola R *et al.* 2002 Abnormalities in glucose regulation during antipsychotic treatment of schizophrenia. Arch Gen Psychiatry 59: 337–345

Niederecker M, Naber D, Riedel R, Perro C, Goebel FD. 1995 Incidence and aetiology of psychotic disorders in HIV infected patients. Nervenartz 66(5): 367–371

Nolan KA, Volavka J, Mohr P, Czobor P. 1999 Psychopathy and violent behaviour among patients with schizophrenia or schizoaffective disorder. Psychiatr Serv 50(6): 787–792

Norfolk, Suffolk and Cambridgeshire Strategic Health Authority. 2003 Independent Inquiry into the Death of David Bennett. Cambridge: Norfolk, Suffolk and Cambridgeshire Strategic Health Authority

Olfson M, Mechanic D, Hansell S, Boyer CA, Walkup J. 1999 Prediction of homelessness within three months of discharge among inpatients with schizophrenia. Psychiatr Serv 50(5): 667–663

Parkman S, Davies S, Leese M, Phelan M, Thornicroft G. 1997 Ethnic differences in satisfaction with mental health services among representative people with psychosis in south London: PRISM study 4. Br J Psychiatry 171: 260–264

Reeves S. 1997 Behavioural misdiagnosis. Nurs Times 93(19): 44–45

Regier DA, Farmer ME, Rae DS et al. 1990 Comorbidity of mental disorders with alcohol and other drug abuse.

Results from the Epidemiologic Catchment Area (ECA) Study. J Am Med Assoc 264: 2511–2518

Ruschena D, Mullen PE, Burgess P et al. 1998 Sudden death in psychiatric patients. Br J Psychiatry 172: 331–336

Ryan MC, Collins P, Thakore JH. 2003 Impaired fasting glucose tolerance in firstepisode, drug-naive patients with schizophrenia. Am J Psychiatry 160: 284–289

Subramaniam M, Chong SA, Pek E. 2003 Diabetes mellitus and impaired glucose tolerance in patients with schizophrenia. Can J Psychiatry 48: 345–347

Thakore JH. 2004 Metabolic disturbance in first-episode schizophrenia. Br J Psychiatry Suppl 47: S76–S79

Thakore J. 2005 Metabolic syndrome and schizophrenia. Br J Psychiatry 186: 455–456

Thakore JH, Mann JN, Vlahos I et al. 2002 Increased visceral fat distribution in drug-naive and drug-free patients with schizophrenia. Int J Obes Relat Metab Disord 26: 137–141

Van Os J, Castle DJ, Takei N, Der G, Murray RM. 1996 Psychotic illnes in ethnic minorities: clarification from the 1991 Census. Psychol Med 26: 203–208

Wessely S, Buchanan A, Reed A et al. 1993 Acting on delusions I: Prevalence. Br J Psychiatry 163: 69–76

11

Therapeutic activities within Psychiatric Intensive Care and Low Secure Units

Faisal Kazi, Brenda Flood and Sarah Hooton

Introduction

Therapeutic activities not only enhance an individual's development, but they can also assist in the management of problematic behaviour and maintenance of a safe environment. The importance of providing therapeutic activities within a Psychiatric Intensive Care Unit (PICU) is highlighted in the National Minimum Standards for General Adult Services in Psychiatric Intensive Care Units and Low Secure Environments:

An effective PICU design will have given the provision of therapeutic activity an equal status to safety and security. (Department of Health 2002a, p. 13)

The range of activities that can be offered within a PICU requires careful consideration in order to meet the acute, complex and challenging needs of the patient population. Clinicians are faced with the task of identifying appropriate strategies and ensuring the necessary structures and systems are in place in order for therapeutic activities to be safely and consistently provided.

This chapter aims to provide clinicians with an introduction to the relevant literature supporting therapeutic activities and presents a practical approach towards developing and maintaning a therapeutic programme within a PICU/Low Secure Unit (LSU). It will explore the benefits and limitations of providing a therapeutic programme and describe how these activities can be effectively implemented within this specialised environment.

Activity

Activities are central to human existence and are vital to meeting basic human needs (Drew and Rugg 2001; Kielhofner and Butler 2002; Law 2002). Meaningful activity, with its intrinsic power to maintain, restore and transform, is fundamental to the health and wellbeing of all humans (Mee and Sumsion 2001). The link between activities, health, wellbeing and quality of life has been well documented in the literature (Hansen and Atchison 2000; Hagedorn 2001; Kelly *et al.* 2001; Creek 2002; Foster 2002; Law 2002; Eklund *et al.* 2003; Mee *et al.* 2004).

When an individual experiences an acute psychiatric illness it is likely that his or her abiltiy to engage in meaningful activities is diminished (Yarwood and Johnstone 2002). Furthermore, patients with mental illness may have a diminished ability to perform daily life tasks successfully. Using activities therapeutically can enable patients to develop and maintain the skills required for healthy functioning.

History of therapeutic activity

The use of activities as a therapeutic tool has long been recognised. Throughout the ages, both in

Psychiatric Intensive Care, 2nd edn., eds. M. Dominic Beer, Stephen M. Pereira and Carol Paton.
Published by Cambridge University Press. © Cambridge Universtiy Press 2008

Eastern and Western culture, there is reference to the belief that activity can both influence and be used to improve mental and physical health and wellbeing (Paterson 2002).

As early as 2600 BC the Chinese taught that disease resulted from organic inactivity and used physical training as therapy; the ancient Egyptians dedicated temples to the treatment of melancholics, where the patient's time was spent in recreational activity; and the ancient Greeks linked mind with body and recommended the use of activity to maintain health and treat mental diseases (Turner 2002).

One of the basic principles of 'moral treatment' which emerged around the beginning of the nineteenth century was the belief in the importance of useful activity and its beneficial effects on mental health (Barthwick *et al.* 2001). The increasing awareness in the value of activity as a treatment modality carried on through the twentieth century.

Activity as a therapeutic tool

Purposeful activity and meaningful occupation can be used as therapeutic tools in the promotion of health and wellbeing (Drew and Rugg 2001). Within a PICU/LSU activity can be used purely to occupy the mind, distracting the individual's attention from disturbing symptoms (e.g. listening to music, board games), or be specifically selected and identified in the individual's care plan to develop and maintain functioning (e.g. relaxation, anger management, cooking, art therapy). Whether an activity is diversional or treatment specific is determined not by what the activity is but how it is used. It is through engagement in activities that patients are able to exercise choice, interact, and adapt to and cope within their environment (Mee and Sumsion 2001).

Some of the benefits patients on a PICU/LSU can experience from engaging in specific activities are outlined below. The benefits of activities can be enhanced when provided within the framework of a wider structured programme.

Benefits of engaging in activities

- Enhance feelings of self-worth
- Maintain present level of functioning
- Provide opportunities for meaningful communication and appropriate socialisation
- Increase ability to solve life stresses
- Increase insight and understanding of mental illness
- Enable orientation to surroundings and reality
- Focus concentration on to productive pursuits
- Facilitate self expression
- Encourage patients to take personal responsibility
- Promote choice
- Maintain a routine and provide a structure
- Provide patients with a purpose and focus to their day, and to their admission
- Increase levels of confidence
- Replace lost roles
- Enable the assessment of a patient's functional performance and mental state over a period of time
- Provide opportunities for developing life skills
- Provide pleasurable experiences
- Promote physical health

Activity and aggression

Activity can not only be used as a therapeutic tool, but also as a means of reducing violence and aggression on a PICU/LSU. Recent studies indicate a direct relationship between engagement in structured activities and reduced levels of violence within inpatient psychiatric units (Shepherd and Lavender 1999; Barlow 2003; Daffern *et al.* 2003; Rutter *et al.* 2004; Secker *et al.* 2004). Furthermore, mental health good practice guidelines have suggested that levels of violence and aggression would be reduced with increased provision of structured activities. Environments with high therapeutic intervention and interaction help diminish disturbance, violence and boredom. Lack of structured activities promotes untoward incidents and creates risks (Department of Health 2002b). Incidents of violence would be reduced if patients were engaged

Monday	Tuesday	Wednesday	Thursday	Friday	Saturday	Sunday
Community Meeting	Craft group	Cooking group	Social skills	Education		
Relaxation	Quiz/Games	Life skills group	Computer sessions	Art therapy	Trip out	Communal meal
Multi gym	Badminton	Multi gym	Art/Craft activities	Pool competition	Video night	

Figure 11.1. A therapeutic programme

in meaningful occupation. Lack of opportunity to participate in therapy and social activities influences the development of violent incidents (Royal College of Psychiatrists College Research Unit, 2001). Provision of activities provides a calming feature in the clinical environment (United Kingdom Central Council for Nursing, Midwifery and Health Visiting 2002). Engaging in therapeutic activities helps to prevent and minimise aggressive and violent behaviour (Department of Health 2004a). These studies and guidelines suggest that the provision of structured, therapeutic activities can directly reduce levels of violence, aggression and untoward incidents within a PICU/LSU.

The therapeutic programme

The provision of a full and purposeful activity and therapy programme is essential for both treatment purposes and as a significant part of the creation of a secure and safe environment. (Tilt *et al.* 2000, p. 6)

The therapeutic programme can be considered to be the overall structure within which activities are provided. It is a combination of planned, structured as well as spontaneous activities which can be both diversional and treatment specific. It includes activities related to self-care, leisure, education and work,

which reflect a balanced lifestyle and can occur on a group or individual basis. These are facilitated by the multidisciplinary team and can occur within the immediate environment, the wider hospital, or involve accessing community facilities. Figure 11.1 provides an example of a unit-wide therapeutic programme within which individual activities such as self-care tasks can be incorporated.

In an 18-month study of one adult acute inpatient unit in England, Barker (2001) found that reducing formal observation and replacing it with a programme of structured activity led to improved quality of care, reduced rates of absconding and self-harm, and reduced staff sickness and staffing costs. It is however important to be cautious and not impose 'aggressive' structured activity programmes (Kelly *et al.* 2001). The therapeutic programme is about the provision of opportunity. The provision of opportunity, not prescription, enables patients to engage in activities of choice which positively affect their sense of subjective wellbeing and mental health (Rebeiro and Cook 1999).

The patient group and the environment

The needs of patients within PICU/LSUs differ from those in open wards due to the consistently greater risk in the behaviour they exhibit, such as violence towards self and others. Other factors closely associated with intensive care patients include: impaired impulse control, decreased tolerance, rapid mood fluctuations, delusional beliefs, hallucinations, poor interpersonal skills, limited concentration, limited cognition, disorientation, damage to property, absconding, increased frustration and irritability, chaotic thoughts and routine, and disturbed sleep patterns.

Hospitals are unfamiliar environments, where there is often limited personal space and privacy, and few opportunities for patients to make choices or have control over their situation. In addition, PICU/LSU patients have other factors to contend with, such as a high staff-to-patient ratio, decreased access to facilities, and a concentration of other highly disturbed individuals on the unit, with possible overcrowding and, in PICUs, rapid turnover. This can result in the patients' presenting negative behaviour in response to the environmental structures and constraints. They may have difficulty establishing rapport, be unable to trust staff, feel disempowered, choose to isolate themselves and may demonstrate increased levels of verbal and physical aggression. This in turn may have an adverse effect on their motivation and level of self worth.

If patients are encouraged to channel their energies into productive pursuits, which have been carefully considered, not only would this lead to increased feelings of self worth and empowerment, but also may have the positive effect of reducing problematic behaviour. The incorporation of therapeutic activities into the ward routine and culture may create an environment that plays a significant part in the management of difficult behaviour, whilst at the same time addressing individual needs. The provision of a therapeutic environment on an inpatient ward is one of the great challenges for psychiatry today (Davenport 2002).

Physical activity and exercise

Strong and established evidence in the literature proves that people with severe and enduring mental health problems have a significantly increased risk of physical illness and premature mortality (Brown *et al.* 1999; Phelan *et al.* 2001; Faulkner *et al.* 2003; Dombrovski and Rosenstock 2004; Bradshaw *et al.* 2005). Poor socio economic and lifestyle factors increase risk of chronic disease for individuals with serious mental illness, such as diabetes and cardiovascular disease (Crone *et al.* 2004; Jones and O'Beney 2004; Greening 2005; Richardson *et al.* 2005). The benefits of exercise on physical health have been proven and are widely established and accepted. However, the DCMS/Strategy Unit (2002) suggest that 95% of people with severe mental illness do not meet national recommendations for physical activity and exercise.

Physical activity and exercise not only help to improve physical health but mental health as well (Scully *et al.* 1998; Fox 2000: Faulkner and Biddle 2001; Edwards 2002; Callaghan 2004). There is evidence to suggest that exercise reduces anxiety, depression and negative mood, and improves self-esteem and cognitive functioning (Lawlor and Hopker 2001; Daley, 2002; Bodin and Martinsen 2004). For people suffering from schizophrenia, physical activity and exercise have also been shown to reduce auditory hallucinations, improve sleep patterns and general behaviour, and improve overall quality of life (Faulkner and Sparkes 1999; Callaghan 2004). From the strong evidence in the literature it is clear that physical activity and exercise can be used therapeutically to improve both the physical and mental health of those suffering from mental illness. Physical activity and exercise may also be useful in helping to reduce problematic behaviours.

Difficulties such as environmental constraints and security issues may hinder the provision of physical activities on a PICU/LSU. However, it is important that any difficulties are addressed as a priority by the clinical and managerial teams. The Department of Health (2002a) highlights the importance of health promotion activities including exercise on a PICU/LSU, stating 'patients should have access to and space for regular exercise with appropriate supervision' (p. 8). Patients on a PICU/LSU may be reluctant to participate in physical activity for a variety of reasons, for example difficulties with concentration or attention, preoccupation with thoughts, apathy or social withdrawal. However, Carless and Douglas (2004 p. 27) suggest the following strategies to facilitate and encourage participation: 'choose a low-intensity physical activity to minimise physical demands; provide a supportive, non-competitive group environment; provide opportunities for personal achievement, success and progression; provide the opportunity for social interaction and exchange'. Further strategies that may be adopted include increasing enjoyment of the activity and promoting the perceived benefits of exercise (Scully *et al.* 1998), exploring the barriers to physical activity, maximising rewards and encouraging goal setting (Reynolds 2001) and having as wide a range of physical activities available as possible (Daley 2002).

The importance of physical activity and exercise in promoting the physical and mental health of people suffering with severe mental illness is becoming increasingly recognised, both nationally and internationally (Department of Health, 2000, 2004b, 2004c; National Institute for Clinical Excellence 2002; World Federation for Mental Health 2004; World Health Organization 2005). It is essential that the provision of physical activity and exercise on a PICU/LSU is treated as a priority. As such it should be included in both the therapeutic programme on a PICU/LSU and the care plans of individuals.

Developing a therapeutic programme

In order to provide a relevant and effective therapeutic programme staff should aim to meet the needs of the patients whilst considering the risk factors and the environmental constraints. This next section will identify and discuss the practical considerations necessary for successful implementation of activities on the ward. This is divided into two interrelated parts, one being the factors required to establish a ward routine, programme or culture and the other focusing on the implementation of specific activities.

Establishing a ward therapeutic programme

The therapeutic programme needs to be an integral part of the overall service provided on the ward, the success of which is significantly affected by the multidisciplinary team's understanding, commitment and facilitation of this fundamental form of treatment. The following points should be considered in order to ensure the successful implementation of a unit programme.

- All staff need to have an understanding of the rationale for engaging in activities to ensure effective support and implementation for this structure. The adoption of a shared philosophy requires leadership and support from the multidisciplinary team, which can be aided by having a clear statement of purpose in the ward's operational policy. An identified individual or individuals with appropriate skills and experience should be responsible for the overall coordination of the programme.
- Patients should receive information upon admission that clearly outlines the principles of the therapeutic programme, and the expectation that they will be required to engage in these activities as part of their treatment during their admission. This can be in the form of a leaflet, which describes the types of activities available, or verbally from the team or named nurse.
- The multidisciplinary team, in conjunction with the patient, should decide on the appropriate activities for the individual based on the assessment findings. This should be discussed in the team's clinical meeting and agreed with the patient, where possible.
- Activity programmes should combine diversional and treatment-specific activities. Each individual should have a specific programme to address areas of need which takes into consideration their current mental state and behaviour, interests, level of functional performance, cultural background and future plans following discharge. This should be documented in the individual's care plan, with a copy of the programme given to the patient.
- The patient's performance within the activities should be regularly reviewed and progress/

Table 11.1. Proposed basic ward structure

9–10 am	Self care tasks:	Washing, dressing, making bed, breakfast
10–12 pm	45-min activity:	Quiz, badminton, art, community meeting, indoor gardening
12–2 pm		Lunch and rest period
2–4 pm	45-min activity:	Life skills group, relaxation, self-awareness, social skills, cooking session
4–6 pm		Dinner and rest period
6–8 pm	Leisure:	Football, pool competition, bingo, board games

changes reported with regard to the individual's mental state, behaviour and level of functioning. This may result in the need to adapt programmes accordingly.

- The daily structure within the unit should be based on the common needs of patients, with specific treatment activities incorporated into this overall approach (Table 11.1).

- Sufficient support at both management level and amongst staff is essential. Adequate staffing levels to ensure that an activity can be facilitated is a basic requirement if the therapeutic programme is to remain consistent. Staff should have dedicated time to provide this activity which includes time to plan, implement and evaluate its effectiveness, and not be expected to undertake other responsibilities for the duration of the activity. Staff not actively engaged in a specific activity can provide valuable support, by ensuring that appropriate patients attend, that noise levels are kept to a minimum and by respecting the need not to disturb patients whilst engaged in an activity.

- There should be adequate opportunity for staff to receive the appropriate training to enable them competently and confidently to provide relevant individual and group activities. Staff should also receive regular supervision from an appropriately qualified member of the team for continued support and guidance.

- During the planning process resource implications should be identified with sufficient provision made for ongoing funds and materials/equipment.

- In order to maintain a high profile and promote the programme, systems should be developed to support it. A weekly programme of unit activities should be displayed in a prominent position and patients should also have their own specific programme. Staff should know what activities are planned and when. This could be built into shift handovers in which the allocation of staff to certain unit activities occurs if not already preplanned.

- Mechanisms should be in place for the multidisciplinary team to plan, evaluate and adapt the overall programme regularly, e.g. a monthly programme planning and review meeting.

This overall framework will enable patients to develop and maintain a routine, which will also assess changes in mental state and behaviour over a period of time. Such a framework will maximise the benefits of both individual and group activities related to self care, activities of daily living, productive and social/leisure pursuits. This not only provides staff with a focus for treatment, but also clearly demonstrates what is expected of patients.

Case history

Bob is a 38-year-old man with a long history of mental health and behavioural problems. During his admission to the PICU, he was frequently prone to violent outbursts directed towards staff and would press panic alarm buttons, much of which the team considered to be attention seeking behaviour. The occupational therapist chose to use an activity (painting) to engage him in a purposeful, non-confrontational way, therefore meeting his immediate need for individual attention and directing his energy towards a task. This demonstrated to the team that Bob was willing and able to engage in a practical activity, during which time no incidents occurred. Whilst the occupational therapist was working with the patient in the communal area the team was aware of the rationale for the activity and maintained an unobtrusive presence to support the activity. The benefits of engaging Bob were acknowledged including the monitoring of his mental state, enabling self-expression and reinforcing socially appropriate behaviour. This approach was continued by other members of the team to assist in his overall management and treatment.

Implementation of therapeutic activities

In order to prepare for activities within the PICU/LSU it is important to take into account the needs of the patient, establish treatment aims with the patient and consider how to adapt an activity to meet individual needs. Preparation for an activity session needs to consider the following five areas: environment, resources, staffing, activity and the patients themselves.

Environment

- The environment plays a significant part in meeting each patient's treatment goals. It should be organised in such a way as to enable patients to function and engage effectively. In many units the environmental design and space available are less than adequate and therefore require innovative techniques to ensure the setting can be made appropriate for that particular activity.
- The overall management of the environment and organisation of the space, including the layout of furniture, should reflect the group aims, patient group and the type of activity. This will have a significant effect on the level of interaction, the patient's sense of inclusion in the activity and the patient's ability to access resources. For example, a room should be at an appropriate temperature and have suitable light to enhance a patient's performance.
- The type of activity and the number of patients will dictate the most suitable location. This is often limited by the availability of space and safety issues. For example, an activity requiring patient concentration and quietness should be within an area where there are few interruptions or noise from the ward, whereas those activities which are social in nature could take place in a communal area.
- Depending on the aims of the activity the facilitator can create a certain type of atmosphere. On

the one hand, if a relaxed and welcoming environment is wanted, tea and fresh fruit/biscuits could be provided; on the other hand, an activity could be presented in a structured way in order to promote a work atmosphere allowing the patients to focus on a specific task.
- Wherever practicable, following appropriate risk assessment, patients should be encouraged to access other environments within the hospital or local community to promote community living skills and reintegration. For example, utilising local leisure and sports centres, shops and cafés.

Resources

- It is important to identify what activities are required prior to the purchase of equipment. The investment in a sufficient range of resources should support the programmed activities and provide choice for patients engaging in diversional activities.
- An allocated budget will be required to maintain the range and availability of resource materials. This should be accessible to the activity facilitators.
- Prior to patients accessing a particular activity it is the clinical team's responsibility to assess the suitability of their using resources required in the activity. The team should assess the patient's level of risk based on their current presentation and previous history, for example of violence, by assessing the patient's level of safety before attending a craft group in which scissors will be available. Staff facilitating the activity should have made the team aware of the equipment used within it; this will assist the team to make an informed decision.
- Patients involved in an activity using equipment such as glue, clay and tools can be closely supervised; the equipment can be locked away before and directly after use, or adapted equipment could be used which minimises the level of risk.

Staffing

- In order to maximise the effectiveness and ensure consistency in the provision of therapeutic

---

Aim

To assist patients to cope more appropriately with stress and tension. To increase patient's level of awareness of the effect stress has on their feelings and behaviours.

Objectives

To provide a safe non-threatening environment for patients to utilise, learn and practise a range of relaxation techniques. To provide opportunities for patients to discuss the effect of stress and the techniques used. To assist patients to generalise relaxation techniques into their everyday lives.

Practical details

Location – Quiet, group room
Time – Monday 2.00–2.30
Facilitator – OT & Nurse
Equipment required – Cassette player and cassettes, relaxation mats
Criteria for group attendance –   Open to patients on ward
                                    Patients should have an interest and/or desire to learn techniques
                                    Patients should be able to attend/concentrate for 30 minutes
                                    Patients' behaviour should not be disruptive to others

Figure 11.2. Activity rationale for a relaxation group

activities, a designated person responsible for progamme coordination and implementation of activities would be most appropriate.

- Staff on shift need to be aware of activities planned and enough people should be made available to directly facilitate or support the activity in terms of calling residents and motivating them to attend. This can be best achieved during staff handovers.
- Continuity and consistency in the provision of activities are important for individuals who have experienced chaotic and disruptive lifestyles prior to admission. Therefore, activities should occur when they have been planned and at the time designated, wherever possible.
- Staff require sufficient time to plan the activity on the day, ensuring the room has been prepared, the equipment is available and the patients have been reminded of the activity.
- Recording of observations made during the activity should be incorporated into the time allocated to the activity.

Case history

A relaxation group was held on the ward each Monday afternoon. It took place in a group room a small distance away from the ward's communal area. Most chairs were moved out of the room, with some left around the edge for those who preferred to sit. Mats were laid on the floor, curtains were drawn and signs informing others that the group was in session placed strategically to ensure minimum disturbance. Staff were aware that the group was occurring and made sure that the ward remained relatively quiet and prevented unnecessary interruptions.

Activity

- The activity selected should be based upon the identified needs of the patient(s). Each activity should have a specific aim, which may be to meet the individual's recognised treatment needs, or for recreational purposes. These aims should be documented in order to ensure staff and patients are aware of why they are engaged in a particular activity. A file could be held centrally with current activity rationales accessible to staff (Figure 11.2).
- In order to monitor a patient's progress throughout their participation in an activity, records must be kept and contain sufficient as well as relevant information on a patient's behaviour, skills and interactions. An example of a form that could be utilised to gather relevant information about a patient's performance is given in Figure 11.3.

Date of activity:_____/_____/_____Name of client:_____Name of activity:_____

Content: *Brief details of format & activity completed*

Motivation: *Willingness to attend, participation in activity, observed level of interest*

Behaviour/Social Skills: *Level & type of interaction, changes in mood/mental state, inappropriate or unsafe behaviours, non-verbal communication*

Cognition: *Level of understanding, ability to follow verbal/written instructions, concentration, memory, problem solving, decision making, literacy & numeracy*

Task Performance: *Assistance required, accuracy, speed/impulsivity, gross motor control, planning, organising and sequencing tasks*

Facilitator:_____ Signature:_____Date:____/____/____

Figure 11.3. Activity progress notes

- The use of individual and group activities depends on the needs of the patient, which should be monitored on an ongoing basis. In some circumstances it may be appropriate for a patient to commence interacting on an individual basis, either because their behaviour is too disruptive or they are not yet able to cope within a group setting. It may be appropriate for other patients to initially undertake activities within a group setting to encourage socialisation and normalisation.
- It is important that activities are both achievable and challenging. If they are too easy or too difficult the patient can experience frustration. This could be perceived as a negative experience for the patient who may be less likely to engage in the future. It is therefore necessary to grade activities in order that the patient can experience success.

Graded activity

Preparing lasagne can be graded at different levels. For example:
1. Purchase a ready-made lasagne, where all the patient has to do is place it in oven, time the meal and serve.
2. Prepare a lasagne using ready-made pasta and cheese sauces.

3. Prepare a cheese sauce using raw ingredients and ready-made pasta sauce.
4. Use all raw ingredients and provide a salad to accompany the meal.

The level of support given by staff would vary throughout this process. Initially this may be more practical and hands on, but gradually become less direct and more supportive in nature.

Patient

- Patients should wherever possible be fully involved in deciding what activities they will participate in and the reasons why. This should be based on the individual's interests and needs, and relate to their cultural beliefs.
- Patients should be informed of what is expected of them in terms of participation in the unit programme upon admission. Initially their involvement in the programme may be minimal or observational in nature. In some circumstances it may be necessary for the team initially to provide external structure/guidelines encouraging the patient to engage. The ultimate aim is to enable the patient to internalise this structure and make informed decisions about attendance at activities.

- A number of methods can be employed to increase the patient's motivation to participate in the therapeutic programme. If patients are fully involved in determining their activity timetable, are aware of the benefits, and are given an individual, personalised copy of this timetable, it is likely to improve their levels of motivation. It may be necessary to remind patients when they are due to attend activities on their timetable. It can be difficult to maintain the balance between rigidly enforcing attendance at an activity and giving up after one refusal by the patient. This is best achieved through negotiation and maintaining respect for the patient's choice.
- The patient's ability to participate in a certain amount and type of activity is affected by their mental state. This should be considered and staff need to maintain realistic expectations of what the patient can practically achieve.

Summary

This chapter has discussed a practical and achievable approach to treatment that can improve the overall quality of care received by the patient. It has outlined how activities used within a PICU/LSU can positively affect the patient's physical and mental health and functioning, the ward atmosphere and the quality of staff interactions.

Some key factors have been highlighted which could assist a PICU/LSU in establishing, implementing and maintaining a ward therapeutic programme. Fundamental to this process is a multidisciplinary team committed to this approach to care. The team should have realistic expectations as to what can be achieved, a clear, staged process of change and a recognition that this process will be gradual and may not always run smoothly. Each service should identify those factors which may preclude the effectiveness of a programme and develop practical solutions to address them.

There are clearly documented benefits of providing therapeutic activities for patients who are admitted to PICUs and LSUs, but these are not always easy to initiate and maintain. It is important to be aware of and to address the potential constraints and limitations within a PICU/LSU. The main difficulties appear to be associated with the environment, the patient group and staff practices/attitudes. Environmental constraints such as the lack of space, poor decor, inadequate resources, and lack of support and availability of staff can all contribute to the difficulties of implementing an activity programme. This requires staff to be flexible and innovative in order to maximise the potential of the service. The often severe nature of the patients' illness and the intense level of input required pose a challenge for staff, which may lead to their becoming demotivated or burnt out. A supportive therapeutic programme structure may assist staff to cope with these challenging needs, by focusing their energies on productive pursuits. It is recognised that considerable time and energy are often employed to maintain control, levels of safety and security. It has been demonstrated in the literature that the provision of therapeutic activities can have a positive effect on an individual's progress and reduce levels of aggression. Review of current practices could allow for an increased emphasis on the provision of activity programmes and therefore contribute to the creation of a more therapeutic and safe environment.

Acknowledgement

A special thank you to Emily Kazi for all her hard work and support in helping to put this chapter together.

REFERENCES

Barker P. 2001 Dismantling formal observation and refocusing nursing activity in acute in-patient psychiatry: a case study. J Psychiatr Mental Health Nurs 8(2): 183–188

Barlow T. 2003 What colour is aggression? Mental Health Pract 7(4): 32–33

Barthwick A, Holman C, Kennard D, McFetridge M, Messruther K, Wilkes J. 2001 Relevance of moral treatment to contemporary mental health care. J Mental Health 10(4): 427–439

Bodin T, Martinsen EW. 2004 Mood and self-efficacy during acute exercise in clinical depression: a randomised, controlled study. J Sport Exerc Psychol 26: 623–633

Bradshaw T, Lovell K, Harris N. 2005 Healthy living interventions and schizophrenia: a systematic review. J Adv Nurs 49(6): 634–654

Brown S, Birtwistle J, Roe L, Thompson C. 1999 The unhealthy lifestyle of people with schizophrenia. Psychol Med 29(3): 697–701

Callaghan P. 2004 Exercise: a neglected intervention in mental health care? J Psychiatr Mental Health Nurs 11: 476–483

Carless D, Douglas K. 2004 A golf programme for people with severe and enduring mental health problems. J Mental Health Promotion 3(4): 26–39

Creek J. 2002 The knowledge base of occupational therapy. In: Creek J (ed) Occupational Therapy and Mental Health, 3rd edn. Edinburgh: Churchill Livingstone

Crone D, Heaney L, Herbert R, Morgan J, Johnston L, Macpherson R. 2004 A comparison of lifestyle behaviour and health perceptions of people with severe mental illness and the general population. J Mental Health Promotion 3(4): 19–25

Daffern M, Mayer MM, Martin T. 2003 A preliminary investigation into patterns of aggression in an Australian forensic psychiatric hospital. J Forensic Psychiatry Psychol 14(1): 67–84

Daley AJ. 2002 Exercise therapy and mental health in clinical population: is exercise therapy a worthwhile intervention? Adv Psychiatr Treat 8: 262–270

Davenport S. 2002 Acute wards: problems and solutions, a rehabilitation approach to in-patient care. Psychiatr Bull 26: 385–388

DCMS/Strategy Unit. 2002 Game Plan: A Strategy for Develivering Government's Sport and Physical Activity Objectives. London: DCMS/Strategy Unit

Department of Health. 2000 National Service Framework: Mental Health. London: HMSO

Department of Health. 2002a National Minimum Standards for General Adult Services in Psychiatric Intensive Care Units (PICU) and Low Secure Environments. London: HMSO

Department of Health. 2002b Adult Acute In-Patient Care Provision. London: HMSO

Department of Health. 2004a Developing Positive Practice to Support the Safe and Therapeutic Management of Aggression and Violence in Mental Health In-Patient Settings. London: HMSO

Department of Health. 2004b At Least Five a Week: Evidence on the Impact of Physical Activity and it's Relationship to Health. London: HMSO

Department of Health. 2004c Choosing Health: Making Healthier Choices Easier. London: HMSO

Dombrovski A, Rosenstock J. 2004 Bridging general medicine and psychiatry: providing general medical and preventative care for the severely mentally ill. Curr Opin Psychiatry 17(6): 523–524

Drew J, Rugg S. 2001 Acivity use in occupational therapy. Br J Occup Ther 64(10): 478–486

Edwards S. 2002 Physical exercise and psychological wellness. Int J Mental Health Promot 4(2): 40–46

Eklund M, Erlandsson LK, Persson D. 2003 Occupational value among individuals with long-term mental illness. Can J Occup Ther 70(5): 276–284

Faulkner G, Biddle S. 2001 Exercise and mental health: it's not just psychology! J Sports Sci 19: 433–444

Faulkner G, Sparkes A. 1999 Exercise as therapy for schizophrenia: an ethnographic study. J Sport Exerc Psychol 21: 52–69

Faulkner G, Soundy AA, Lloyd K. 2003 Schizophrenia and weight management: a systematic review of interventions to control weight. Acta Psychiatr Scand 108(5): 324–332

Foster M. 2002 Theoretical frameworks. In: Turner A, Foster M, Johnson S (eds) Occupational Therapy and Physical Dysfunction: Principle Skills and Practice, 5th edn. Edinburgh: Churchill Livingstone

Fox KR. 2000 Physical activity and mental health promotion: the natural partnership. Int J Mental Health Promot 2(1): 4–12

Greening J. 2005 Physical health of patients in rehabilitation and recovery: a survey of case note records. Psychiatr Bull 29: 210–212

Hagedorn R. 2001 Foundations for Practice in Occupational Therapy, 3rd edn. Edinburgh: Churchill Livingstone

Hansen RA, Atchison B (eds). 2000 Conditions in Occupational Therapy, Effect on Occupational Performance, 2nd edn. Philadelphia: Lippincott, Williams and Wilkins

Jones M, O'Beney C. 2004 Promoting mental health through physical activity: examples from practice. J Mental Health Promot 3(1): 39–48

Kelly S, McKenna H, Parahoo K, Dusoir A. 2001 The relationship between involvement in activities and quality of life for people with severe and enduring mental illness. J Psychiatr Mental Health Nurs 8: 139–146

Kielhofner G, Butler J (eds). 2002 A Model of Human Occupation: Theory and Application. Philadelphia: Lippincott, Williams and Wilkins

Law M. 2002 Participation in the occupations of everyday life. Am J Occup Ther 56(6): 640–649

Lawlor D, Hopker SW. 2001 The effectiveness of exercise as an intervention in the management of depression: systematic review and meta-regression analysis of randomised controlled trials. Br Med J 322(7289): 763–767

Mee J, Sumsion T. 2001 Mental health clients confirm the motivating power of occupation. Br J Occup Ther 64(3): 121–128

Mee J, Sumsion T, Craik C. 2004 Mental health clients confirm the value of occupation in building competence and self-identity. Br J Occup Ther 67(5): 225–233

National Institute for Clinical Excellence. 2002 Schizophrenia, Core Interventions in the Treatment and Management of Schizophrenia in Primary and Secondary Care. Clinical Guideline 1. London: NICE

Paterson CF. 2002 A short history of occupational therapy in psychiatry. In: Creek J (ed) Occupational Therapy and Mental Health, 3rd edn. Edinburgh: Churchill Livingstone

Phelan M, Stradins L, Morrison S. 2001 Physical health of people with severe mental illness: can be improved if primary care and mental health professionals pay attention to it. Br Med J 322(7284): 443–444

Rebeiro KL, Cook JV. 1999 Opportunity, not prescription: an exploratory study of the experience of occupational engagement. Can J Occup Ther 66(4): 176–187

Reynolds F. 2001 Strategies for facilitating physical activity and wellbeing: a health promotion perspective. Br J Occup Ther 64(7): 330–336

Richardson CR, Faulkner G, McDevitt J, Skrinar GS, Hutchinson DS, Piette JD. 2005 Integrating physical activity into mental health services for persons with serious mental illness. Psychiatr Serv 56: 324–331

Royal College of Psychiatrists College Research Unit. 2001 National Audit of the Management of Violence in Mental Health Settings Final Report: Year 2. London: Royal College of Psychiatrists

Rutter S, Gudjonsson G, Rabe-Hesketh S. 2004 Violent incidents in a medium secure unit: the characteristics of persistent perpetrators of violence. J Forensic Psychiatry Psychol 15(2): 293–302

Scully D, Kremer J, Meade MM, Graham R, Dudgeon K. 1998 Physical exercise and psychological well being: a critical review. Br J Sports Med 32: 111–120

Secker J, Benson A, Balfe E, Lipsedge M, Robinson S, Walker J. 2004 Understanding the social context of violent and aggressive incidents on an in-patient unit. J Psychiatr Mental Health Nurs 11(2): 172–178

Shepherd M, Lavender T. 1999 Putting aggression into context: an investigation into contextual factors influencing the rate of aggressive incidents in a psychiatric hospital. J Mental Health 8(2): 159–170

Tilt R, Perry B, Martin C, Maguire N, Preston M. 2000 Report of the Review of Security at the High Security Hospitals. London: Department of Health

Turner A. 2002 History and philosophy of occupational therapy. In: Turner A, Foster M, Johnson S (eds) Occupational Therapy and Physical Dysfunction: Principle Skills and Practice, 5th edn. Edinburgh: Churchill Livingstone

United Kingdom Central Council for Nursing, Midwifery and Health Visiting. 2002 The Recognition, Prevention and Therapeutic Management of Violence in Mental Health Care. London: UKCC

World Federation for Mental Health. 2004 The Relationship Between Physical and Mental Health: Co-occuring Disorders. Alexandria: World Federation for Mental Health

World Health Organization. 2005 Promoting Mental Health: Concepts, Emerging Evidence, Practice. Geneva: World Health Organization

Yarwood L, Johnstone V. 2002 Acute psychiatry. In: Creek J (ed) Occupational Therapy and Mental Health, 3rd edn. Edinburgh: Churchill Livingstone

12

Risk assessment and management

Stephen M. Pereira, Sabrina Pietromartire and Maurice Lipsedge

The violent patient

Introduction

Many view risk assessment as being firmly within the realm of forensic mental health practitioners. In everyday practice, however, all mental health practitioners knowingly or unknowingly pay attention to those factors that give rise to concern, either in the patient's history or at presentation. Indeed, the Care Programme Approach (Department of Health 1992) requires the assessment of need including risk. The area of risk assessment has been one of increasing interest in the light of numerous Government initiatives such as the supervision register (Department of Health and Home Office 1994), supervised discharge (Secretary of State for Health 1997), Clinical Governance, the National Service Framework for Mental Health (Secretary of State for Health 1997), the Home Office paper 'Managing Dangerous People With Severe Personality Disorder' (Kapur 2000). Proposals for Policy Development (July 1999; Department of Health 1999c) and the proposed Mental Health Bill which has since been abandoned in its current form.

Mention of a formal risk assessment often arouses anxieties in staff carrying out the assessment. 'Risk assessment is surrounded by an aura of mystique, which it does not deserve. The basis for risk management is a thorough clinical assessment, which any multidisciplinary team should be able to undertake' (Maden 2003).

This chapter focuses on those issues relevant to everyday practice encountered by Psychiatric Intensive Care Unit (PICU) multidisciplinary teams. De-institutionalisation has led to a larger number of potentially high-risk patients living in the community, some not in receipt of adequately resourced care. The development of teams such as assertive outreach or intensive case management teams has gone some way towards addressing this problem. Owing to a shortage of inpatient beds, especially in inner cities, largely those who are seriously at risk to others or themselves are usually admitted to these beds. Thus, there has been increased preoccupation with risk identification of patients. It is important to get this right as often as possible, not least because at least half of reported incidents of assault are thought by victims to be avoidable (Aiken 1984).

Various inquiries into homicides and serious incidents comment on the inability of services to manage seriously disturbed individuals with difficult behaviour and the lack of appropriate facilities for this group, e.g. the Clunis Inquiry (1994). Various other shortcomings have been identified: poor or absent consultant supervision; poor communication of important information within the team and other relevant people (including relatives); lack of opportunities for training in risk assessment and inadequate resources of space and of trained staff

Psychiatric Intensive Care, 2nd edn., eds. M. Dominic Beer, Stephen M. Pereira and Carol Paton.
Published by Cambridge University Press. © Cambridge University Press 2008

(Birley 1996). It is impossible to conclude whether there is a real or apparent increase in violence. Increased awareness, fear of litigation and better methods of recording and reporting may account for higher figures in recent times. However, a review by Taylor and Gunn (1999) concluded that, over a 38-year period, there was little fluctuation in the numbers of people with a mental illness committing criminal homicide. In the UK, the Confidential Inquiry into Suicide and Homicide (Appleby et al. 1999, 2001) found that about two thirds of perpetrators of homicide had a diagnosis of mental disorder based on life history but most do not have severe mental illness or a history of contact with mental health services (Shaw et al. 1999). Shaw et al.'s data correspond to around forty homicides per year by people who have been in contact with mental health services in the previous 12 months. Shaw et al.'s study was based on a total of 718 homicides reported to the inquiry. Discussion of risk assessment invariably involves risk to self, although risk to others is a larger public preoccupation.

Whilst it is clear that violent people are more likely to demonstrate symptoms of mental disorder and that those who are mentally disordered are more likely to be violent, it is important to put these findings into perspective. Swanson's Epidemiologic Catchment Area study shows that 4%–5% of violent acts are committed by persons with major mental illness. A literature review carried about by Walsh et al. (2002) indicated similarly that less than 10% of societal violence is attributable to schizophrenia and that comorbid substance misuse significantly increases the risk. The Confidential Inquiry (Appleby et al. 1999) found that of 500 homicides for whom psychiatric reports were available (out of a total of 718 reported homicides, 1996–1997), 102 were in contact with mental health services at some time; however, only 71 had a mental disorder. The commonest diagnosis was personality disorder (20 cases) Alcohol and drug misuse was common. Moran et al. (2003) concluded that comorbid personality disorder is independently associated with an increased risk of violent behaviour in psychosis and suggested that personality assessment should be part of the early routine assessment of all psychiatric patients.

Maden (1996) in his excellent review advocates the importance of distinguishing between the assessment of dangerousness and that of risk. Violence researchers (e.g. Steadman et al. 1993) also urge mental health professionals to be concerned with risk, rather than dangerousness for the following reasons. Firstly, risk can be objectively assessed; secondly, the context in which the risk behaviour occurs can be considered; thirdly, risk can be subdivided into further manageable components; and finally risk is not static, and therefore lends itself to be managed over time.

The PICU clinician is often asked to make an assessment of risk at various stages:

- At the community interface, e.g. police stations, Accidents and Emergency departments, Section 136 rooms (prisons, courts)
- At the inpatient interface, e.g. acute and other inpatient facilities
- Within the PICU, e.g. at admission, ongoing assessments, considering leave arrangements
- At the point of discharge from the PICU

The ability to carry out a comprehensive risk assessment is often compromised by the urgency of the request for admission to the PICU and the acuteness of the patient's behavioural disturbance. Some other factors that can influence a thorough risk assessment and the subsequent decision to admit or not are:

- Training and experience of the assessor
- Availability of clinical information
- Knowledge of local service, e.g. training, experience of staff managing the situation
- Availability of local resources

Table 12.1 is not meant to represent an exhaustive list of risk factors associated with violence, but such factors are important to consider when assessing patients at the community interface.

The relationships between the factors and violence tend to be complex. For example, with respect to gender, men are more violent than women in the general population, but this may not be the case among psychiatric inpatients. Krakowsi et al. (2004) found that during the period studied, similar percentages of female and male inpatients carried out physical assaults, with women tending to have

Table 12.1. Risk factors associated with violence

Demographic or personal history
- Youth, male gender
- A history of violent behaviour
- Association with a subculture prone to violence
- Previous use of weapons
- Previous dangerous impulsive acts
- Denial of previous established dangerous acts
- Evidence of rootlessness or 'social restlessness'
- Known personal trigger factors present
- Evidence of recent stress, especially loss or threat of loss
- Stated threat of violence
- Carers report concerns
- One or more of the above together with:
  - cruelty to animals
  - reckless driving
  - history of bedwetting
  - loss of a parent before age 8

Clinical variables
- Alcohol or other substance misuse, irrespective of diagnosis
- Diagnosis: Table 12.2 lists some mental disorders which may be associated with violence
- Active symptoms of schizophrenia or mania, in particular if:
  - delusions or hallucinations are focused on a particular person
  - there is specific preoccupation with violence
  - there are delusions of control particularly with a violent theme
  - there is agitation, excitement, overt hostility or suspiciousness
  - command hallucinations
- Poor collaboration with suggested treatments
- Antisocial, explosive or impulsive personality traits
- Organic dysfunction
- Drug effects (disinhibition, akathisia)

Situational factors
- Extent of social support
- Immediate availability of a weapon
- Access to potential victim
- Limit setting (for example, staff members setting parameters for activities, choices, etc.)
- Staff attitudes

Modified from NICE (2005).

higher rates of 'early assaults' (within the first 10 days of admission). Their findings also suggested that positive psychotic symptoms were more likely to result in assaults in women than in men. Physical assaults in the community were however more common in men and were associated with substance abuse, property crime and a history of school truancy.

Swanson *et al.* (1990), in a massive survey of the general population called the Epidemiologic Catchment Area study in the USA, found that delusional symptoms, independent of diagnosis, appear to have a significant association with violence. Patients with a combination of delusions and alcohol abuse had a high risk of violence. Other community surveys (e.g. Link and Stueve 1994) showed similar findings. The delusions that were particularly relevant included delusions of influence and control, e.g. that one's mind was dominated by forces beyond one's control, thoughts were being inserted into one's mind and there were people who wished to do one harm. Studies vary in their findings regarding the association between violence and command-type auditory hallucinations. If the individual can identify and access a specific person or entity as a 'target', then risk is clearly increased. As regards reported violent thoughts, data from the MacArthur Risk Assessment Study (Monahan *et al.* 2001) revealed that violent inpatients reported violent thoughts toward others twice as commonly as did controls.

The relevance of 'symptom-consistent' violence is in determining not only the risk of future violent behaviour but also the contexts in which this is most likely to occur and it may help identify those at increased risk of becoming targets of this violence.

Violent behaviour in patients with schizophrenia is a poorly defined and broad concept. It may be useful to use subcategories such as suggested by Krakowski *et al.* (2004). They found that violent patients could be allocated to two main groups: 'transiently violent patients' in whom violent behaviour only occurred during a well-defined period of acute decompensation, and 'persistently violent patients' in whom there was no limitation of violent behaviour to a short time period.

Table 12.2. *DSM-IV TR* categories which include violence and aggression

1. Alcohol-related disorders	9. Intermittent explosive disorder
2. Amphetamine intoxication	10. Mental retardation
3. Inhalant intoxication	11. Conduct disorder
4. Phencyclidine intoxication	12. Oppositional defiant disorder
5. Antisocial personality disorder	13. Post-traumatic stress disorder
6. Borderline personality disorder	14. Personality change due to a general medical condition, aggressive type
7. Dementia	15. Sexual sadism
8. Delirium	16. Schizophrenia, paranoid type

Some questions to assist a risk assessment framework

General factors

Has all the required relevant information been gathered?

Do other professionals or agencies need to be involved?

Harm factors

Harm that has occurred, or that is being threatened

Description and frequency of the threat or act or thought or fantasy (is this provoked or spontaneous)? What risk is being considered, e.g. harm to self or others? How serious is the potential harm?

How serious was the act/s (or if committed did the patient express remorse)?

Why is the harm being considered or, if committed, what is the reason for the act?

What is the *intent?*

Who or what is at risk?

Is there a concrete plan, e.g. when, where?

Does the patient have access to instruments of harm?

What is the likelihood of harm occurring?

Diagnostic factors

Does the patient suffer from a mental illness?

How active are the features of the patient's illness?

Does the patient have an associated substance abuse? Why does the patient use the substance? What are its effects on the patient?

Does the person suffer from a personality disorder, e.g. antisocial, borderline, sadistic?

Does the patient suffer from developmental or acquired brain damage or disorder?

Predispositional/historical factors

Does the patient have a previous history of violence?

Are there any relevant childhood or familial factors?

Does the patient suffer from chronic anger, hostility, resentment, low tolerance for frustration, have difficulty in delaying gratification, a sadistic orientation?

Does the patient have a history of loss of control?

Is the patient impulsive?

Has the patient exhibited remorse for his/her past acts?

Has further information been sought from the police?

Contextual factors

Where and how do they usually spend their time?

What factors are likely to increase or decrease risk?

Does the patient have stress factors, e.g. loss, frustration, provocation?

What are the patient's usual coping strategies?

Does the patient feel well supported by family and/or professional carers?

In what context did past violent occur?

In an inpatient ward:

- is the ward overcrowded?
- does it lack clear leadership, training, experience and morale?

Is the patient frank and cooperative or guarded, irritable, defensive?

Is the patient overaroused, agitated and excited?

Is the patient compliant with prescribed treatments?

- is the patient on the appropriate medication, taking an appropriate dose?
- is the patient engaging with nursing, occupational therapy, psychological interventions?

How disruptive/dangerous is the patient's current behaviour?

Prediction of risk of violence is very difficult. A reasonable degree of success can be achieved in short-term prediction, i.e. the near future, but not so for longer-term violence prediction. Published research so far does not provide any clear consensus on criteria that would be clinically useful across the different varieties of clinical settings. In addition these difficulties arise due to variations in the period covered, choice of predictor items, patient sampling, level of detail provided in the studies, methods of analysis and the way in which available actuarial scales are used. An up to date understanding of approaches to violence risk prediction is however important. It has become increasingly vital to develop as accurate a means as possible of assessing risk. This is important not only for the protection of others but also for the protection of individuals who would otherwise be inaccurately assessed as posing a risk to others.

Approaches to violence risk assessment

Unaided clinical risk assessment

In day to day practice, clinicians have tended to use case formulation approaches to risk assessment. Clinical case formulations can provide very useful information specific to the individual such as the context in which violent behaviour tends to occur. Formulations are subjective and different clinicians may of course come up with very different formulations. There is however some evidence to suggest that clinical assessments may be more accurately predictive of violence than expected. Fuller and Cowan (1999) found that multidisciplinary team risk predictions were comparable with actuarial risk predictions.

Actuarial risk assessment tools

Some tools are useful screening tools, helping clinicians to ensure that all important factors are explored. Other tools explore specific areas which may have been highlighted as potential risk factors for violence in the relevant individual during generic risk assessment or clinical assessment (e.g. impulsivity). Actuarial tools are fraught with methodological difficulties, including; conceptual difficulties, e.g. definition of violence; they measure different target behaviours, e.g. internally/externally directed violence; they lack flexibility; they are not truly generalisable; and there is a need for access to detailed accurate information. Most such tools do not take into account individual circumstances (including rare risk factors or protective factors) and do not clarify the motivation for past behaviour. Despite these deficits, actuarial risk assessment tools are increasingly in use in clinical settings.

Tools include: The Violence Risk Appraisal Guide (VRAG); Quinsey et al. 1998. The PCL-R, Dangerous Behaviour Rating Scale, Novaco Anger Scale, Barratt's Impulsivity Scale, Maudsley Assessment of Delusions Schedule, Staff Observation Aggression Scale, Overt Aggression Scale, Global Aggression Scale, Hostility and Direction of Hostility Questionnaire and Buss-Durkee Hostility Inventory, Minnesota Multiphasic Personality Inventory, Monroe Episodic Dyscontrol Scale, State-Trait Anger Expression Scale, and Brown-Goodwin Inventory. For a review of some of these measures, see Mak and Koning (1995), Monahan and Steadman (1994) and Dolan and Doyle (2000).

The iterative classification tree

This tool was developed in the MacArthur Violence Assessment Study. The iterative classification tree (ICT) may be more accurate than many other current approaches used to assess risk among inpatients in acute psychiatric facilities but use of the ICT method and its scoring is complex, necessitating the use of computer software (Monahan *et al.* 2005).

Structured clinical guides

The Historical/Clinical/Risk Management 20-item scale (HCR-20) (Webster *et al.* 1997) can be described as a structured clinical guide. There is a manual that helpfully explains how and when to use this tool. It is a twenty-item tool including ten (past) historical, five (current) clinical and five (future) risk management variables and the PCL-R is incorporated into it. It has been validated in North American samples and has been shown to have good inter-rater reliability. Dr Kevin Douglas and associates (2006) provide continually updated information relating to the HCR-20, which is accessible on the World Wide Web (www.violence-risk.com/hcr20annotated.pdf).

Limited funds and resources may limit the use of the above tools in acute psychiatric settings. The cost:benefit ratio is different in forensic services, where a battery of standardised assessments should be routine (Maden 2003).

Various systems have been set up in an attempt to help professionals and organisations assess and manage risk. Risk Assessment Management and Audit Systems known as RAMAS (O'Rourke *et al.* 2001) was developed with Department of Health funding with the aim of providing better protection for the public whilst improving care planning, and the treatment and management of people posing a risk to themselves or others. The Clinical Assessment of Risk Decision Support (CARDS) system (2002), developed at the Institute of Psychiatry London, is a clinical decision support system to aid clinicians in their assessment and management of the risk of violence and suicide in adults of working age using mental health services (Watts *et al.* 2002).

The growing list of tools and systems can contribute to feelings of anxiety and confusion in mental health professionals tasked with assessing risk. Professionals have to be guided by their trust's and unit's policies and protocols with respect to risk assessment and management, but may find the above resources useful in broadening their knowledge base and skills. There is no gold standard risk assessment tool.

NB. Obtaining collateral information, a detailed history, carrying out a detailed mental state examination and reviewing past case notes are important for a good risk assessment. A formulation providing an understanding of the individual's difficulties and potential risks posed, as well as the protective factors and skills the patient has should be compiled using the information gleaned from the assessment, theory and research.

Events that indicate imminent violence in psychiatric settings

The rate of violence towards mental health workers is much higher than in any other occupation. Psychiatric nurses are particularly at risk. A review by Whittington (1994) indicated that 90% of assaults by psychiatric patients are directed at nurses. This figure is not surprising given their role as direct, round-the-clock caregivers and is a significant occupational risk. Rates of violence against psychiatrists range from 32% to 42%. Jones (1985) found that of assaults in psychiatric facilities, 65% were against staff and 32% were directed at other patients or property.

Various attempts have been made to examine the accuracy of patient behaviour as a predictor of imminent violence. Powell *et al.* (1994) examined antecedents for a thousand incidents in three psychiatric hospitals over a 13-month period. They allocated incidents to fifteen categories of antecedents. The most common antecedents were:
- Patient agitation or disturbance
- Restrictions being placed on patients associated with the routine hospital regime
- Provocation by other patients, relatives, visitors

Interestingly, they found that incidents arising from staff members' initiating contact with patients were very rare. The study also confirmed the experience of most PICU clinicians that small numbers of largely detained patients were involved in a high number of incidents. These patients were more likely to commit assaults after certain incidents, e.g. self-harm, absconding and arson. Whittington and Patterson (1996) studied verbal and non-verbal behaviour immediately prior to assault. These included: verbal abuse, high overall activity and standing uncomfortably close. However, many of these behaviours were also exhibited by patients who did not assault staff members. There is, on the other hand, general agreement amongst researchers that only a small number of assaults occur in the absence of any behavioural predictors (3% of the sample in the Whittington Study). The clinical practice guidelines (CPG) also identified possible antecedents of violence. Some other researchers (e.g. Aiken 1984; Lanza 1988) believe that the highest predictor for assault is what has been variously described as the 'pre-assaultative tension state' or the 'acute excitement phase'. These cues may seem obvious, but go unheeded on many occasions. Taken together with the experience of many clinicians, it may be suggested that the above factors in younger male patients who are more acutely ill, e.g. floridly psychotic and under-medicated, may lead them to present with higher rates of violence.

Some factors leading to violence in PICU

Sheridan et al. (1990) identified some of these factors in inpatient settings that apply equally to PICUs. These include:

- Patient–staff conflict (e.g. limit setting, denial of privileges)
- Conflict with other patients
- Patient's personal problems (e.g. money, family, social problems)
- Events internal to patients (e.g. delusions, hallucinations, confusion)

McNeil and Binder (1994), in their study of 330 patients admitted to a locked short stay unit, explored the relationship between acute psychiatric symptoms, diagnosis and short-term risk of violence. The proportions of violence by diagnosis were: schizophrenia 36%, mania 28%, organic psychosis 27%, the rest 12%. A complex analysis of BPRS (Brief Psychiatric Rating Score) and the OAS (Overt Aggression Scale) showed three summary scores significantly associated with violence. These were hostile-suspiciousness, agitation-excitement and thinking disturbance. Palmstierna and Wistedt (1990) found that risk factors for aggressive behaviour are of limited value in predicting the violent behaviour of acute involuntarily admitted patients. The only predictor of some value in the immediate future (first 8 days) was previous damage to property or person; and, in the near future (first 28 days), use of drugs other than alcohol.

Derived from available literature and clinical experience, some of the features are summarised below.

Cues suggestive of imminent violence

Physical cues

These are largely features of motor overactivity and include:

- Agitation, arousal, restlessness, pacing
- Physical tension, rigid posture, erratic movements
- Threatening gestures or stance
- Glaring, breathlessness, aggressive to objects (e.g. thumping tables, walls) or self (e.g. banging head)

Mood cues

- 'Irritable', 'upset', angry, 'high' or elated, lability of mood

Speech cues

- Verbal threats, abuse, swearing
- Complaining, demanding or refusal to communicate
- Loud and pressured speech

Thought and perceptual cues

- Inability to concentrate or register information
- Unclear or disordered thought processes

- Bizarre, paranoid, persecutory, violent thoughts and delusions
- Active hallucinations, usually auditory, sometimes visual
- Preoccupation with violent themes in thinking
- Confusion, disorientation

Boundary cues
- Perception by patient that his/her own space/boundaries or privacy is being violated
- Persistent intrusion by patient of others' personal space, e.g. standing very close
- Insistence that demands be met immediately, however unrealistic

Contextual and past cues
- Early warning signs elicited from previous episodes of violence
- Current reports from carers, other patients or self of angry feelings, unmet demands
- Current use of illicit substances or alcohol
- Poor frustration tolerance and other coping strategies

Therapeutic cues
- Breakdown in rapport
- Uncooperativeness, lack of encouragement
- Usually worsening mental state
- Failure to respond to reassurance, de-escalation, time out or other previously successful, agreed strategies.

Risk management

There is acknowledgement from various inquiry panels that, even in the best run service, the possibility remains that something may go wrong. The UK National Confidential Inquiry into Homicides (Shaw *et al.* 1999) recognised that mentally ill patients committed only a small proportion of homicides annually and that these patients were only a small fraction of the total number of psychiatric patients. It also called for recognition of the limitations to what

treatment of mental illness alone could achieve in preventing homicides.

The key issue, however, remains that, whilst one may not be able to eliminate the risk of a serious untoward incident, various systems can be put into place to reduce the risk of these occurring. 'Inquiries into homicides by psychiatric patients suggest that, when things do go wrong, it is usually because of basic failures in procedure. If services are based on good clinical practice, most risk can be safely managed' (Maden 1996). Some of the systems referred to above are further discussed in Chapter 2, Management of Acutely Disturbed Behaviour, and Chapter 23, Managing the Psychiatric Intensive Care Unit.

Reith (1998) identified four major themes that were consistently lacking in care provided to violent patients:

1. Thoroughness (detailed and accurate recording of information)
2. Communication and liaison (proper inter-agency cooperation and real team working)
3. Listening to all members of the clinical team (recognising and valuing the contribution of all staff, especially junior members, who are in contact with the patient)
4. Listening to those closest to the patient (careful attention being paid to the experience and understanding of relatives and carers)

Some of these issues have also been highlighted by the Department of Health UK (1995), in Building Bridges, 'The key principle of risk assessment is to use all available sources of information . . .', and in the Blom-Cooper Inquiry (1995), 'Professionals need to be trained to trust the experienced judgement of close family rather than rely on their own impressions made at one isolated assessment', to name but two.

The National Confidential Inquiry in its full report, Safer Services (Appelby 2000), make thirty-two recommendations for changes in clinical practice. These include: training in risk assessment, documentation, use of specific drug and psychological treatments and changes in the Mental Health Act to allow compulsory treatment, e.g. in the community.

In the PICU setting, risk management should be considered in multiple domains, as now described.

The patient domain

With a view towards adequately managing risk on the PICU, as much information as possible should be obtained via referral forms, and full discussion with the referring service prior to admission. Urgent clinical need takes priority over this requirement but this should very much be the exception rather than the rule.

Standardised assessment forms, incorporating a clinical risk assessment framework and some objective measures, help contribute towards obtaining a fuller picture. This also reduces the risk of idiosyncratic PICU assessments based on personality, judgmental attitudes and level of training on the part of the assessor. Response times to requests for admission to the PICU should be derived by local discussion with contracted referrers. This gives a clear idea as to the type of risk being managed and over a defined period of time. Clinical experience shows that disturbance is moderated over a period of time by initiated treatment strategies including appropriate nursing interventions, adequate medication regimens and appropriate placements. This is especially true for disturbance due to mental illness, but not necessarily so for those with personality disorders, co-morbid substance misuse, acquired or developmental brain disorders and treatment-resistant conditions.

Those patients considered unsuitable for admission to the PICU should be discussed further in detail with the referring teams. This would serve the purpose of providing a second multidisciplinary team's opinion and advice regarding management of the patient. These opinions should be accepted in the spirit in which they are given rather than, 'we don't require them to tell us what to do', or viewed as being undermining of the care plan in place. Feedback should be provided to referrers as soon as possible for those who are accepted or not by the PICU. Clinical situations can change rapidly. All PICU assessments should be flexible to acknowledge this.

Once admitted to the PICU, multidisciplinary protocols derived from the most up-to-date guidance from peer bodies, research, audit and code of practice should govern all clinical practice. Some of the areas thus regulated are outlined below. Risk assessment should occur as often as is required in the PICU, clearly documented, with at least one or two full multidisciplinary team risk reviews involving referrers and all involved carers.

The discharge from the PICU should contain clear guidance regarding identified risk factors, the context in which risk behaviours occur, and suggested multidisciplinary strategies to manage them. It is essential that referrers at the very least attend pre-discharge reviews of their patients. This ensures a smooth transition of care back to the catchment area wards. Unless PICUs are adequately resourced with community or assertive outreach services, discharge should always occur back to the catchment area wards to enable full planning and delivery of previously identified care needs by the referring catchment area teams. Whenever patients are transferred to or from a PICU, the PICU should adhere to a clear transfer protocol. Handwritten communication of risk according to a predetermined risk protocol and format can be helpful on a more immediate basis at the time of transfer.

Every service should identify the small group of mentally ill patients who are most at risk, especially to others, when relapsing in the community. Doing so enables the service to fast track admissions to the appropriate secure facility or environment. However, good practice would suggest this should be to the acute open inpatient ward in the first instance, with appropriate safeguards, e.g. predetermined medication and nursing strategies, to prevent labelling and thus stigmatisation of this group of patients as always being violent. In a significant number of cases, even such patients usually settle down on admission to the open ward.

The staff domain

The PICU can be particularly effective in safely modifying the outcome of violent, destructive acts, once they have started. However, the real expertise of PICU clinicians should be in the area of early identification of violent, aggressive thoughts, feelings and behaviour, thereby preventing their occurrence at best, or reducing their frequency at the very least.

All staff in the PICU should be trained to recognise the early warning signs predisposing to violence. This entails drawing up individual risk assessment profiles. In order to do this, crucial information should be gleaned from past notes, discussion with referrers, other professional carers and relatives. This should be as detailed and as accurate as possible. Particular attention is paid to psychopathology, personality factors, coping strategies, past violence (see 'A framework for risk management' below). This should be incorporated in multidisciplinary team care plans.

The ability to identify risk factors in itself is insufficient to manage violence within the PICU. Staff should be able to respond to the many crises that develop in an effective and professional manner. For example, there is evidence to show that training in the methods of control and restraint (C&R) can lead to a reduction in violent behaviour and injury to both staff and patients. Reasons suggested include greater confidence engendered in staff by such training, enabling them to defuse situations before they escalate (Anonymous 1976; Lion 1977). Before employing C&R, other strategies such as time out, talking down and de-escalation techniques (see Chapter 3) should be considered. This presumes that staff teams possess skills in verbal and behavioural interventions and are able to react to patients in a non-provocative manner (Tardiff and Sweillam 1982).

Thus a balance is required between professionalism, confident management and the rigid judgmental authoritarian attitudes that may develop. This in itself may predispose to further violence. Overcontrolling, authoritarian staff rarely socialise with patients and have little person to person contact with them, unless the interaction involves limit setting or confrontation (Sanson-Fisher *et al.* 1979; Hodges *et al.* 1986). 'Fear, counter-transference difficulties, denial, and unrecognized provocative behaviour by the therapist or staff may interfere with good clini-

cal judgment. The therapist and staff may distance themselves from the patient, ignore threats, or overreact and overcontrol' (Berg *et al.* 2000). Being able to identify issues relevant to counter-transference, e.g. a professional's negative feelings towards a patient, especially with chronically disturbed and personality-disordered or dual-diagnosis patients can play an important role in provocation and therefore prevention of patient violence.

Ensuring an appropriate mix of skills and staff gender has a role in risk management. Reports from both psychiatric and forensic hospitals show that employing female staff on male wards (Levy and Hartocollis 1976) or male staff in a female-only PICU at Rampton High Security Hospital (Carton and Larkin 1991) led to a reduction in violent incidents.

Clear evidence-based protocols are required in the use of rapid tranquillisation and emergency medication (see Chapter 4) as part of an effective risk management plan. Distinctions need to be drawn between short-term and long-term usage of medication in risk management, e.g. administration of benzodiazepines as required in schizophrenic patients is significantly high. It is possible that staff resort to medication too easily and increasing non-medication techniques may reduce the need for such prescriptions (Paton *et al.* 2000).

The multidisciplinary domain

Psychological therapies are effective in reducing levels of violence. For example, cognitive behavioural therapy is effective for anger problems (Beck and Fernandez 1998). Some patients respond to a primarily behavioural programme. Talking and listening must be regarded as active interventions, as they are greatly valued by patients (Royal College of Psychiatrists 1998). All PICUs should have dedicated input from a psychologist, not only to help develop effective interventions for patients, but also to provide regular support and supervision to staff working in this high-risk subspecialty. The role of an occupational therapist in the PICU is discussed elsewhere in the book (see Chapter 11). The role of the pharmacist in advising medication strategies and planning medication reviews is a very important one. Dedicated input from social workers or support workers is crucial in helping to understand family dynamics, social stresses and supports and in providing practical help. This goes a long way to allaying short-term anxiety and irritability, reduces provocation and helps long-term planning of care at an early stage. The important contributions made by other professional carers and relatives in risk assessment and management cannot be overemphasised. Their involvement is mandatory in planning care.

The environmental domain

Several factors affect how the therapeutic milieu can influence effective management of risk. These include the design, quality, comfort of accommodation, as well as staff support and patient participation in decision making, e.g. community meetings and patient autonomy. It may be suggested that the milieu is one of the most important factors influencing the outcome of treatment. Psychotic patients (e.g. in PICUs) seem to benefit primarily from a milieu with a high level of support, practical orientation, order and organisation (Frilis 1986). This may help to maintain a low level of anger and aggression.

Drinkwater and Gudjonsson (1989) found that for the majority of patients observed on the ward, 89% of their day consisted of no planned activities. She reported that the frequency of violent incidents was, on average, four times higher during periods without planned activities, in addition to other prohibited behaviours, e.g. being verbally abusive, breaking ward rules. It has been suggested that wards with low levels of planned activities and staff–patient interaction appear to foster violence.

Although seclusion rooms are used as part of a risk management plan, a significant number of PICUs do not have these. No strong evidence-based conclusions can be derived from the literature advocating or diminishing the usefulness of this practice. If employed, staff should have rigorous training to prevent the situation from escalating to a level requiring seclusion and in the monitoring standards expected once a patient is in seclusion. NICE recommend that there should be a designated area or room used only

for reducing arousal and agitation. If the unit has a seclusion room, this area should be in addition to that.

The organisational domain

The main features are summarised in the risk management framework below. This includes clear management support of clinical staff in ensuring a safe and clinically effective environment for patients. Firm backing from managers leads to a high morale amongst staff. Organisational responsibilities include training, specification of responsibilities, appraisal of performance and job stability (Royal College of Psychiatrists 1998).

Thomas and Bell (1998) suggested there is a chance of reducing the levels of violence and preventing its occurrence by working together with those who use mental health services and by addressing current inadequacies in the system.

Developing policies, e.g. prosecution of violent patients, should be carefully considered by organisations. With the growing number of violent patients being admitted to hospital, a principled, uniform, rational deterrent response needs to be in place to protect other patients and staff. Most carers find this very difficult to do for ethical, legal and professional considerations.

Drinkwater and Gudjonsson (1989) suggest the following advantages in reporting serious assaults on staff:

- It highlights the seriousness of the offence to the patient
- It ensures that the offence is properly recorded and investigated by an independent authority
- It is the court who decides the appropriate outcome for criminal offences, not the clinical team
- It enables staff to apply for compensation for personal injuries, e.g. to the Criminal Injuries Compensation Board
- It helps maintain staff morale, which tends to be poor in settings where physical assaults are common

There are some arguments against having such a policy. Some would consider such policies as being radical, open to abuse, affecting patient

Table 12.3. Important PICU multidisciplinary team skills to assist risk management

1. Initiate, communicate, develop rapport and a caring professional relationship with patients
2. Listen effectively, communicate clearly
3. Learn to identify verbal and non-verbal cues
4. Write concise, easily understood, legible case notes
5. Validate perceptions
6. Create a therapeutic milieu by individual and collective participation in programmes
7. Develop easily available and clearly understood risk management plans
8. Watch for signs of negative attitudes to patients, environmental stresses and examine own coping strategies
9. Pay attention to personal and professional development
10. Ask for help in managing difficult situations

confidentiality and that violent attacks are an occupational hazard that staff members should learn to accept. Although some contend that prosecuting a patient is never justified, this position is unwarranted (Appelbaum and Appelbaum 1991). Having such a policy regarding persecution of patients prevents inconsistent, idiosyncratic decision making and sends a clear message to habitually violent patients.

It is important that PICU teams develop a culture of change and learning (Table 12.3). Mason and Chandley (1999) suggest that units which have such cultures not only quickly develop strategies that keep them abreast of recent advances in their field but also, 'become places in which it is pleasurable to work and morale is high. They *offer* job opportunities and experience and there is a feeling of worth in the establishment'.

A framework for risk management

Harm factors

- Well rehearsed, clearly understood
- Management of acute disturbance protocols, displayed/easily available

- Experienced, trained staff delivering well rehearsed interventions, e.g. de-escalation
- Regular reviews by keyworker and the multidisciplinary team of the risk assessment and management plan
- Clear action plan, communicated to all appropriate individuals, within and outside teams, organisations
- Critical incident analysis after all events

Diagnostic factors

- Review of diagnosis and associated conditions
- Comprehensive and thorough case notes review of past history, adverse incidents and response to interventions
- Highlighted risk factors, early warning signs of relapse with patients
- Easy accessibility of such information involving high-risk individuals especially when seen in emergency settings, e.g. community Accident and Emergency

Predispositional/historical factors

- Past history of violence (descriptions of act/s, intent, remorse, weapons used if any, severity of injury, outcome), expression of remorse
- Childhood factors (brutality or deprivation, decreased warmth affection in the home, early loss of parent, fire setting, bed wetting, cruelty to animals)
- Psychological profiles of high-risk individuals, e.g. anger, self view as a victim, resentful of authority, recklessness, impulsivity

Contextual factors

Particular attention is paid to:
- Ward design and safety issues (e.g. lines of observation), suitability of placement and secure areas on wards
- Alarm systems and rehearsed contingency plans
- A well-structured therapeutic milieu

- Ongoing risk assessment of ward environment (physical environment and other patients)
- Careful assessment of immediate and longer-term social supports
- Accessibility to named and experienced link workers to fast-track known violent patients to appropriate care
- Accessibility to longer-term risk minimisation strategies, e.g. short- and long-term psychotherapies

Organisational and management factors

- Well-developed policies, procedures, protocols covering all areas of clinical practice *including and reinforcing the NHS zero violence tolerance policy*
- Well-defined, regularly updated management policies and leadership in areas of risk strategy
- Collaboration with service users in planning clinical environments, policies, monitoring practices
- Regular availability and monitoring of staff training, e.g. risk assessment and management, morale, multidisciplinary working
- Policies sensitive to patient care in relation to overcrowding, individuality and choice, privacy, gender and ethnic mix, ward layout and safe activity areas
- Central recording and regular clinical audit, e.g. seclusion, control and restraint, adverse incidents
- Well-developed liaison with local services, e.g. police, forensic services
- *Robust procedures for supporting staff members who have been a victim of violence*

Potential victim factors

- If there are specific groups of people or specific individuals at risk, appropriate steps should be taken to communicate and reduce risk
- In the community, the family, friends and acquaintances of individuals suffering from psychotic illness are most at risk. The assessment of relationships and dynamics and involvement and support of these 'at risk' individuals may be useful, in particular in cases where symptom resolution

in response to treatment is incomplete (Johnston *et al.* 2003)

The suicidal patient

Introduction

Suicide has been the focus of some interest in recent times with the Department of Health's Saving Lives: Our Healthier Nation setting the target of reducing the death rate from suicide by at least one-fifth by 2010. In support of this objective, guidelines and strategies such as the National Service Framework: Mental Health (Department of Health 1999b), the National Suicide Prevention Strategy for England (Department of Health 2002c) and NICE guidelines for the short-term physical and psychological management and secondary prevention of self-harm in primary and secondary care (NICE 2004) were developed.

The following are some key findings regarding inpatient suicides from the National Confidential Inquiry into Suicide and Homicide by People with Mental illness (Appleby *et al.* 1996, 2001):

- Inpatients accounted for 16% of suicide inquiry cases in England and Wales; 9% of inpatient suicides occured on locked wards
- Of all inpatient suicides, 31% took place on the ward. The majority of the rest occurred during authorised leave, with only a minority occurring following absconding from the ward
- Inpatient suicides, particularly those occurring on the ward, were most likely to be by hanging, most commonly from a curtain rail and using a belt as a ligature
- Around one-quarter of inpatient suicides occurred during the first week of the admission
- Around one-fifth of inpatient suicides were under non-routine observation (constant or intermittent)
- Mental health teams more often regarded inpatient suicides as preventable

Although staff tend to view inpatient suicides as preventable, accurately identifying those at high risk is difficult. Powell *et al.* (2000) attempted to identify risks specific to inpatients and to evaluate their predictive power. They found five factors significantly associated with suicide: planned suicide attempt, actual suicide attempt, recent bereavement, presence of delusions, chronic mental illness and family history of suicide. Once this was known, the cases were reviewed to see how accurately the suicides could be predicted. Only two of the patients who committed suicide had a predicted risk of suicide above 5%. So although several factors were identified that were strongly associated with suicide, their clinical utility is limited by low sensitivity and specificity.

A rolling in-house training programme on suicide awareness and prevention will reduce the frequency of false-negative predictions. It is salutary to recall that many of the suicides reported to the Confidential Inquiry (Appleby *et al.* 1999) were totally unexpected by medical and nursing staff.

Violent and self-destructive behaviour can, of course, co-exist and, as with predictions of violence, forecasts of deliberate self-harm can be safely made only for fairly short periods. By the same token, risk must be reviewed in the light of changes and symptoms and alterations in the personal, domestic, social and legal circumstances of the patient. As with predictions of violence, a realistic short time frame and ongoing reviews are essential.

Completed suicide is a relatively rare event and many patients on the PICU will have identifiable risk factors such as co-morbidity, personality disorders or a past history of deliberate self-harm. The high rate of false-positive predictions might demotivate staff by creating a sense of complacency or of frustration at ostensibly unnecessary restrictions on patients and the imposition of a regime of intrusive surveillance. It is hoped that specific guidelines will reduce the risk of a counter productively excessive caution on the one hand and a casual recklessness on the other. Reduction of the risk of suicide in the PICU requires vigilant awareness of the various factors that might increase the frequency of deliberate self-harm. Recognised risk factors include:
- Declared intent
- A previous history of deliberate self-harm
- Clinical risk factors
- 'Malignant alienation'
- Demographic and social factors
- Physical features of the unit

Declared suicidal intentions

A threat to harm oneself should never be disregarded. Even the most transparently 'manipulative' threat has to be assessed in the context of the patient's current mental state, preoccupations, frustrations and personal and social circumstances. Conversely, the absence of any declared suicidal intention does not mean that the risk is negligible.

For example, patients with persecutory delusions and threatening auditory hallucinations sometimes kill themselves as a way of escaping from imaginary torturers and executioners, even in the absence of a frank depressive illness.

Previous history of deliberate self-harm

It is dangerous to assume that there is little risk just because a particular patient has survived numerous previous episodes of deliberate self-harm (DSH). Indeed, 1% of patients who harm themselves will go on to commit suicide within a year, while the risk of subsequent suicide during the 10 years after an episode of deliberate self-harm is 30 times higher than in the general population.

Clinical risk factors

A 30-year cohort comparison of suicide attempters carried out by Henriques *et al.* (2002) found that present-day suicide attempters exhibited greater levels of psychopathology on every major variable assessed compared with a sample evaluated between 1970 and 1973. This could be an indication of challenges facing mental health services.

The National Confidential Inquiry into suicide and homicide by people with mental illness found the most common diagnoses amongst those who committed suicide to be depression, schizophrenia, personality disorder and alcohol or drug dependence.

Suicide occurs in 15% of patients with *bipolar-affective* disorder and 10% of people with schizophrenia. In schizophrenia, the risk of suicide is often associated in young people (especially men) with a fear of deterioration, and also after a recent discharge and development of insight. In bipolar disorder, Slama *et al.* (2004) found early age at onset, a high number of depressive episodes, a history of antidepressant-induced mania, co-morbid alcohol abuse, suicidal behaviour and a family history of suicidal behaviour to be risk factors for suicide.

As well as the relatively well-known risk factors for suicide in depression, it is important to be aware that marked anxiety in a depressed patient may be a warning sign and that delusional depressed patients are at greater risk of suicide than non-delusional depressed patients (Busch *et al.* 2003).

Alcohol and drug addiction also have a well-known association with suicide (King 1994). Data collated by Goldberg *et al.* (2001) suggest a five- to tenfold increased risk for attempting suicide among alcohol abusers above and beyond the effects of psychiatric co-morbidity.

'Malignant alienation' (Watts and Morgan 1994)

Just as the quality of the relationship between patients and staff can be a strong predictor of violence (Beauford *et al.* 1997), and the initial therapeutic alliance helps in evaluating a psychiatric patient's risk of violence, so the lack of a therapeutic alliance also correlates with a higher risk of suicide. 'Malignant alienation' describes a potentially lethal distancing of the patient from staff, from other patients and from relatives. This is particularly likely to happen with patients who are regarded as manipulative or attention-seeking.

Demographic and social risk factors

Although suicide is commonest in the elderly, there has been a significant increase in suicide in young men over the past 15 years (Hawton *et al.* 1997). Other risk factors include divorce, unemployment and recent bereavement. Further demographic and social factors worth noting are that suicide is more common in men, in those aged over 45, in those who are divorced, single or widowed, and that it is associated with unemployment and retirement. Highest rates are in social classes I and V. Other associations have been made with broken homes in childhood, loss of role, mental and physical illness, and social disorganisation, including criminality, drug and alcohol misuse.

Different ethnicities may carry with them different risk and protective factors relating to suicide. The National Confidential Inquiry (Appleby *et al.* 1999, 2001) found that 5% of suicides were from an ethnic minority group. Individuals from ethnic minorities who committed suicide usually had severe mental illness; three quarters of black Caribbean suicides had a diagnosis of schizophrenia.

Physical safety features of the unit

Structures such as brackets or curtain rails should not be weight-bearing whilst false ceilings should not provide easy access to electric wiring. Windows must be made of unbreakable glass and stairwells have to be made safe. Obviously exit from the unit has to be controlled.

Search procedures have to be implemented according to clear guidelines to remove potentially dangerous objects such as scissors and lighters.

Evaluation and management of short-term suicide risk

- Evaluate past and recent deliberate self-harm and declared intention and preparations.
- Assess mental state and look for despair, pessimism, anhedonia, morbid guilt, severe insomnia, self-neglect, agitation and panic attacks.
- Patients with a history of violence should be assessed for suicidal ideation and those who are suicidal assessed for potential for violence to others.
- Tools such as the Beck Hopelessness Scale and The Reasons for Living Scale may contribute to a more complete risk assessment.

- Consider recent adverse life events.
- Identify current stressors such as overcrowding, bullying, the effects of detention on relationships.
- Assess the quality of relationships with staff and others. Has the patient established a working alliance with the key worker or any other member of the team?
- The patient should be explicitly encouraged to approach staff when distressed and to discuss suicidal ideas openly.
- Frequently review mental state.
- Use nursing observation levels appropriate to current risk.
- Reduce/eliminate access to means of suicide.
- Prevent absconding.
- Ensure that the service user receives appropriate treatment for their mental illness (including appropriate medication, psychological assistance, electroconvulsive therapy).
- Monitor compliance with medication (not stockpiling).
- Manage difficulties relating to alcohol or other substance misuse/dependence.
- Document management plans, decisions and rationale. Ensure that the patient is allocated to the appropriate level of Care Programme Approach and that documents are complete and up to date.
- Encourage and facilitate communication with carers (with the service user's consent).
- Any incidents (e.g. self-harm) should be followed promptly by multidisciplinary team review and open communication with carers.

Note the following cautions (Morgan and Stanton 1997; NIMHE 2004):

- The period shortly after admission carries a high risk of deliberate self-harm.
- Extra vigilance is also required during shift handovers.
- With a misleading clinical improvement and temporary amelioration of distress, but without resolution of stress factors, be aware of the possibility of a reluctance to talk specifically about suicide (the patient's level of distress might fluctuate markedly throughout the day).

Observation

Intensive, supportive observation allows close monitoring of behaviour and mental state. The level of supportive observation has to be agreed jointly by the patient's key worker together with medical and other members of the team. It must be recorded and passed on to all the unit staff as well as to the patient. The level of observation can be intensified unilaterally by the nursing staff and reviewed at every change of nursing shift as well and regularly by senior nursing and medical staff.

On the one hand, repeatedly asking patients the same questions with each change of staff can have an obvious alienating effect. On the other hand, one-to-one, special or continuous care observation provides an opportunity for staff to work intensively with the suicidal patient using a cognitive approach to suicidal preoccupations. See helpful guidelines on cognitive therapy for suicidal behaviour (Weishaar and Beck 1990).

The Good Practice Statement of the CRAG/SCOTMEG Working Group with Mental Illness (1995) provides clear guidelines on nursing observation. The Department of Health (1999a) has since issued Practice Guidance: Safe and Supportive Observation of Patients at Risk; Mental Health Nursing, Addressing Acute Concerns.

Leave

Risk assessment should always be carried out prior to granting leave in patients who are recovering from illness. Patients under any form of increased observation should not be allowed leave or time off the ward (National Institute of Mental Health in England 2004).

Summary

Suicide is a relatively rare event on PICUs and highly suicidal patients are less commonly seen than are aggressive, violent patients. Nonetheless, a comprehensive multidisciplinary approach to the assessment and management of suicide risk is an important aspect of the service provided by PICUs.

Acknowledgements

We would like to thank Dr Santosh R. Mudholkar, specialist registrar in forensic psychiatry, North London Forensic Service for his helpful advice and contributions.

REFERENCES

Aiken GJM. 1984 Assaults on staff in a locked ward: predictions and consequences. Med Sci Law 24: 199–207

Anonymous. 1976 Gold award. A program for the prevention of and management of disturbed behaviour. Hosp Community Psychiatry 27: 724–727

Appelbaum KL, Appelbaum PS. 1991 A model hospital policy on prosecuting patients for presumptively criminal acts. Hosp Community Psychiatry 42: 1233–1237

Appelby L. 2000. Safer services: conclusions from the report of the National Confidential Inquiry. Adv Psychiatr Treat 6: 5–15

Appleby L, Shaw J, Amos J et al. 1999 Safer Services: Report of the National Confidential Inquiry into Suicide and Homicide by People with Mental Illness. London: Stationery Office

Appleby L, Shaw J, Sherratt J et al. 2001 Safety First: Report of the National Confidential Inquiry into Suicide and Homicide by People with Mental Illness. London: Stationery Office

Beauford JE, McNiel DE, Binder RL. 1997 Utility of the initial therapeutic alliance in evaluating psychiatric patients' risk of violence. Am J Psychiatry 154: 1272–1276

Beck R, Fernandez E. 1998 Cognitive behaviour therapy in the treatment of anger: a meta-analysis. Cogn Ther Res 22: 63–74

Berg AZ, Bell CC, Tupin J. 2000 Clinical Safety: assessing and managing the violent patient. New Dir Mental Health Serv 86: 9–29

Birley J. 1996 Homicide and suicide by the mentally ill. J Forensic Psychiatry 7: 234–237

Blom-Cooper L. 1995 The Falling shadow – One Patient's Mental Health Care 1978–1993. Report of the Committee of Inquiry into the Events Leading up to and Surrounding the Fatal Incident at the Edith Morgan Centre, Torbay on 1 September 1993 (Chair: Louis Blom-Cooper). London: Duckworth

Blumenthal S, Lavender T. 2000. Violence and Mental Disorder. A Critical Aid to the Assessment and Management of Risk. Philadelphia: Jessica Kingsley

Borum R. (1998) Improving the clinical practice of violence risk assessment: technology, guidelines, and training. Am Psychol 51: 945–956

Busch KA, Fawcett J, Jacobs DG. 2003 Clinical correlates of inpatient suicide. J Clin Psychiatry 64: 1

Carton G, Larkin E. 1991 Reducing violence in a Special Hospital. Nurs Stand 5(17): 29–31

Castle K, Duberstein PR, Meldrum S, Conner MSK, Conwell Y. 2004 Risk factors for suicide in blacks and whites: an analysis of data from the 1993 National Mortality Followback Survey. Am J Psychiatry 161: 452–458

Clinical Assessment of Risk Decision Support (CARDS). 2002 Health Services Research Department. London: Institute of Psychiatry

Clunis Inquiry. 1994 The Report of the Inquiry into the Care and Treatment of Christopher Clunis (Chair: Jean Ritchie QC). London: HMSO

CRAG/SCOTMEG Working Group on Mental Illness. 1995 Final Report. Nursing Observation of Acutely Ill Psychiatric Patients in Hospital: A Good Practice Statement. Edinburgh: Clinical Resource Audit Group

Department of Health. 1992 The Health of the Nation. Strategy for Health in England. London: HMSO

Department of Health. 1995 Building Bridges – A Guide to Arrangements for Interagency Working for the Care and Protection of Severely Mentally Ill People. London: HMSO, p. 88

Department of Health. 1999a Practice Guidance: Safe and Supportive Observation of Patients at Risk; Mental Health Nursing, "Addressing Acute Concerns" (June 1999)

Department of Health. 1999b National Service Framework: Mental Health. London: Department of Health

Department of Health. 1999c Managing Dangerous People with Severe Personality Disorder. Proposals for Policy Development. London: HMSO

Department of Health. 2002a Mental Health Policy Implementation Guide: Adult Acute Inpatient Care Provision. London: Department of Health

Department of Health. 2002b National Minimum Standards for Psychiatric Intensive Care Units and Low Secure Units. London: Department of Health

Department of Health. 2002c National Suicide Prevention Strategy for England. London: Department of Health

Department of Health and Home Office. 1994 Report of the Department of Health and Home Office Working Group on Psychopathic Disorder. London: Department of Health and Home Office

Doctor R. 2004 Psychodynamic lessons in risk assessment and management. Adv Psychiatr Treat (2004) 10: 267–276

Dolan M, Doyle M. 2000 Violence risk prediction: clinical and actuarial measures and the role of the Psychopathy Checklist. Br J Psychiatry 177: 303–311

Douglas KS, Guy LS, Weir J. 2006 HCR-20 Violence risk assessment scheme: overview and annotated bibliography. Burnaby, British Columbia: Department of Psychology, Simon Fraser University

Drinkwater J, Gudjonsson GH. 1989 The nature of violence in psychiatric hosptials. In: Howell K, Hollin CR (eds) Clinical Approaches to Violence. New York: John Wiley and Sons

Feeney A. 2003. Dangerous severe personality disorder. Adv Psychiatr 9: 349–358

Frilis S. 1986 Characteristics of a good ward atmosphere. Acta Psychiatr Scand 74: 469–473

Fuller J, Cowan J. 1999 Risk assessment in a multidisciplinary forensic setting: clinical judgement revisited. J Forensic Psychiatry 10: 276–289

Goldberg FG, Singer TM, Garno JL. 2001 Suicidality and substance abuse in affective disorders. J Clin Psychiatry 62 [Suppl. 25]

Gordon H. 2002 Suicide in secure psychiatric facilities. Adv Psychiatr Treat 8: 408–417

Hare R. 2003 Manual for the Hare Psychopathy Checklist – Revised, Version 2. Toronto, Ontario: Multi-Health Systems

Hawton K, Fagg J, Simkin S, Bale E, Bond A. 1997 Trends in deliberate self-harm in Oxford, 1985–1995. Br J Psychiatry 171: 556–560

Hawton K, Houston K, Hae C, Townsend E, Harris L. 2003 Comorbidity of axis 1 and axis II disorders in patients who attempted suicide. Am J Psychiatry 160: 1494–1500

Henriques GR, Brown GK, Berk MS, Beck AT. 2002 Marked increases in psychopathology found in a 30-year cohort comparison of suicide attempters. Psychol Med 34: 833–841

Hodges V, Sanford D, Elzinga R. 1986 The role of ward structure on nursing staffing behaviours: an observational study of three psychiatric wards. Acta Psychiatr Scand 73: 6–11

Hollin CR. 2001 The Essential Handbook of Offender Assessment and Treatment. Chichester: John Wiley and Sons Ltd

Jenkins MG, Rocke LG, McNicholl BP, Hughes DM. 1998 Violence and verbal abuse against staff in accident and emergency departments: a survey of consultants in the UK and the Republic of Ireland. J Accid Emerg Med 15: 262–265

Johnston I, Crim M, Taylor PJ. 2003 Mental disorders and serious violence. J Clin Psychiatry 64: 819–824

Jones MK. 1985 Patient violence: report of 200 incidents. J Psychosoc Nurs Ment Health Serv 23(6): 12–17

Junginger J, McGuire L. 2004 Current research on serious mental illness and rates of violence. Schizophr Bull 30: 21–22

Kapur N. 2000 Evaluating risk. Adv Psychiatr Treat 6: 399–406

King E. 1994 Suicide in the mentally ill: an epidemiological sample and implications for clinicians. Br J Psychiatry 165: 658–663

King EA, Baldwin KDS, Sinclair JMA, Campbell MJ. 2001 The Wessex Recent In-Patient Suicide Study, 2. Case-control study of 59 in-patient suicides. Br J Psychiatry 178: 537–542

Krakowski M, Czobor P. 2004 Gender difference in violent behaviours: relationship to clinical symptoms and psychological factors. Am J Psychiatry 161: 459–465

Krakowski M, Czobor P, Chou JC. 1999 Course of violence in patients with schizophrenia: relationship to clinical symptoms. Schizophr Bull 25(3): 505–517

Lanza ML. 1988 Factors relevant to patient assault. Issues Mental Health Nurs 9: 239–257

Levy P, Hartocollis P. 1976 Nursing aides and patient violence. Am J Psychiatry 133(4): 429–431

Link BG, Stueve A. 1994 Psychotic symptoms and the violent/illegal behaviour of mental patients compared to community controls. In: Monahan J, Steadman HJ (eds) Violence and Mental Disorder: Developments in Risk Assessment. Chicago: University of Chicago Press, pp. 137–160

Lion JR. 1977 Training for battle: thoughts on managing aggressive patients. Hosp Community Psychiatry 38(8): 875–882

Lipsedge M. 2000 Clinical risk management in psychiatry. In: Vincent C (ed) Clinical Risk Management, 2nd edn. London: BMJ Publishing

Maden A. 1996 Risk assessment in psychiatry. Br J Hosp Med 56: 78–82

Maden A. 2003 Standardised risk assessment: why all the fuss? [Editorial] Psychiatr Bull 27: 201–204

Mak M, Koning PD. 1995 Clinical research in aggressive patients, pitfalls in study design and measurement of aggression. Prog Neuropsychopharmacol Biol Psychiatr 19: 993–1017

Mason T, Chandley M. 1999 Managing Violence and Aggression. A Manual for Nurses and Health Care Workers. New York: Churchill Livingstone

McNeil DE, Binder RL. 1994 The relationship between acute psychiatric symptoms, diagnosis and short term risk of violence. Hosp Community Psychiatry 45: 133–137

McNeil DE, Eisner JP, Binder RL. 2000 The relationship between command hallucinations and violence. Psychiatr Serv 51(10): 1288–1292

Monahan J, Steadman HJ. 1994 Violence and Mental Disorder: Developments in Risk Assessment. Chicago: The University of Chicago Press

Monahan J, Henry J, Silver E et al. 2001 Rethinking Risk Assessment. The MacArthur Study of Mental Disorder and Violence

Monahan J, Steadman H, Robbins P, Appelbaum, P et al. 2005 An actuarial model of violence risk assessment for persons with mental disorders. Psychiatr Serv 56: 810–815

Moran P, Walsh E, Tyrer P, Burns T, Creed F, Fahy T. 2003 Impact of comorbid personality disorder on violence in psychosis. Report from the UK700 trial. Br J Psychiatry 182: 129–134

Morgan HG, Stanton R. 1997 Suicide among psychiatric inpatients in a changing clinical scene. Br J Psychiatry 171: 561–563

National Institute of Mental Health in England (NIMHE). 2004 Toolkit for Suicide Prevention. London: Department of Health

NICE. 2004 Guidelines for the Short-Term Physical and Psychological Management and Secondary Prevention of Self-Harm in Primary and Secondary Care. Developed by the National Collaborating Centre for Mental Health. London: National Institute for Clinical Excellence

NICE. 2005 Violence: The Short Term Management of Disturbed/Violent Behaviour in Inpatient Psychiatric Settings and Emergency Departments. Clinical Guideline CG25. London: National Institute for Clinical Excellence

Oquendo MA, Ellis SP, Greenwald S, Malone KM, Weissman MM, Mann JJ. 2001. Ethnic and sex differences in suicide rates relative to major depression in the United States. Am J Psychiatry 158: 1652–1658

O'Rourke M, Hammond S, Bucknall M. 2001 Multi-Agency Risk Management: Safeguarding Public Safety and Individual Care. RAMAS report available online at www.ramas.co.uk/rptmultia.pdf

Palmstierna T, Wistedt B. 1990 Risk factors for aggressive behaviour are of limited value in predicting the violent behaviour of acute involuntarily admitted patients. Acta Psychiatr Scand 81: 152–155

Paton C, Banham S, Whitmore J. 2000 Benzodiazepines in schizophrenia. Psychiatr Bull 24: 113–115

Powell G, Caan W, Crowe M. 1994 What events precede violent incidents in Psychiatric Hospitals? Br J Psychiatry 165: 107–112

Powell J, Geddes J, Deeks J, Goldacre M, Hawton K. 2000 Suicide in psychiatric hospital in-patients: risk factors and their predictive power. Br J Psychiatry 176: 266–272

Quinsey VL, Harris GT, Rice ME, Cormier C. 1998 Violent offenders: Appraising and Managing Risk. Washington, DC: American Psychiatric Association Press

Reith M. 1998 Risk assessment and management: lessons from mental health inquiry reports. Med Sci Law 38(3): 89–93

Rice ME, Harris GT, Quinsey VL. 2000 The apraisal of violence risk. Curr Opin Psychiatry 15: 589–593

Royal College of Psychiatrists. 1998 Management of Imminent Violence: Clinical Practice Guidelines to Support Mental Health Services: OP 41. London: Gaskell Publications

Saarinen P, Lehtonen J, Lönnqvist J. 1999 Suicide risk in schizophrenia: an analysis of 17 consecutive suicides. Schizophr Bull 25: 533–542

Sanson-Fisher RW, Poole D, Thompson V. 1979 Behavioural patterns within a general hospital psychiatric unit: an observational study. Behav Res Ther 17: 317–332

Secretary of State for Health. 1997 The New NHS. London: HMSO

Shaw J, Appleby L, Amos T et al. 1999. Mental disorder and clinical care in people convicted of homicide: national clinical survey. Br Med J 318: 1240–1244

Sheridan M, Henrion R, Robinson L, Baxter V. 1990 Precipitants of violence in a psychiatric inpatient setting. Hosp Community Psychiatry 41: 776–780

Slama F, Bellivier F, Henry C et al. 2004 Bipolar patients with suicidal behaviour: toward the identification of a clinical subgroup. J Clin Psychiatry 64: 1035–1039

Snowden P. 2001 Substance misuse and violence: the scope and limitations of forensic psychiatry's role. Adv Psychiatr Treat 7: 189–197

Steadman HJ, Monahan J, Robbins P *et al.* 1993 From dangerousness to risk assessment: implications for appropriate research strategies. In: Hodgins S (ed) Crime and Mental Disorder. London: Sage Publications, pp. 39–62

Swanson JW, Holzer CE, Ganju VM, Jono RT. 1990 Violence and psychiatric disorder in the community: evidence from the Epidemiologic Catchment Area Surveys. Hosp Community Psychiatry 41: 761–770

Tardiff K. 1999 Assessment and Management of Violent Patients, 2nd edn. Washington, DC: American Psychiatric Publishing Group

Tardiff K, Sweillam A. 1982 Assaultative behaviour among chronic patients. Am J Psychiatry 139: 212–215

Taylor P, Gunn J. 1999 Homicides by people with mental illness: myth and reality. Br J Psychiatry 174: 9–14

Thomas B, Bell F. 1998 Bitter sweet sympathy: staff support after violence. Mental Health Pract 1: 6–10

Walsh E, Buchanan A, Fahy T. 2002 Violence and schizophrenia: examining the evidence. Br J Psychiatry 180: 490–495

Watts D, Morgan HG. 1994 Malignant alienation. Br J Psychiatry 164: 11–15

Watts D, Bindman J, Slade M, Thorncroft G. 2002 The development and evaluation of CARD (Clinical Assessment of Risk Decision Support). Final Report. London: Department of Health

Webster CD, Douglas KS, Eaves D, Hart SD. 1997 HCR-20: Assessing Risk for Violence, version 2. Burnaby, British Columbia: Mental Health, Law and Policy Institute, Simon Fraser University

Weishaar ME, Beck AT. 1990 The suicidal patient: how should the therapist respond? In: Hawton K, Cowen P (eds.) Dilemmas and Difficulties in the Management of Psychiatric Patients. Oxford: Oxford Medical Publications

Whittington R. 1994 Violence in psychiatric hospitals. In: Wykes T (ed) Violence and Healthcare Professionals. London: Chapman and Hall, pp. 23–43

Whittington R, Patterson P. 1996 Verbal and non-verbal behaviour immediately prior to aggression by mentally disordered people: enhancing the assessment of risk. J Psychiatr Mental Health Nurs 3: 47–54

PART II

Interface issues

13

The provision of intensive care in forensic psychiatry

Harvey Gordon

In some countries, the practice of forensic psychiatry is confined to providing psychiatric evaluation to the court (Harding 1993). In England and Wales, forensic psychiatrists are involved in the assessment and treatment of patients who have been charged with an offence or convicted by a court and, since the 1959 Mental Health Act, patients may be transferred to forensic psychiatric units without being charged with any offence. Most of these patients would now be detained on Section 3 of the 1983 Mental Health Act, though a few may be subject to Section 2 of the same Act. Consequently, when the Reed Committee reported (Department of Health and Home Office 1992), it covered not only mentally abnormal offenders, but also 'those requiring similar services'.

In reality, therefore, there is an overlap between general and forensic psychiatry rather than any sharp demarcation. It can indeed be arbitrary whether or not a patient in the community or a psychiatric hospital is charged with a criminal offence (James and Hamilton 1991; Cripps *et al.* 1995). Most patients admitted to regional secure units or Special Hospitals have previously received treatment in general psychiatric hospitals (Parker 1973; Cope and Ndegwa 1990; Murray 1996). Considerable tension may exist between general and forensic psychiatrists, and related health professionals, as to which patients are accepted for transfer into forensic psychiatric units, and then subsequently back to the general psychiatric sector, though liaison is better in some areas compared to others. Such professional border disputes must contribute little benefit to patients who may find themselves caught between differences of perspective between clinicians. The issue was indeed identified at the time of the genesis of medium secure units by the Butler Committee (Home Office and Department of Health and Social Security 1975). That report reflected a contemporaneous one by the Department of Health and Social Security (1974) on security in psychiatric hospitals, which concluded that medium secure units were needed for patients presenting with severely disruptive behaviour, with a diagnosis of mental illness, mental handicap or psychopathic or severe personality disorder. Admission to a medium secure unit would be decided by multidisciplinary assessment, taking account of the potential risk to others and risk of self injury, and the prospects of response to treatment.

In practice, patients on Section 3 of the 1983 Mental Health Act, if psychotically disturbed, may be located in intensive care units in general psychiatric hospitals (Mortimer 1995), medium secure units (Kennedy *et al.* 1995a, 1995b) and in Special Hospitals (Grounds *et al.* 1993a).

Violence by patients in psychiatric hospitals is common (Crighton 1995) though its severity tends to rise with the level of security provided (Larkin *et al.* 1988). Most psychiatric hospitals have found it necessary to provide intensive care facilities in order to separate the more violent and disturbed group

Psychiatric Intensive Care, 2nd edn., eds. M. Dominic Beer, Stephen M. Pereira and Carol Paton.
Published by Cambridge University Press. © Cambridge University Press 2008

from the more behaviourally stable majority (Ford and Whiffin 1991; Beer *et al.* 1997; Allan *et al.* 1998). Risk of harm to fellow patients and staff, potential for self-harm, absconding behaviour, and the tendency for any unit's functioning to be adversely affected by the degree of restrictions or resources needed for the most disturbed patients have led to the provision of locked facilities in general psychiatry.

Intensive care units in general psychiatric hospitals have their counterparts in intensive or special care areas or units in medium secure facilities and in Special Hospitals. Whilst the literature on intensive care units in general psychiatry is extensive, that pertaining to intensive or special care in forensic psychiatry is sparse. A history of violence to some degree is characteristic of virtually all patients admitted to forensic psychiatric units, the ethos of which is the assessment and treatment of the mental disorder and its associated violence and antisocial behaviour.

Studies of regional secure units in England and Wales have described a broad range of patient variables (Higgins 1981; Faulk and Taylor 1984; Bullard and Bond 1988; Rix and Seymour 1988; Cope and Ndegwa 1990; Higgo and Shetty 1991; Sugarman and Collins 1992; Torpy and Hall 1993; Kaul 1994; Cripps *et al.* 1995; James 1996; Murray 1996; Mohan *et al.* 1997; Brown *et al.* 2001; Ricketts *et al.* 2001; Maden *et al.* 1999; Edwards *et al.* 2002). Only one study has investigated the use of an intensive care unit within a medium security, unit, that being the Edenfield Centre in Prestwich Hospital, Manchester (Dolan and Lawson 2001). Studies reflecting the use of intensive or special care facilities in Special Hospitals are also relatively few in number (Larkin *et al.* 1988; Coldwell and Naismith 1989; Carton and Larkin 1991; Mason and Chandley 1995; Brook and Coorey 1996; Gordon *et al.* 1998).

Many medium secure units have provided an intensive care area, e.g. the Denis Hill Unit in the Bethlem Royal Hospital, which can be brought into effect with extra nursing staff when required. Other medium secure units have more permanent intensive care wards, such as the Shaftesbury Clinic, the Reaside Clinic and the Three Bridges Unit. Patients may be transferred into the intensive care unit from elsewhere in the medium secure unit or directly, if appropriate, when admitted. It is assumed that placement in the intensive care facility can be harmoniously negotiated but at present this is not known. Health professionals, especially nursing staff in intensive care units, in general psychiatry are known to often feel professionally isolated (Zigmond 1995), but in the hitherto relatively small medium secure units perhaps more mutual understanding regarding patient location has been developed. In the Edenfield Centre study (Dolan and Lawson 2001), the decision to admit into the intensive care unit was primarily a nursing one for patients presenting as challenging or unmanageable on the main wards. Clearly an intensive care facility, whether in general or forensic psychiatry, should provide an effective service to its feeder units, with the understanding that patients should stay no longer in intensive care than is necessary.

The majority of patients admitted to medium secure units suffer from schizophrenia or a related psychosis (Higgins 1981; Faulk and Taylor 1984; Bullard and Bond 1988; James 1996; Murray 1996). Although it was originally felt that some patients with personality disorder would be suitable for medium secure units, most are disinclined to admit such patients other than by transfer from Special Hospitals and then only after extra careful assessment (Faulk and Taylor 1984; Bullard and Bond 1988), though one partial exception is the Trent regional secure unit, which is disposed towards admission of offender patients with a diagnosis of personality disorder on assessment sections under Part III of the 1983 Mental Health Act (Kaul 1994). The avoidance by medium secure units of many patients with personality disorder is not necessarily inappropriate however, as the more severe group of personality-disordered patients can be highly disruptive unless in a well-contained therapeutic environment providing an extended length of stay. Then again, blanket rejection of patients on the basis of diagnosis alone is of doubtful ethical soundness. The Government's decision to ensure that people with personality disorder are assessed and treated (National Institute for Mental Health for England 2003) (albeit in appropriate facilities) is an opportunity for psychiatric health care professionals to assist therapeutically with what is a needy albeit difficult patient group. Government determination in this regard has been necessary in order to overcome the more negative views towards personality disorder held by most general (Cawthra and Gibb 1998) and many forensic psychiatrists (Cope 1993). The main clinical and ethical concern by psychiatrists in regard to personality disorder is that admission of such patients to psychiatric facilities would have more of a preventive detention function than one of therapeutic gain (Haddock *et al.* 2001). In forensic psychiatry co-morbidity in patients is now virtually the norm (Coid *et al.* 1999; Snowden 2001), such that elements of personality disorder are likely to be present in patients in medium and high secure units even where the substantive diagnosis is one of mental illness.

The limitations of general psychiatric facilities and medium secure units have been outlined in regard to the types of patients they find too difficult to manage successfully. Coid (1991), in a survey of the private sector, found that the group of patients most difficult to place in the public sector were those presenting with persistently challenging behaviour, those on Section 3 of the 1983 Mental Health Act, and those suffering from severe schizophrenia, mild or moderate mental handicap or brain damage. Murray (1996), in a review of all the medium secure units in England, found that these units had proved unable to provide adequately for those offender patients requiring medium security over a long period of time, i.e. several years, and separately the problematic non-forensic patients on Section 3 of the 1983 Mental Health Act, most of whom had schizophrenic illnesses that were more resistant to treatment than usual. Now almost 30 years since the Butler Report the issue of the provision of facilities for the persistently disturbed psychotic outside the Special Hospitals remains unresolved, and one of the parameters always provided by Special Hospitals, namely extended length of stay, is found to be necessary. However, the provision of long-term medium security may prove far more complex in practice than in theory (Taylor *et al.* 1996).

Whether patients located for periods in intensive care areas in medium security resemble those difficult-to-place patients described by Coid (1991) or are those referred to by Murray (1996) is not currently known. Neither is it known whether these are the same group who find themselves transferred from medium to maximum security, though clinical impression suggests this might be the case. Coid and Kahtan (2000) found that 25% of transfers to Special Hospitals were from medium secure units, many being non-offender patients on Section 3 of the Mental Health Act 1983. Bullard and Bond (1988), in their study of a precursor to the Reaside Clinic, found that 10% (seven cases) of their patient group required transfer to a Special Hospital, four of the seven being young female patients with a diagnosis of personality disorder, two of whom also had a degree of mental impairment. Higgo and Shetty (1991), in a study of the Scott Clinic in Liverpool, found that, over a 6-year period, about 10% of patients leaving the unit were transferred to a Special Hospital. Cope and Ward (1993), in the Reaside Clinic, found that almost one-third of patients transferred there from a Special Hospital required transfer back to the Special Hospital, noting a special concern about the risks associated with patients legally categorised as psychopaths with a propensity towards sexual violence. However, the overt dangerousness of that group would be more likely to manifest itself in the community than in hospital, and indeed the violence perpetrated by a patient in the community may not in all cases correlate with that in hospital (Gordon *et al.* 1998).

Dolan and Lawson's study (2001) of the Edenfield Centre found that the intensive care unit was used more for the prevention of probable or impending violence than as a response to it, an approach which indeed seems most sensible. The study also indicated that the Edenfield intensive care unit had been used to locate female patients prone to self-harm who required higher levels of observation, and a separate group of female patients who were pregnant in which condition they may have been at greater risk if in the main wards of the medium secure unit. A history of alcohol abuse was also a factor associated with location in the intensive care unit. Substance abuse generally now poses a major challenge to the integrity and safety of general and forensic psychiatric services and effective strategies are needed for both treatment and prevention (Gordon and Haider 2004).

The Special Hospitals have been the subject of extensive professional and public review and criticism over recent decades (Department of Health and Social Security 1980; Bluglass 1992; Department of Health 1992; Department of Health and Home Office 1992; Special Hospitals Service Authority 1993; Fallon *et al.* 1999). However, they continue to provide sizeable proportions of patients who could be safely managed elsewhere in lesser degrees of security if such were available (Maden *et al.* 1995). Around the time of the Butler Report, Tidmarsh (1974) referred to the impression that the Special Hospitals were having to accept patients who previously would have been treated in general psychiatric hospitals. The Special Hospitals had continued to provide humane asylum in some cases, a concept which became unpopular but has stood the test of time even if its optimum modern characteristics may take a different form, at least for the group who are not a serious danger to the public (Munetz *et al.* 1996). The role of the therapeutic environment is also a concept still adhered to theoretically, but not always fully appreciated in practice, in general and forensic psychiatry (Cohen and Khan 1990).

Larkin *et al.* (1988), in a study in Rampton, found that the rate of serious violence within the hospital was significantly higher than in general psychiatry. He found the highest rates were in Rampton's female intensive care unit, though reasons for that were unclear. A follow-up study by Carton and Larkin (1991) found that the acquisition of skills in the use of control and restraint techniques had led to a reduction in the levels of serious violence.

Larkin *et al.*'s study (1988) pointedly illustrates that most units in Special Hospitals are segregated by gender, compared to the widespread integration hitherto available elsewhere in psychiatry (Special Hospitals Service Authority 1991; Taylor and Swann 1999). A return however after 30 years or more (Gordon 1999) towards units in psychiatry, segregated by gender for patients will render the Special Hospitals similar to mainstream psychiatry, which

is also returning to a degree of segregation (Department of Health 2002).

Coldwell and Naismith (1989), in what was then Park Lane Hospital for male patients only (subsequently Ashworth Hospital), found an excess of patients in their male special care ward who were detained on Section 3 of the 1983 Mental Health Act; albeit this excess did not reach statistical significance. A similar finding is reported by Gordon *et al.* (1998) in a study at Broadmoor Hospital, where it applied both to male and female patients in their respective special care units. It therefore seems that patients on Section 3 who are behaviourally disturbed in general psychiatric hospitals or regional secure units who require transfer to Special Hospitals tend to remain disturbed at least for a period of time. The clinical state of such patients seems to be somewhat independent of the environment in which they receive treatment, though in due course improvement does occur. The absence of unrealistic expectations of length of stay for these patients may here be a positive benefit, allowing the patient to improve at his or her own pace. However, this need not preclude the construction of appropriate alternative long-term secure facilities for such patients elsewhere (Taylor *et al.* 1996). Such facilities need to provide not only a lengthy placement, but also a flexibility and a range of therapeutic facilities within a secure perimeter. The availability of clozapine has in some cases ameliorated the chronicity of active psychosis and its associated behaviour disturbance, with some evidence of reduced levels of violence, but not all patients will take clozapine or respond to it.

The special care units in Special Hospitals are the buffer zones of psychiatry, the outer limits of the therapeutic stratosphere. It is of considerable note that the study in Broadmoor Hospital showed that the special care units were used mainly by patients with chronic schizophrenia or a related psychosis, the proportion of transfers into them of psychopathic patients being low, especially for males. Within a secure psychiatric hospital, most of the violent incidents are perpetrated by the acutely or chronic mentally ill. This is, however, more so for male patients than for female patients for whom borderline personality disorder also accounts for sizeable numbers of transfers into special care and is reminiscent of Bullard and Bond's study (1988), in which several female borderline patients required transfer to a Special Hospital. The disruption by psychopaths in hospital tends to be much more covert, whilst schizophrenic violence is more blatant, disinhibited and frequent.

The operational problems in the special care units in Special Hospitals have focused around two different groups with differing lengths of stay. The average length of stay in special care in the Broadmoor study was about 4 months for females and about 6 months for males. A significant minority continued to show protracted challenging behaviour in excess of 2 years, with a few cases even beyond 5 years or more. Mason and Chandley (1995) in Ashworth Hospital have described these persistently challenging cases. Most of these patients suffer from a chronic schizophrenic illness, though there may be an occasional case of exceptional difficulty where there is superadded brain damage. Efforts to reduce seclusion for these patients is understandable (Special Hospitals Service Authority 1995), but the notion that seclusion could be abolished for this group is based on ideological and clinical naivety. In two particularly rare cases known to the author, seclusion has been reduced only by the controversial use of mechanical restraint to allow the patient to get up safely (Gordon *et al.* 1999). However, these are unusual cases and most patients in special care units in Special Hospitals can usually be transferred back to an ordinary ward in the hospital within a reasonable time. A length of stay of 4–6 months in most cases may seem rather long in comparison to length of stay in general psychiatry, but it is not unduly long when considered in the context of the average length of stay in a Special Hospital, which is about 8 years (Grounds *et al.* 1993b).

Some advantages accrue by separating the more chronic group from those requiring only shorter periods in special care. Brook and Coorey (1996) described the opening in Ashworth Hospital of such an acute intensive care unit in September 1994 in an attempt to have a more consistent environment for the separate more chronically disturbed group. Similar changes were made at Broadmoor Hospital in January 1997, although in practice blending of the two groups still tends to occur.

Over the last 30 years the numbers of special care beds in the Special Hospitals have seemingly tended to decrease in excess of the reduction in the overall numbers of beds there. It is unlikely that this reflects a real reduction in the level of aggressive disturbance and is probably more determined by the need to improve public acceptability. A further change, at least in Broadmoor Hospital, has been that up until the late 1990s, the special care units tended to accept referrals liberally, essentially affording the decision to admit not with the Consultant and team for the special care unit itself, but with the referring team if it was felt that the patient could no longer be safely manageable in its ward. Such a system worked well and avoided the many problems and indeed errors associated with a process of assessment which results not infrequently in refusing to take the patient for reasons which are far from persuasive. The special care units in Special Hospitals, or the intensive care units in general psychiatry or in medium secure units, can be seen as a vital resource available to the rest of the hospital, albeit not one to be abused, but in my view such abuse was uncommon. The current author is sceptical that assessment for transfer to special or intensive care can be based on any real objective criteria, and prefers a system driven by the referring team rather than the receiving one. The corollary of this however is that a patient must remain in special care for only as long as is necessary, the decision on which being made by dialogue and attempted consensus, and arbitration when consensus cannot be reached.

On occasions, a patient may preferably be transferred when ready from special or intensive care, not back to the original referring ward but to another ward, especially when traumatic memories of an adverse incident on the referring ward may still be raw. 'Blacklisting' however of patients is unacceptable.

A major issue for special care units in Special Hospitals is their reputation as 'punishment wards'.

Similar concerns have been expressed in regard to intensive care units in general psychiatric hospitals (Ford and Whiffin 1991; Zigmond 1995). Whether such punitive impressions can be entirely avoided may be doubtful, even if the clinicians working in such units do not employ such a philosophy of care. Regular liaison with the units from which the patient has been transferred to special care, close sharing of relevant information with managers, and encouragement of visiting by legal and other legitimate agencies with an interest in mental health are helpful.

Although forensic psychiatry's focus is on the violent patient, some patients in forensic psychiatric units of medium or maximum security pose a greater threat than others either in the short term or on a more protracted basis. The provision of an intensive or special care facility allows the more stable group within the hospital to undertake their treatment and rehabilitation without undue excessive restrictions. Additionally the more disturbed and dangerous patient may be located in a unit more appropriate to his or her needs and that of others. It is vital, however, that, once sufficient progress has been achieved, the patient returns to a more liberal area of the hospital. In the author's experience, achieving that requires close cooperation with medical colleagues and related health professionals as well as a degree of patience but also firmness and determination, without which an intensive or special care facility can become an injustice in some cases.

REFERENCES

Allan ER, Brown RC, Laury G. 1998 Planning a psychiatric intensive care unit. Hosp Community Psychiatry 39(1): 81–83

Beer MD, Paton C, Pereira S. 1997 Hot beds of general psychiatry: a national survey of psychiatric intensive care units. Psychiatr Bull 21: 142–144

Bluglass R. 1992 The Special Hospitals should be closed. Br Med J 305: 323–324

Brook R, Coorey PR. 1996 An acute ICU in a maximum secure hospital. Psychiatr Bull 20: 306–311

Brown CSH, Lloyd KR, Donovan M. 2001 Trends in admissions to a regional secure unit (1983–1997). Med Sci Law 41: 35–40

Bullard H, Bond M. 1988 Secure units: why they are needed? Med Sci Law 28(4): 312–318

Carton G, Larkin E. 1991 Reducing violence in a Special Hospital. Nurs Stand 5(17): 29–31

Cawthra R, Gibb R. 1998 Severe personality disorder – whose responsibility? Br J Psychiatry 173: 8–10

Cohen S, Khan A. 1990 Antipsychotic effect of milieu in the acute treatment of schizophrenia. Gen Hosp Psychiatry 12: 248–251

Coid JW. 1991 A survey of patients from five health districts receiving special care in the private sector. Psychiatr Bull 15: 257–262

Coid J, Kahtan N. 2000 Are Special Hospitals needed? J Forensic Psychiatry 11(1): 17–35

Coid J, Kahtan N, Gault S, Jarman B. 1999 Patients with personality disorder admitted to secure forensic psychiatric services. Br J Psychiatry 175: 528–536

Coldwell JB, Naismith LJ. 1989 Violent incidents on special care wards in a Special Hospital. Med. Sci Law 29(2): 116–123

Cope R. 1993 A survey of forensic psychiatrists' views on psychopathic disorder. J Forensic Psychiatry 4: 215–235

Cope R, Ndegwa D. 1990 Ethnic differences in admission to a regional secure unit. J Forensic Psychiatry 3: 368–378

Cope R, Ward M. 1993 What happens to Special Hospital patients admitted to medium security? J Forensic Psychiatry 4(1): 13–24

Crighton J. 1995 A review of psychiatric inpatient violence. In: Crighton J (ed) Psychiatric Patient Violence: Risk and Response. London: Duckworth

Cripps J, Duffield G, James D. 1995 Bridging the gap in secure provision: evaluation of a new local combined locked forensic/intensive care unit. J Forensic Psychiatry 6(1): 77–91

Department of Health. 1992 Report of the Committee of Inquiry into Complaints about Ashworth Hospital. Cm-2028–1 and 2. London: HMSO

Department of Health. 2002 Women's Mental Health: Into the Mainstream. Strategic Development of Mental Health Care for Women. London: Department of Health

Department of Health and Home Office. 1992 Review of Health and Social Services for Mentally Disordered Offenders and Others Requiring Similar Services, Final Summary Report. CM2088. London: HMSO

Department of Health and Social Security. 1974 Revised Report of the Working Party on Security in NHS Psychiatric Hospitals (Glancy Report). London: HMSO

Department of Health and Social Security. 1980 Report of the Committee of Inquiry into Rampton Hospital. Cmnd 8073. London: HMSO

Dolan M, Lawson A. 2001 A psychiatric intensive care unit in a medium security unit. J. Forensic Psychiatry 12(3): 684–693

Edwards J, Steed P, Murray K. 2002 Clinical and forensic outcome 2 years and 5 years after admission to a medium secure unit. J Forensic Psychiatry 13(1): 68–87

Fallon P, Bluglass R, Edwards B, Daniels D. 1999 The Report of the Committee of Inquiry into the Personality Disorders Unit, Ashworth Special Hospital. Cmnd 4194. London: Stationery Office

Faulk M, Taylor J. 1984 The Wessex interim secure unit. Issues Crimin Legal Psychol 6: 47–57

Ford I, Whiffin M. 1991 The role of the psychiatric ICU. Nurs Times 87(51): 47–49

Gordon H. 1999 International perspectives on relationships and sexuality in secure institutions. In: Taylor PJ, Swan T (ed) Couples in Care and Custody. Oxford: Butterworth-Heinemann, pp. 188–199

Gordon H, Hammond S, Veeramani R. 1998 Special care units in Special Hospitals. J. Forensic Psychiatry 9(3): 571–587

Gordon H, Hindley N, Marsden A, Shirayogi M. 1999 The use of mechanical restraint in the management of psychiatric patients: is it ever appropriate? J Forensic Psychiatry 10(1): 173–186

Gordon H, Haider D. 2004 The use of 'drug dogs' in psychiatry. Psychiatr Bull 28(6): 196–198

Grounds A, Gunn J, Mullen P, Taylor P. 1993a Secure institutions: their characteristics and problems. In: Gunn J, Taylor PJ (eds) Forensic Psychiatry: Clinical, Legal and Ethical Issues. Oxford: Butterworth-Heinemann

Grounds A, Snowden P, Taylor P, Basson J, Gunn J. 1993b Forensic psychiatry in the National Health Service of England and Wales. In: Gunn J, Taylor PJ (eds) Forensic Psychiatry: Clinical, Legal and Ethical Issues. Oxford: Butterworth-Heinemann

Haddock A, Snowden P, Dolan M, Parker J, Rees H. 2001 Managing dangerous people with severe personality disorder: a survey of forensic psychaitrists' opinions. Psychiatr Bull 25: 293–296

Harding T. 1993 A comparative survey of medico-legal systems. In: Gunn J, Taylor PJ (eds) Forensic Psychiatry: Clinical, Legal and Ethical Issues. Oxford: Butterworth-Heinemann

Higgins J. 1981 Four years experience of an interim secure unit. Br Med J 282: 889–893

Higgo R, Shetty G. 1991 Four years experience of a regional secure unit. J Forensic Psychiatry 2(2): 202–210

Home Office and Department of Health and Social Security. 1975 Report of the Committee on Mentally Abnormal Offenders (Butler Report). Cmnd 6244. London: HMSO

James A. 1996 Suicide reduction in medium security. J Forensic Psychiatry 7(2): 406–412

James DV, Hamilton LW. 1991 The Clerkenwell scheme: assessing efficacy and cost of a psychiatric liaison service to a magistrates' court. Br Med J 303: 282–285

Kaul A. 1994 Interim hospital order – a regional secure unit experience. Med Sci Law 34(3): 233–236

Kennedy J, Wilson C, Cope R. 1995a Long stay patients in a regional secure unit. J Forensic Psychiatry 6: 541–551

Kennedy J, Harrison J, Hills T, Bluglass R. 1995b Analysis of violent incidents on an RSU. Med Sci Law 35(3): 255–260

Larkin E, Murtagh S, Jones S. 1988 A preliminary study of violent incidents in a Special Hospital (Rampton). Br J Psychiatry 153: 226–231

Maden A, Rutter S, McClintock T, Friendship C, Gunn J. 1999 Outcome of admission to a medium secure psychiatric unit. I. Short and long term outcome. Br J Psychiatry 175: 321–335

Maden T, Curle C, Meux C, Burrow S, Gunn J. 1995 Treatment and Security Needs of Special Hospital Patients. London: Whurr

Mason T, Chandley M. 1995 The chronically assaultive patient: benchmarking best practices. Psychiatr Care 2(5): 180–183

Mohan D, Murray K, Taylor P, Steed P. 1997 Developments in the use of regional secure unit beds over a 12 year period. J Forensic Psychiatry 8(2): 321–335

Mortimer A. 1995 Reducing violence on a secure ward. Psychiatr Bull 19: 605–608

Munetz MR, Peterson GA, Vandershie PW. 1996 Safer houses for patients who need asylum. Psychiatr Serv 47(2): 117

Murray K. 1996 The use of beds in NHS medium secure units in England. J Forensic Psychiatry 7(3): 504–524

National Institute for Mental Health for England. 2003 Personality Disorder: No Longer a Diagnosis of Exclusion. Policy Implementation Guidance for the Development of Services for People with Personality Disorder. Gateway reference 105. London: NIMH(E)

Parker E. 1973 An Inquiry into the Reliability of Special Hospital Case Records with Reference to the Recording of

Previous Psychiatric Hospitalisations and Criminal Histories. London: Special Hospitals Research Unit, Department of Health and Social Security

Ricketts D, Carnell H, Davies S, Kaul A, Duggan C. 2001 First admissions to a regional secure unit over a 16 year period: changes in demographic and service characteristics. J Forensic Psychiatry 12: 78–89

Rix G, Seymour D. 1988 Violent incidents on a Regional Secure Unit. J Adv Nurs 13: 746–751

Snowden P. 2001 Substance misuse and violence: the scope and limitations of forensic psychiatry's role. Adv Psychiatr Treat 7: 189–197

Special Hospitals Service Authority. 1991 Advisory Committee on Facilities for Married Patients within Special Hospitals. Interim Report. London: Special Hospitals Service Authority

Special Hospitals Service Authority. 1993 Report of the Committee of Inquiry into the Death of Orville Blackwood and a Review of the Deaths of Two Other Afro-Caribbean Patients: Big, Black and Dangerous? London: Special Hospitals Service Authority

Special Hospitals Service Authority. 1995 Service Strategies for Secure Care. London: Special Hospitals Service Authority

Sugarman P, Collins P. 1992 Informal admission to secure units: a paradoxical situation? J Forensic Psychiatry 3(3): 477–485

Taylor PJ, Swan T. 1999 Couples in Care and Custody. Oxford: Butterworth-Heinemann

Taylor PJ, Maden A, Jones D. 1996 Long-term medium security hospital units: a service gap of the 1990s. Crim Behav Mental Health 6: 213–229

Tidmarsh D. 1974 Secure hospital units [Letter]. Br Med J 4(5939): 286

Torpy D, Hall M. 1993 Violent incidents in a secure unit. J Forensic Psychiatry 4(3): 517–544

Zigmond A. 1995 Special care wards: are they special? Psychiatr Bull 19: 310–312

14

The interface with forensic services

James Anderson

Introduction

Psychiatric intensive care is at the interface with forensic psychiatric services because they share a common clinical problem – violence. This is the behavioural disability which characterises the majority of patients within the forensic psychiatric service. Knowing how to evaluate violence, and quantify the risk of future violence, is the essence of risk assessment. Knowing when to refer a particular patient to forensic psychiatric services is an important part of effective risk management. Understanding what services are offered by forensic psychiatry is a necessary precondition to using that service effectively.

The aim of this chapter is to provide guidelines to those working outside forensic psychiatry on what is and what is not available within that service. The assessment of dangerousness is discussed elsewhere, but dangerousness in terms of risk to others is pivotal to an evaluation of a patient's need for secure care. It is therefore vital to know whether that patient warrants referral to forensic psychiatric services.

It is unrealistic, given existing resources, to imagine that forensic psychiatric services could, or should, manage all those patients who are violent. But knowing which patient should be managed in a more secure setting, whether that be intensive care or the local medium secure unit, is our current concern. However, there are no absolute rules or fixed access criteria; local services vary and are in a state of flux, developing new services for old problems. Many facilities at one time provided within the old asylums are being re-invented and re-named.

The Butler Committee Report (1975), which was particularly influential and which provoked the modern development of regional secure units, recognised that there was 'a yawning gap' between the Special Hospitals (maximum secure) and the 'increasingly liberal asylums.' The latter were shutting beds and could offer less in terms of secure facilities than they had hitherto. Thirty years later we still have that gap and, despite the continuing fall in total psychiatric bed numbers, there are now more people aged 15–44 years in psychiatric hospitals than there were 20 years ago. This increase is most pronounced among young men who account for over 40% more hospital episodes than they did 20 years ago (Department of Health 1995). It is young men, both in the community at large and amongst the mentally ill, who account for most violence (Walmesley 1986). It is also this group that are associated with drug and alcohol abuse – a factor which, in conjunction with serious mental illness, significantly increases the risk of violent behaviour (Monahan and Steadman 1994). However, the relationship between schizophrenia, substance abuse and violence is not uniform: it is suggested that for a substantial proportion of men with schizophrenia, substance abuse is only part of a syndrome of antisocial behaviour that

Psychiatric Intensive Care, 2nd edn., eds. M. Dominic Beer, Stephen M. Pereira and Carol Paton.
Published by Cambridge University Press. © Cambridge University Press 2008

characterises them from a young age and through-out their lives. For others who display no antisocial behaviour before the onset of schizophrenia, substance abuse and intoxication may exacerbate the symptoms of schizophrenia (Hodgins *et al.* 1998).

Care pathways for violence in mental illness

It is the need to safely manage violence in the context of mental illness which prompts admission to secure wards – whether in the general psychiatric service or within forensic psychiatric services. Most of the violently mentally ill have a schizophreniform psychosis. While the relationship between schizophrenia and violence has long been recognised, the inter-relationship between antisocial personality disorder (ASPD), substance abuse, schizophrenia and violence has not. This relationship is beginning to emerge as providing useful markers to the type of care pathways different individuals are likely to require over their lifetime. It is already possible to anticipate individuals who are at high risk of developing ASPD and schizophrenia; it is arguable whether early intervention to treat their conduct problems in childhood may ameliorate their risk of developing violent schizophrenia if not of developing schizophrenia itself.

Epidemiological studies on offenders who develop major mental illness have shown that there are two distinct groups – early starters, who begin offending in adolescence before symptoms of mental illness are manifest, and late starters, who only begin to offend once the disorder is present (Tengström *et al.* 2001). Early starters are convicted of more crimes – both violent and non-violent – than the late starters (Hodgins *et al.* 1996, 1998). They have higher scores on Hare's Psychopathy Check List (Hodgins *et al.* 1998). They have a higher level of social functioning (Schanda *et al.* 1992; Hodgins *et al.* 1998), which is itself related to antisocial behaviour including substance abuse (Halle *et al.* 1995; Laroche *et al.* 1995) and aggressive behaviour (Léveéillée 1994; Rasmussen *et al.* 1995).

A recent meta-analysis showed that historical variables were the best predictors of future criminal-ity among those with major mental illness (Bonta *et al.* 1998). Future risk of violence can be usefully evaluated through predictor instruments e.g. HCR 20 (Webster *et al.* 1997; Douglas *et al.* 2006) and VRAG (Quinsey *et al.* 1998). Both highlight the necessity of accurately documenting the age of onset and history of antisocial behaviour in order to make valid assessments of the risk of future violence.

The incidence of antisocial behaviour is also higher in those who subsequently develop major mental illness than it is in the population who do not (Hodgins *et al.* 1998; Mullen *et al.* 2000) Whether this increased incidence of criminality is a consequence of the neurobiological deficits of schizophrenia or whether it represents a completely discrete issue with its own determinants is, as yet, unknown. What is known is that if the risk of violence that is associated with schizophrenia is to be effectively reduced then the influence of the attitudes, neurobiological deficits and associated behaviours (e.g. substance abuse) that characterise ASPD need to be evaluated and addressed.

Dichotamous attitudes that have tended to separate ASPD and mental illness as completely distinct problems – the one being outside the medical domain and beyond therapeutic intervention, the other bona fide illness – are no longer justified or acceptable. Programmes designed for those who have both ASPD and mental illness that recognise their special needs – substance abuse, inadequate life and social skills, antisocial attitudes and behaviour – can work (Heilbrun and Peters 2000; Hodgins and Müller-Isberner 2000). Such approaches, in conjunction with intense supervision post discharge, compulsory powers for readmission if necessary and, rehousing outside previous neighbourhoods, represent the approach to management needed. These strategies are now well established in forensic psychiatric services; the challenge for general and forensic services alike is to match services to the individuals that require them, and to provide them. This requires yet further integration of forensic and general psychiatric services in order to achieve what amounts to a tall order.

Nonetheless this is the expectation of current UK Government policy. While recognising that specific services for the care and treatment of personality disorder at all levels of psychiatric provision are limited, new legislation and services are in development. For example, 140 new beds are opening in Broadmoor and Rampton Maximum secure hospitals for the treatment of dangerous severe personality disorder.[a] This inevitably represents a highly selected group where a clear functional link exists between their personality disorder and their offending and who pose a very high risk to the public (it is estimated that only 10% of those currently in maximum security fulfil these criteria). A similar provision now exists in HMP Whitemoor and HMP Frankland, again with 140 beds. While local and regional forensic services treat many patients with co-morbidity – where aspects of personality disorder present alongside major mental illness, there is very little dedicated infrastructure for the assessment and treatment of personality disorder per se. Arnold Lodge in Leicester is a notable exception. Equally, there are few dedicated facilities available within general psychiatric services although some exist: the intensive Psychological Treatment Service, Dorset, and Paddington Outreach Treatment Team. An overview of effective treatment models, planned legislation and National Health Service policy on developing treatment facilities in forensic and general psychiatric services is available through the Department of Health (UK) websites (www.doh.gov.uk and www.nimhe.org.uk).

The medium secure unit – forensic psychiatric services at the interface with general psychiatry

The medium secure unit is the hub of forensic psychiatric services in most districts. It is the inpatient facility, the academic base and the home base for most community forensic psychiatric services. In response to the Butler Report medium secure units were developed to take patients who were persistent absconders, who represented a risk to the public, who were seriously disruptive to hospital regimes or who exhibited persistent and impulsive violence – these being the criteria originally considered in a working party set up by the UK Ministry of Health in 1961 (cited in Eastman 1993). Since the first medium secure units were built there has been increasing awareness of the psychiatric needs of the mentally disordered offender (Reed Committee 1992) and increased public concern about community care of the mentally ill. Whether justified or not, there is a perception of increasing risk to the public from the mentally ill in the community. This has provoked a flurry of legislation ostensibly to tighten professional procedure in community care. There has been a corresponding increase in the awareness and concern about risk in the general psychiatric patient population (Milmis Project Group 1995). The Milmis Project has demonstrated increasing bed occupancy, falling bed numbers, a high level of assaults and sexual harassment by patients of other patients or staff, premature discharges and a dependence on secure facilities in the private sector.

The composition of patients within the medium secure unit reflects these various demands. Although there is some regional variation, by far the majority of inpatients come from prison or the courts. Fewer than 25% come from general psychiatric services, and fewer than 10% from Special Hospitals (Gunn

---

[a] Dangerous severe personality disorder is a non-clinical designation that has developed from UK legislative proposals. It has led to a number of clinical initiatives some of which are described. The criteria that must be established to meet the admission criteria for DSPD are:
 1. An assessment confirming that they are more likely than not to reoffend.
 2. A severe personality disorder. Severity is defined according to two measures. Personality disorder is diagnosed using the DSM IV system, and psychopathy is measured using the Psychopathy checklist – Revised (PCL-R). The assessment is based on structured clinical judgement, using the following guidelines. A PCL-R score of 30 or above defines a severe personality disorder. As an alternative, a PCL-R score of 25–29 is sufficient if there is another personality disorder diagnosis as well as antisocial personality disorder (which will always be present with a PCL-R score in this range). Finally patients may qualify with a lower PCL-R score if they have two or more DSM IV personality disorders from different clusters. For example, there may be a borderline personality disorder in association with paranoid or antisocial personality disorder. (www.dspdprogramme.gov.uk).
 3. A functional link between the personality disorder and the risk.

and Taylor 1993). These relative ratios remain largely unchanged although the severity of offending leading to admission has increased (Ricketts *et al.* 2001). This has increased pressure on the medium secure services, as has the increased pressure from the maximum secure service to reduce their patient population by moving patients down the secure 'ladder'. The overall consequence has been a continuing squeeze on the beds available.

Forensic psychiatric services are developing to meet these differing demands. They include:

• *Inpatient facilities.* Bed numbers are increasing and services are becoming more specialised. There is an awareness of the need for long-term medium security (a provision which at the moment is limited and variable across different districts). There is recognition of a need for low secure beds, as well as challenging behaviour and intensive care facilities. Some UK National Health Service Trusts are developing these latter facilities within the forensic directorate; others are separate. However they are developed, it is important that clear clinical boundaries are established to ensure that patients are appropriately placed.

• *Community forensic psychiatric services* are developing in recognition of the commonality of many patients in general and forensic psychiatric services, particularly those patients who are recognised as potentially dangerous but may not have offended. These community-based services can offer advice and expertise in risk assessment and management. Adopting a strategy of assertive outreach for patients who are recognised as potentially dangerous if untreated will, it is hoped, ameliorate the risk of violent behaviour to others – whether such patients are being rehabilitated following previous admission to the medium secure unit, or identified as potentially dangerous by the general service. How community services are developing is variable: in some areas in the UK 'parallel' forensic community psychiatric services are developing alongside generic services. This contrasts with 'integrated' services in which forensic specialists work within community mental health teams. Key characteristics of parallel teams include having their own team base, separate referral meetings, a specialist management line, specialist supervision, protected funding, forensic psychology, good links with the criminal justice system and capped caseloads. Integrated teams are distinguished by their close links with community mental health services and acceptance of more referrals from primary care. The parallel model may be able to deliver a more specialised treatment programme to a select few; however, there is concern that it may discourage non-forensic clinicians from developing risk assessment and risk management skills (Mohan *et al.* 2004).

• *Court diversion schemes* have developed in recognition of the frequency with which the mentally ill become involved in the Criminal Justice System. Once involved, they often experience unacceptable delay before they receive hospital treatment while languishing in prison. Court diversion schemes have been established in many parts of the country in order to identify the mentally ill within the Criminal Justice System and expedite their transfer to appropriate psychiatric facilities (James and Hamilton 1991). However, a recent review has demonstrated that it is a minority of schemes that are effectively achieving these aims. What is recommended is a comprehensive diversion service which would include police station liaison; community psychiatric nurses (CPN) – led and linked to community mental health teams; improved remand prison reception screening; and greater participation of the NHS in providing health care to prisons (Reid and Lyne 1997; James 1999).

• *Forensic psychiatry in prison.* Most forensic psychiatric services attempt to provide regular liaison with their local prisons. This is in recognition of the level of psychiatric morbidity in both the remand and sentenced prisoner populations (Gunn *et al.* 1991; Brooke *et al.* 1996). Unfortunately for many schizophrenic patients in the inner city, prison is an established part of their itinerary. If such patients are to be well managed, it is important that general and forensic psychiatrists alike acknowledge this reality. Trying to provide an integrated service that monitors the psychiatric population in the community, psychiatric hospitals, the courts and prison can reduce the distress that results when the seriously mentally ill are committed to prison. Nonetheless there is evidence that much psychiatric morbidity in prison remains undetected. Where it is detected, the nature of the prison regime and actions of the courts can make effective delivery of care difficult, many patients being discharged from court before psychiatric contact is established (Birmingham *et al.* 1998). A recent development in the UK is a change in the responsibility for the commissioning of health care from the prison department to the primary care trusts (PCTs) to the National Health Service (from 2006). This will hopefully raise the standard of prison health care, but it will also increase the pressure on medium secure inpatient services to comply with pre-set standards for transfer of prisoners requiring mental health care.

The forensic psychiatric service therefore has a wide constituency ranging from patients in Special Hospital, patients in prison and attending court, outpatients and patients within the general psychiatric service. The latter include those considered a serious enough risk to warrant forensic psychiatric management, or having special treatment needs particular to forensic psychiatry, e.g. sexual offending, morbid jealousy, etc. Obviously the service can offer advice on the suitability of referral of a particular patient and clearly, if indicated, offer a bed for patient admission. If the clinical criteria for admission are met, but no bed is available locally, the patient may be admitted to a private medium secure unit. What the service clearly cannot do is manage all patients who exhibit violent behaviour.

Guidelines on access to inpatient forensic care

With the burgeoning of costs for the treatment of mentally disordered offenders, a need has arisen to identify more rigorously the factors that characterise those requiring forensic secure services. In some parts of the UK this has led to the formalisation of access criteria to forensic services (Eastman and Bellamy 1998). These criteria can only provide guidelines but they do help to encourage a consistent approach within the service and provide referral guidelines to external agencies. However, there are limitations to such an approach: admission policies must to some extent reflect the local context, although there is a need to establish clearly delineated clinical boundaries between different types and levels of secure facilities. Unfortunately the reality is that analysis of admission criteria to medium secure units across the UK has shown a woeful lack of consistency of approach (Grounds *et al.* 2004).

The most common reasons for the general psychiatric services to request forensic psychiatric advice are:

• to obtain a risk assessment
• to transfer a patient to the medium secure unit

The approach to risk assessment is described in a number of excellent reviews (Gunn and Taylor 1993; Royal College of Psychiatrists 1996) and I commend these (Figure 14.1). The latter is published as a pocket-sized booklet and is an invaluable companion. The protocol for risk assessment is described as follows:

The standard psychiatric assessment *including* the following:

• History
• Developmental history with particular focus on *childhood behavioural disorder*
• Evaluation of *personality disorder(s)*
  • Previous convictions, *violence* and/or suicidal behaviour
  • Evidence of rootlessness or 'social restlessness', e.g. few relationships, frequent changes of address or employment
  • Evidence of *poor compliance* with treatment or disengagement from psychiatric aftercare
  • Presence of *substance misuse* or other potential disinhibiting factors, e.g. a social background promoting violence
  • Identification of any precipitants and any changes in mental state or behaviour that have occurred prior to violence and/or relapse

- Are the risk factors stable or have any changed recently?
  - Evidence of recent severe stress, particularly of loss events or the threat of loss
  - Evidence of recent discontinuation of medication
- Environment
  - Does the patient have access to potential victims, particularly victims identified in mental state abnormalities?
- Mental state
  - Evidence of any threat/control override symptoms: firmly held beliefs or persecution by others (persecutory delusions), or of mind or body being controlled or interfered with by external forces (delusions of passivity)
  - Emotions related to violence, e.g. irritability, anger, hostility, suspiciousness
  - Specific threats made by the patient

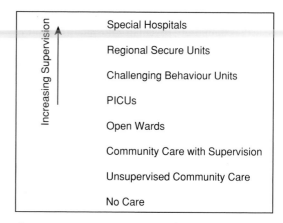

Figure 14.1. A hierarchy of supervision and security within the English Hospital System (from Gunn and Taylor 1993)

Conclusion

A formulation should be made based on these and all other items of history and mental state. The formulation should, as far as possible, specify factors likely to increase the risk of dangerous behaviour and those likely to decrease it. The formulation should aim to answer the following questions:

- How serious is the risk?
- Is the risk specific or general?
- How immediate is the risk?
- How volatile is the risk?
- What specific treatment, and which management plan, can best reduce the risk?

I would elaborate one aspect of this protocol and that is the evaluation of potential violence because this dictates where in the hierarchy of supervision and security the patient should be managed.

By and large, it is violence and the risk of further serious violence that determine the patient's admission to forensic psychiatric facilities. This is true of the offender and non-offender populations alike. It is true that on occasions the courts or the Mental Health Unit at the British Ministry of Justice will dictate the level of security a patient requires, regard-

less of clinical need, but that is relatively unusual. It remains the case that the seriousness of a patient's violent behaviour will dictate the level of security that a patient requires.

Admission assessment therefore focuses on violence in the context of a full risk assessment. In evaluating previous violence (and by implication risk of future violence) it is important to obtain as much information as possible about previous behaviour including: previous criminal record, witness statements, arresting officers' statements, etc. However, a significant minority of patients show highly dangerous behaviour not 'officially recognised' or processed through the Criminal Justice System, prior to their admission. It is then necessary to establish the gravity of the patient's current violent behaviour. This is relatively easy if they are subject to criminal proceedings because it will be stated as the charge. However, it is important to attempt to re-create the details of the offence as accurately as possible. This is not only because the charge may underestimate (or less commonly overestimate) the seriousness of what took place, but also because a charge as such gives little information about motivation for the offence. For instance, 'attempted murder' gives little information about motivation: the stabbing of a young man by another outside a pub at 11.30 p.m. on Saturday night in the context of an alcohol-inflamed argument has very different implications to the near strangling of a young woman by a young man in the context of a sadistic sexual assault.

If the patient has not offended but has been violent in the community or in hospital, it is important to obtain as much detail of that violence as possible: from the patient, family and friends, GP, social workers, nursing staff, etc.

To assess violence, therefore:

- Obtain the arresting officer's statement (by ringing the police station in which he was charged)
- Read witness statements (sometimes these are difficult to obtain, but should be provided by the Crown Prosecution Service or solicitors, if you are providing a psychiatric report)
- Speak to witnesses
- Speak to family or friends, GP, social worker, nursing staff

The index offence, or the 'equivalent' behaviour associated with the patient's admission to hospital, can be ranked in severity. It can also be quantified by its frequency. Behaviour should be evaluated in the patient's life-span of violent behaviour and conclusions drawn about whether there is a changing pattern of offending or violence.

Secure care admission criteria (from Eastman and Bellamy 1998)

Behaviour category 1

- Murder
- Manslaughter
- Attempted murder
- Infanticide
- Arson with intent to endanger life
- Rape (against men or women)

Behaviour category 2

- Aiding or abetting suicide
- Administering poison
- Arson with recklessness towards life
- Contact sexual offending (not rape but including attempted rape)
- False imprisonment (e.g. kidnapping)

- Grevious bodily harm (GBH)
- Possession of a firearm
- Robbery
- Threats to kill
- Wounding with intent to cause GBH

Behaviour category 3

- Actual bodily harm (ABH)
- Affray
- Aggravated burglary
- Arson (no recklessness or intention to endanger life)
- Attempted assault
- Blackmail
- Breaking and entering
- Burglary
- Common assault
- Criminal damage
- Deception
- Forgery
- Fraud
- Going equipped to steal
- Handling stolen property
- Non-contact sexual offences
- Possession of an offensive weapon
- Public nuisance offences
- Public order offences
- Theft
- Trespass

Offences can be categorised according to seriousness (as above) and this schema can be adopted to provide guidelines to access different levels of security (Eastman and Bellamy 1998). The major determinant of acceptance to admission in the non-offender population is also violence. Offen and Taylor (1985) found violence was the precipitant to referral in all but thirteen (18%) of their series of referrals to an interim secure unit. The more serious the violence, the more likely it was that a bed would be made available. Treasaden (1985) found in a review of four Interim Secure Units (ISUs) that violence was the behavioural indication for admission in the majority (67%–83%) with fire-raising (19%–24%) and sexual behaviour (3%–10%) also found. More recently the three global measures of dangerousness, severity of mental illness, and personality disorder were analysed as to their influence on an individuals needing medium security. That need increased as severity of mental illness and the level of dangerousness increased. Patients with personality disorder (irrespective of severity) had just under three times the odds of needing medium security than patients not thought to have personality disorder (Melzer *et al.* 2004)

Violent behaviour in the non-offender population can be ranked in terms of its equivalent in the offence categories described above. As a rule of thumb, offences of violence equivalent to category 1 will require admission to medium or maximum secure care – the major factor determining which of the two is the level of continuing risk. Offences or violence equivalent to offence Category 2 can generally be managed in medium secure care. Offences of Category 3 can generally be managed in low secure care. In all cases the major additional factor to the level of security required is the continuing risk of such behaviour.

This approach is summarised in Figure 14.2.

So violence is categorised in terms of *severity* and quantified in terms of *frequency*. Risk of repeated violence in the short and longer term is also assessed. Furthermore if there is *specific pathology* that predicts serious violence (whether or not that has taken place to date), this may indicate the need for secure care, e.g. morbid jealousy. The risk of violence taking place on the unit itself should be considered, i.e. what level of continuing risk does that patient pose and to whom?

If the patient should *abscond* from hospital, it must be decided if he or she represents a *serious, immediate risk* to the general public, or only to named individuals. If it is named individuals only, do those individuals live nearby or not?

Another major consideration in assessing a patient's need for specialist forensic involvement is the *psychopathology* they exhibit. Forensic psychiatry has developed specialised interest and skill in the management of particular disorders. Sexual pathology, for instance, is almost exclusively dealt with by forensic psychiatry. Other pathologies are also more commonly encountered by forensic psychia-

trists, because of their association with offending and dangerous behaviour, e.g. morbid jealousy, erotomania and sadistic fantasies.

Personality disorder, which will often preclude a patient's admission to general psychiatric services, will not necessarily preclude them from forensic psychiatric care. It is often the presence of personality disorder in conjunction with serious mental illness that perpetuates the risk of violence. This conjunction of mental illness and personality disorder may be an indication for admission to medium secure care. However, it is notable that very few patients are detained in medium secure care under the legal category of psychopathic disorder, the majority being designated as mentally ill. This contrasts with a Special Hospital, where approximately 25% of patients are detained under the legal category psychopathic disorder (Dell and Robertson 1988). However, this picture is changing with the development of specialist facilities for the assessment and treatment of dangerous severe personality disorder and other facilities in lower levels of security (as above).

Other *co-morbid factors* include drug and alcohol abuse; those with diagnosed drug and alcohol misuse are much more likely to be violent than those with mental illness alone.

The majority of patients in medium secure care are detained under criminal sections of the Mental Health Act, and many of them under *restriction orders*. The increasing number of patients subject to restriction orders has had significant impact on the ability to discharge patients. Unfortunately there is some evidence that this has increased the average duration of admission, the net result being that, despite increasing numbers of medium secure beds, it remains as difficult to admit a patient as it was 10 years ago (Brown *et al.* 2001). The influence of the Mental Health Unit, at the Ministry of Justice in determining where a patient is admitted from prison can override clinical decisions on the patient's security needs. In other words the Ministry of Justice can dictate that a patient be admitted to medium secure care even if the clinicians involved feel that his or her risk to others does not warrant this. Certainly in maximum secure hospitals there are patients who are considered too high a *political profile* to allow

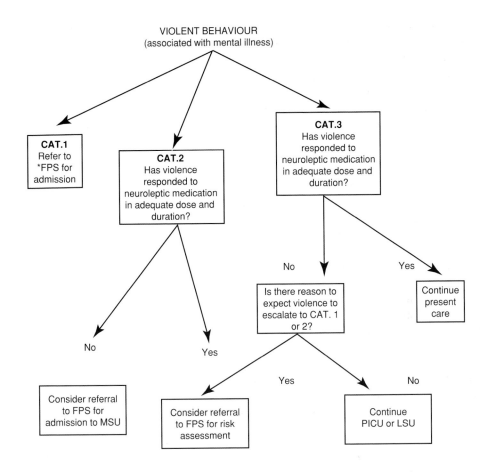

VIOLENT BEHAVIOUR
(associated with mental illness)

CAT.1
Refer to
*FPS for
admission

CAT.2
Has violence
responded to
neuroleptic medication
in adequate dose and
duration?

CAT.3
Has violence
responded to
neuroleptic medication
in adequate dose and
duration?

No   Yes

Is there reason to
expect violence to
escalate to CAT. 1
or 2?

Continue
present
care

No   Yes

Yes   No

Consider referral
to FPS for
admission to MSU

Consider referral
to FPS for risk
assessment

Continue
PICU or LSU

*FPS Forensic Psychiatric Services

Figure 14.2. Guidelines on access to different levels of secure care

their care in lower levels of security. Furthermore it is not just the patient's risk to others if they should abscond that should be considered, but also whether they have *dangerous friends* who might execute an escape attempt, possibly exposing staff and other patients to risk.

Although an attempt should be made to determine the patient's security needs on current clinical grounds, this judgement may be influenced by previous experience of that patient in other settings. It is surprising how many extremely disturbed patients settle rapidly, without any change in medication, when they move into a more secure environment.

How to make a referral

First and foremost, know what you want: advice, moral support, a risk assessment or a transfer? Advice can be enormously reassuring, and as a matter of principle good liaison between general and forensic psychiatric services helps to establish a culture of dialogue which itself tends to facilitate good working relationships and discourages entrenched protectionist attitudes and policies. Nonetheless it has its drawbacks: advice is informal and inevitably does not represent a formal risk assessment. Forensic psychiatrists can be hesitant about making judgements without undertaking a formal assessment if a potentially violent patient is released on the basis of such a judgement.

If you feel the patient is inappropriately placed in psychiatric intensive care and warrants admission to medium secure care, make the case persuasively.

1. Provide a full history with as much supportive information as possible, e.g. informant history, arresting officer's statement, previous criminal record, witness statements.
2. Provide a multiaxial diagnostic formulation.
3. Detail treatment to date and indications for referral including:
   • Violence category of index offence or equivalent behaviour
   • Perceived risk of continued violence including seriousness of risk, whether risk is specific or general, whether risk is immediate, how volatile the risk is

Conclusion

In the previous edition of this book, a call was made for the greater integration of general and forensic psychiatric services. This is happening as a result of an awareness of shared clinical responsibilities, greater understanding of the relationship between offending and major mental illness and political directives. Perhaps the challenge to be addressed before the next edition is to counter the pessimistic perception that still exists about the treatability of personality disorder. If collectively we are to manage the violence associated with major mental illness, we need to develop the necessary skills and services to achieve this.

Acknowledgements

I am grateful to Dr Nigel Eastman for permission to reproduce the Behaviour Gravity Categories from Admission Criteria to Secure Services Schedule (ACSeSS) (Eastman and Bellamy 1998). Other aspects of the evaluation of violence risk are also derived from ACSeSS and from discussion with Dr Eastman.

REFERENCES

Birmingham L, Mason D, Grubin D. 1998 A Follow-up study of disordered men remanded to prison. Crim Behav Ment Health 8: 202–213

Bonta J, Law M, Hanson K. 1998 The prediction of criminal and violent recidivism among mentally disordered offenders: a meta-analysis. Psychol Bull 123: 123–142

Brooke D, Taylor C, Gunn J, Maden A. 1996 Point prevalence of mental disorder in unconvicted male prisoners in England and Wales. Br Med J 313: 1524–1527

Brown CS, Lloyd KR, Donovan M. 2001 Trends in admissions to a regional secure unit (1983–1997). Med Sci Law 41(1): 35–40

Butler Committee Report. 1975 Better Services for the Mentally Ill. London: Home Office/DHSS

Dell S, Robertson G. 1988 Sentenced to Hospital. [Maudsley Monograph No. 32]. Oxford: Oxford University Press

Department of Health. 1995 Mental Health in England. London: Department of Health

Douglas KG, Guy LS, Weir J. 2006 HCR-20 Violence Risk Assessment Scheme: overview and annotated bibliography. Burnaby, British Columbia: Department of Psychology, Simon Fraser University

Eastman NLG. 1993 Forensic psychiatric services in Britain. Int J Law Psychiatry 16: 1–26

Eastman NLG, Bellamy S. 1998 Admission criteria to secure services and service definitions. Unpublished

Grounds A, Melzer D, Fryers T, Brugha T. 2004 What determines access to medium secure psychiatric provision? J Forensic Psychiatry Psychol 15: 1–6

Gunn J, Taylor PJ. 1993 Forensic Psychiatry Clinical Legal and Ethical Issues. London: Butterworth-Heinemann, pp. 624–640, 716

Gunn J, Maden A, Swinton M. 1991 Treatment needs of prisoners with psychiatric disorders. Br Med J 300: 338–341

Hallé P, Fiset S, Hodgins S et al. 1995 Profil Neuropsychologique de Personnes Atteintes de Schizophrénie Avec ou Sans Trouble d'Abus, de Drogues ou d'Alcool." Poster presented at Société Québécoise de la Recherche en Psychologie, Ottawa, Canada, 1995

Heilbrun K, Peters L. 2000 The efficacy of community treatment programs. In: Hodgins S, Müller-Isberner R. (eds) Violence, Crime and Mentally Disordered Offenders: Concepts and Methods for Effective Treatment and Prevention. London UK: Wiley, pp. 187–210

Hodgins S, and Müller-Isberner R. (eds) 2000 Violence, Crime and Mentally Disordered Offenders: Concepts and

Methods for Effective Treatment and Prevention. London: Wiley

Hodgins S, Toupin J, Côté G. 1996 Schizophrenia and antisocial personaltiy disorder: a criminal combination. In: Schlesinger LB. (ed) Explorations in Criminal Psychopathology: Clinical Syndromes with Forensic Implications. Springfield, Ill.: Charles C. Thomas, pp. 217–237

Hodgins S, Côté G, Toupin J. 1998 Major mental disorders and crime: an aetiologic hypothesis. In: Cooke D, Forth A, Hare RD (eds) Psychopathy: Theory, Research and Implications for Society Dordrecht: Kluwer Academic, pp. 231–256

James D. 1999 Court Diverson at ten years: can it work, does it work and has it a future? J Forensic Psychiatry, 10: 507–524

James DV, Hamilton LW. 1991 Assessing efficacy and cost of a psychiatric liaison service to a magistrates' court. Br Med J 303: 282–285

Laroche I, Hodgins S, Toupin J. 1995 Liens entre les symptômes et le fonctionnement social chez des personnes souffrant de schizophrénie ou de trouble affectif majeur. Can J Psychiatry 40: 27–34

Léveillée S. 1994 Evaluation multidimensionelle du reseau de support social de sujts schizophrenes. Thése de doctorat, Université de Montréal

Melzer D, Tom B, Brugha T. 2004 Access to medium secure psychiatric care in England and Wales. 1. A national survey of admission assessments. J Forensic Psychiatry Psychol 15: 7–31

Milmis Project Group. 1995 Monitoring Inner London mental illness services. Psychiatr Bull 19: 276–280

Mohan R, Slade N, Fahy T. 2004 Clinical characteristics of community forensic mental health services. Psychiatr Serv 55(11): 1294–1298

Monahan J, Steadman HJ. 1994 Violence and Mental Illness. Chicago: University of Chicago Press

Mullen PE, Burgess P, Wallace C, Palmer S, Ruschena D. 2000 Community care and criminal offending in schizophrenia. Lancet 355: 614–617

Offen L, Taylor PJ. 1985 Violence and resources: factors determining admission to an interim secure unit. Med Sci Law 25: 165–171

Quinsey VL, Harris GT, Rice ME, Cornier CA. 1998 Violent Offenders – Appraising and Managing Risk. Washington, DC: American Psychological Association

Rasmussen K, Levander S, Sletvold H. 1995 Aggressive and non-aggressive schizophrenics: symptom profile and neuropsychological differences. Psychol Crime Law 15: 119–129

Reed Committee. 1992 Review of Health and Social Services for Mentally Disordered Offenders and Others Requiring Similar Services. London: DOH/Home Office

Reid J, Lyne M. 1997 The Quality of healthcare in prisons: results of a year's programme of semi-structured inspections. Br Med J 315: 1420–1424

Ricketts D, Carnell H, Davies S, Kaul A, Duggan C. 2001 First admissions to a regional secure unit over a sixteen year period: changes in demographic and service characteristics. J Forensic Psychiatry 12 (1): 78–89

Royal College of Psychiatrists. 1996 Assessment and Clinical Management of Risk of Harm to Other People. Council Report CR53. London: Royal College of Psychiatrists

Schanda H, Fodes P, Topitz A, Knecht G. 1992 Premorbid adjustment of schizophrenic criminal offenders. Acta Psychiatr Scand 86: 121–126

Tengström A, Hodgins S, Kullgren G. 2001 Men with schizophrenia who behave violently: the usefulness of an early versus late start offender typology. Schizophr Bull 27 (2): 205–218

Treasaden IH. 1985 Current practice in interim secure units. In: Goslin L. (ed) Secure Provision. London: Tavistock

Walmesley R. 1986 Personal Violence. Home Office Research Study No. 89. London: HMSO

Webster CD, Douglas KS, Eaves D, Hart SD. 1997 HCR-20: Assessing Risk for Violence, version 2. Burnaby: Mental Health, Law and Policy Institute, Simon Fraser University

15

Supporting people with learning disabilities on general psychiatric wards, PICUs and LSUs

Andrew Flynn

Introduction

The syndrome of cognitive and social impairments known as 'learning disability' (LD) is an important vulnerability factor for developing serious psychiatric disorders. When people with LD need acute psychiatric admission this is frequently to general psychiatric wards where they are often under the care of general adult psychiatrists and mental health nurses who often have little knowledge or training in looking after psychiatric disturbance in this group. Common mental illnesses may have unfamiliar presentations, there may be idiosyncratic responses to treatment and it may not even be clear how conventional treatments should be applied. The psychiatric care of people with LD can become further complicated by boundary disputes between general adult and LD services, who frequently misunderstand one another's roles, expertise and resources.

This chapter will look at some of the principal challenges that generic mental health professionals (including psychiatrists, nurses and psychologists) face in looking after people with LD as inpatients, whether that is on the acute ward or, occasionally, in highly specialised settings such as the Psychiatric Intensive Care Unit (PICU). It is not an exhaustive account of the specialist psychiatric aspects of LD but highlights recurrent themes that concern general mental health professionals and for which advice is most often sought. The chapter is written mainly

with patients with so-called mild LD (the group with which general psychiatric services most often come into contact) in mind.

Defining learning disability

ICD-10 continues to refer to LD by the now archaic term of 'mental retardation'. Although, at least for clinical purposes, the terms are synonymous there is scope for occasional confusion: in the USA for example 'learning disability' usually refers to *specific* cognitive impairments such as dyslexia.

Both ICD-10 and DSM-IV base the diagnosis of LD on three essential components, all of which need to be demonstrable to justify the diagnosis, as shown in Box 15.1

Box 15.1. Essential features of LD

Evidence of significant intellectual *impairment*

+

Evidence of significant difficulties in *adaptive function* arising from that impairment

+

Impairment arising in the *developmental period*

---

1. **There should be evidence of significant generalised intellectual impairment**

This is usually expressed in terms of an intelligence quotient (IQ) score significantly below the

Psychiatric Intensive Care, 2nd edn., eds. M. Dominic Beer, Stephen M. Pereira and Carol Paton.
Published by Cambridge University Press. © Cambridge University Press 2008.

population average. There are a number of different psychometric instruments used to estimate IQ, the most widely used being the Wechsler Adult Intelligence Scale (WAIS). These scales are purposely designed to yield a population mean score of 100 and a normal distribution with a score of 70 (the usually accepted threshold for significantly below-average performance) lying two standard deviations below that mean. IQ tests look at performance across a variety of tasks that are broadly grouped into 'performance' and 'verbal' subscales that can be scored separately or combined into a single 'full scale' score, the figure frequently referred to when making judgements about overall degree of impairment.

2. **This impairment results in significant problems in 'adaptive functioning'**

   This refers to the various day-to-day activities that are presumed to depend on general intelligence. It particularly refers to performance on the basic building blocks of everyday life including self-care, awareness of personal safety, managing money and independent travel but also includes social problem-solving and interpersonal understanding.

3. **These problems are established in the developmental period**

   Regardless of cause (genetic, traumatic, psychosocial or otherwise) the intellectual impairment should be present since childhood, and certainly before later adolescence (taken by most to mean 18 years of age).

ICD-10 specifies four levels of LD: mild, moderate, severe and profound. Mild LD is associated with a measured IQ of 50–69. Patients with mild LD will generally have had some special educational provision at school (usually as part of a statement of special educational need), and some (but not all) will have attended specialist schools. Whereas the more severe degrees of LD are usually recognised in preschool years, mild LD is often only revealed when children are introduced to mainstream educational environments and begin to fall behind or develop reactive behavioural problems. Occasionally mild LD is not recognised until secondary school. Many

adults with mild LD, depending crucially on personal characteristics (such as temperament, other health problems, and particularly the effects of mental illness), local social factors (especially family support) and wider social issues (such as employment rates in general and availability of certain types of job in particular), are, in the words of ICD-10, 'able to work and maintain good social relationships and contribute to society'.

These contextual factors mean that the correlation between IQ (however measured) and overall personal functioning for people with mild LD is rather modest. For example, a recent study (Dacey *et al.* 1999) explored the relationship between IQ (measured by the Stanford Binet-IV test) and the domain subscales of the Vineland Adaptive Behaviour Scale (a commonly used measure of functional ability in LD research) in people with mild and moderate LD. Subscale correlations varied between a high of 0.65 (communication skills) to a low of 0.37 (daily living skills) with the skills of socialisation and adaptation falling in between.

The disparities in performance in everyday life for any given IQ score mean that prevalence rates for mild LD show marked regional variation. Although approximately 2% of the overall population will have a measured IQ between 50 and 69, prevalence rates for learning *disability* as opposed to intellectual *impairment* have been estimated to be as low as 2.97 per 1000 in Wessex, UK, but as high as 77.91 per 1000 in Rose County, USA (Fryers 1997).

For this and other, technical, reasons full-scale IQ scores alone are rather poor arbiters of eligibility for services despite the reassuring feel of objectivity attached to them. The diagnosis of mild LD, whilst showing an important association with IQ, inevitably requires broader psychosocial and developmental inquiry for it to be made with conviction. Recent guidelines published by the British Psychological Society and downloadable from the society's website (http://www.bps.org.uk, Learning Disabilities: Definitions and Contexts.) summarise the practicalities of assessment in more detail. Helpful and accessible critical appraisals of IQ testing and the clinical diagnosis of LD have recently been published in the psychiatric (Carpenter 2002) and psychological (Whitaker 2003) literature.

Special issues in psychiatric assessment

Communication

Barriers to effective communication arguably constitute the biggest challenge to effective psychiatric assessment and treatment. This is particularly the case with *verbal* communication, the channel most often used in routine clinical practice. Almost all patients with mild LD will be able to take part in verbal exchanges but the extent and nature of this vary considerably reflecting an individual's balance between *expressive* and *receptive* (understanding) skills.

Receptive problems may arise because of *hearing impairment* (with a prevalence of about 10% in mild LD) but are more commonly due to *limited vocabulary*, deficits in *working memory* (so that long phrases cannot be held effectively in mind), difficulties with *sustained attention* (including that due to social anxiety when confronted by an authority figure such as a doctor) and misunderstandings due to *concrete thinking* and related difficulties with abstract thinking (so that statements are interpreted in overly literal ways sometimes with major emotional or behavioural consequences).

The capacity for verbal expression is also variable, frequently for similar reasons. In addition some people with LD may be hampered by difficulties with *speech* (as opposed to language) *production* e.g. many adults with Down's syndrome have large tongues that can make articulation difficult.

Of course, similar communication problems are seen in other patient groups (e.g. chronic schizophrenics) and, at least qualitatively, will be familiar to most generically trained psychiatrists and their colleagues. However, there are some special difficulties that do seem to occur more often in LD work and can lead to errors in assessment.

Acquiescence and suggestibility

These aspects of communication have attracted particular attention in people with mild LD, especially because of their relevance for police interviewing. 'Acquiescence' is the tendency to answer 'yes' to questions even if the person means 'no' or doesn't actually know the answer. 'Suggestibility' is a little different, and has been defined by Gudjonsson and Clare (1986) as the extent to which someone comes to accept messages communicated during an interview. It comprises yielding to leading questions and shifting an initial response following negative feedback and results in the person shaping their story according to cues (verbal and non-verbal) from the interviewer. The patient may come to accept the story that has been shaped as the true account.

Both acquiescence and suggestibility may result from a desire by the interviewee to give answers he or she thinks will please or impress the interviewer. This is a particular risk when vulnerable individuals are confronted by interviewers they feel intimidated by, or who are of special status (like a doctor, especially one in a smart suit), whose esteem may be desired. Alternatively, it will occur because of tiredness, hunger, pain and the like, and the person wants to get through the interview as quickly as they can. Finally, acquiescence and suggestibility can reflect attempts to make up for lack of knowledge (and perhaps not wanting to appear stupid) or to fill in gaps in episodic memory (confabulation).

Gaps between expression and understanding

It often happens that someone's skill at verbal expression outstrips their ability to understand. This can easily give an illusory impression of linguistic competence. The style of speech is chatty (cocktail party speech) but its fragility only becomes apparent when the person is asked to elaborate on specific points. In many cases this communicative style serves an important psychological purpose for the person, minimising the outward appearance of an LD and preserving self-esteem for those where appearing 'normal' is important. Mismatches of this sort can also be seen with reading skills, where someone may be able to read text out loud but have little comprehension of its content.

Concept formation

Concepts such as time are often shakily held so that narrative accounts can become jumbled and events compressed in time. Other concepts such as property and the location and function of internal bodily organs may also be poorly formed. Categories may become overextended (e.g. the term depression coming to mean all unpleasant mood states) or overly restricted (as occurs in concrete thinking) compared with conventional use.

'Autistic' communication impairments

Characteristic impairments of communication are one of the core defining features of the autistic spectrum disorders (considered below). Echolalia, both immediate and delayed, is common, as are repetitiveness (often extreme, with the person having great difficulty switching between themes) and the use of rote-learned stock phrases that sound out of place in conversation. From time to time pronominal reversal is observed, with the second or third person used when the 'I' form is appropriate. Words are frequently used in overly precise ways that can make speech seem pedantic. Related to this is the observation that autistic individuals regularly make literal interpretations that fail to understand the flexible, metaphorical and often inaccurate use of language by other people (with the result that phrases such as 'I'd like to take a blood sample, can you give me your arm?' can cause considerable confusion and distress). Non-verbal aspects of communication also cause difficulties for autistic people, with the use and appreciation of gesture and facial expression generally diminished. Even where speech may seem superficially normal, there are problems with communicative reciprocity and the pragmatics of social communication. The autistic person frequently does not appreciate the mechanics of turn taking in the conversational round or the needs of the other person for particular types of information to make the encounter understandable and does not understand why others may get tired or frustrated listening to an overlong or overinclusive monologue.

The clinical interview

Clinical interviews generally require *significant involvement from an informant*, ideally one who has a good relationship with the interviewee, who can corroborate aspects of an account (or fill in important gaps) and also act as an emotional support. The interviewer needs to feel comfortable using a *flexible approach*, arranging several *shorter assessment sessions* instead of a single prolonged one (the traditional psychiatric hour can be particularly demanding for patients with LD and may be experienced as aversive or even intolerable), trying to *make the setting and personal approach as friendly as possible* and getting *background information* before the interview begins (providing a framework with anchor points around which the patient can be helped to structure their account). The interviewer should be prepared to *simplify language* and especially *avoid jargon* and be *careful in the use of metaphor* (which is frequently misunderstood or misconstrued). *Sentences should be short* (conveying a single idea at a time) and use the *active rather than passive voice* (for example, 'did you go to make the tea?' rather than 'was the tea made by you?'). The interviewer should be prepared to *rephrase questions* often and *regularly check understanding* if an answer is slow in coming or seems to lack appropriate content. *Open-ended questions* helpfully introduce avenues of inquiry but need to be followed by more *closed questions*, and even *'yes-no'* questions sooner than is usual for non-learning disabled patients.

Box 15.2. Interviewing people with LD

- Involve a key informant
- Gather information in advance
- Shorter sessions with limited scope of enquiry
- Simplify sentence structure and avoid jargon
- Use metaphor and humour with care
- 'Active voice' in sentence construction
- Visual aids
- Rephrasing and checking

Diagnosing psychiatric disorder

Psychiatric disorders are over-represented in people with LD. Prevalence rates vary between studies but on average are increased fourfold compared with the general population (Bernal and Hollins 1995). However, many clinically significant psychiatric problems in LD are either not easily explained in terms of diagnosis or not conveniently classifiable as such. It is therefore common for specialist LD psychiatrists to use broader notions such as 'mental health need' to organise their work.

Learning difficulty is an important psychiatric vulnerability factor, in no small part because the predisposing factors for mental ill health in the general population are more common in LD. Mild LD is strongly associated with economic and social disadvantage: rates of all forms of abuse and exploitation are more common (both in childhood and adult life), and cognitive and communicative problems undermine coping and problem solving. Mild LD in particular is an extremely stressful condition, individuals being much more aware of their difficulties and sensitive to the effects of stigma than those with more severe LD.

A number of psychiatric disorders appear as part of specific genetic syndromes (and causes of LD) and represent *behavioural phenotypes*. Examples include pathological overeating and proneness to Prader-Willi syndrome (partial deletion of chromosome 15), hyperactive and autistic-like behaviour in Fragile X syndrome (expansion of a portion of the X-chromosome involving CGG repeats in the FMR-1 gene, and the most common inherited cause of LD) and autistic behaviours in tuberous sclerosis (an autosomal-dominant disorder with significant physical, neurological and psychiatric morbidity). The study of behavioural phenotypes is a rapidly expanding area, extending outside the field of LD to include behavioural genetics in general. Despite this, it is disappointing that the knowledge available to date has little to say about the *differential* management of these disorders or the types of therapeutic assumption that can be made by knowing that a clinical problem may be part of a behavioural phenotype. Patients and carers often value these labels because they provide causal explanations that avoid blame on upbringing (a worry that haunts many families), act as gateways to syndrome-specific support organisations and peer networks and occasionally justify genetic counselling. Behavioural phenotypes have been extensively reviewed by O'Brien and Yule (1995).

Epilepsy is common in people with LD and, again as with the general population, is an important risk factor for psychiatric disorder. Epilepsy may form part of a wider pattern of neurological impairments, is itself a stigmatising condition and its treatment may have psychiatric adverse effects. These include psychosis with vigabatrin, paradoxical overarousal with phenobarbitone (principally in children), and sedation or confusional states with valproate, carbamazepine and phenytoin.

Psychiatric disorder or 'challenging behaviour'?

Diagnostic overshadowing is the erroneous ascription of emotional or behavioural disturbance in someone with LD to the LD itself (Bernal and Hollins 1995). Problems of diagnostic overshadowing are not unique to LD and similar difficulties are encountered with the assessment of patients with personality disorder or substance misuse.

In contrast, *challenging behaviour* belongs to a different realm of discourse to the language of psychiatric diagnosis. Eric Emerson has provided the most frequently quoted definition:

Severely challenging behaviour refers to culturally abnormal behaviour of such an intensity, frequency or duration that the physical safety of the person or others is likely to be placed in serious jeopardy, or behaviour which is likely to seriously limit use of, or result in the person being denied access to, ordinary community facilities. (Emerson 1995)

This definition emphasises the broadness of what might constitute a challenging behaviour and the need to specify the nature of the challenge, including the wide-ranging personal and social consequences of behavioural disturbance. Challenging behaviour is seen as a social construction, partly dictated by the perceptions of observers (including their acceptance or toleration of behaviour or 'deviance'), partly with the topography of the behaviour itself, and partly with its 'social fit' (the types of opportunities the behaviour precludes access to). Although serious aggression and self-harm generally *do* constitute challenging behaviours, so also do social withdrawal, apathy and self-neglect.

Prevalence rates of severe challenging behaviour vary according to a number of risk factors (Emerson 1998), being relatively more frequent in males, between the ages of 15 and 35, with more severe intellectual impairment, associated with sensory and physical disability and occurring in conjunction with specific syndromes (e.g. autistic spectrum disorders). Prospective studies show that the most severe challenging behaviours appear early in life and are strongly persistent over time.

Psychosis in LD

The full range of psychotic illnesses found in the general population also occurs in people with LD, particularly mild LD, and may occur more frequently. Schizophrenia for instance is believed to have a prevalence of 3%–4%, showing a possible inverse relationship with IQ (Turner 1989), although current diagnostic criteria mean that it cannot be reliably diagnosed below an IQ of about 45. There is continuing controversy about the relationship between schizophrenia and autism (see below). Finally, schizophrenia with its own pattern of cognitive impairments is itself an important cause of 'acquired learning disability'.

Although patients with LD can develop hallucinations and delusions in readily recognisable ways, identifying and interpreting these phenomena can be difficult for the specialist and generalist alike. Despite the frequency with which diagnostic difficulties arise (and the discussions they provoke amongst clinicians), there is remarkably little published literature (empirical or otherwise) on the subject. What follows is a guide based on clinical experience.

> **Box 15.3.** Differential diagnosis of 'psychotic' phenomena in LD patients
>
> - Genuine disclosure (e.g. of abuse)
> - Concrete or rigid interpretations of events
> - Fantasy or wish-fulfilment
> - Self-talk (vocalising thoughts)
> - Imaginary friends
> - Vivid auditory or visual imagery

Take, for example, *delusional thinking*. Well-formed and systematised delusional thinking is relatively uncommon and delusions may present in simpler or less sophisticated ways than is usually seen in general psychiatry. This may be because of difficulty with expressing complicated beliefs but can also reflect problems with complex concept formation in general, as shown in the following case study.

Case Study

John, a 25-year-old man with mild-to-moderate LD, was seen at the day centre he had attended for some years. Staff had noticed that John had become dishevelled and was avoiding mixing with people, preferring to remain on his own at meal times and during group activities. On occasion he would shout out at staff and had even been physically aggressive, behaviour that was considered unusual for him. The visiting psychiatrist spent some time gathering history with the day centre manager. He then arranged to see John in a quiet room with a staff member with whom John previously had a good relationship and whom he still seemed to trust. Though initially appearing guarded and a little suspicious of the psychiatrist, John finally began talking about how people were teasing and picking on him and this made him angry, though he preferred to give his answers to the staff member. He found it hard to give specific examples but was obviously distressed about things and was adamant in his conviction. The psychiatrist was aware that he needed to simplify his use of language considerably and begin talking about more neutral themes (such as how long John had been going to the centre and what sessions he liked best) before John started to open up. Subsequently the staff member told the psychiatrist that he thought it unlikely that John was being victimised as he normally got on well with everyone.

Context is especially important in making judgements about delusional thinking. Although in the above example there are sufficient other abnormalities to weight an assessment in favour of a diagnosis of psychosis, nonetheless there can remain considerable room for doubt and uncertainty even with extensive history taking and mental state examination. Alternative explanations for apparent delusional thinking are:

1. **Disclosure:** in the above example it remains a possibility that other centre users *really are* bullying John. This could easily give rise to the same pattern of withdrawal and irritability for readily understandable reasons. Despite increased awareness and vigilance in the wake of a number of scandals in hospitals and care homes, people with LD are highly vulnerable to exploitation and abuse of all varieties. Although services often (and sadly with good reason even these days) become preoccupied with concerns about possible abuse perpetrated by staff members or carers, the majority of such incidents occur between service users. With the possible exception of clearly bizarre or utterly implausible ideation, the possibility that a patient is making an important disclosure needs to be kept in mind and may well need to be revisited.
2. **Concrete and rigid thinking:** people with LD may be particularly prone to misinterpreting the communications or actions of others because of inflexible styles of thinking. Comments intended to be innocent or humorous may be taken literally and personally.
3. **Fantasy and wish-fulfilment:** patients give rather elaborate accounts with a rather grandiose quality

about achievements of events in their lives that seem highly unlikely but leave the impression that they serve to prop up a fragile sense of self, or are told as a way of establishing status in a group of peers who are likely to accept the story as true.

Case Study

Carl, a 30-year-old man with mild-to-moderate LD, was assessed for counselling sessions following a series of altercations at his day centre. In the course of these Carl told a story that he had been the drummer for a famous pop group, had worked as a *DJ* at a nightclub in Ibiza and had tracked down and killed John Lennon's assassin as an act of retribution because Lennon was his idol. The counsellor independently ascertained that Carl was a big music fan and had built up a large collection of records that he listened to at home avidly. He was especially fond of the Beetles and had a large John Lennon poster over his bed. She also discovered that Carl was a lonely young man who lived with his elderly mother and who had no friends and almost no social life outside his day centre. At the day centre he often got into fights and was seen as something of a bully. In a subsequent session the counsellor challenged Carl's stories. Although he initially continued to defend them he later admitted that sometimes he made things up to impress people. He was anxious that none of his peers should find out.

The assessment of *hallucination* is similarly complicated by other psychological phenomena, often with a strong developmental flavour. *Self-talk*, for example, is frequent in people with LD and, when accompanied by behavioural problems, often provokes referral for assessment for possible psychosis. Self-talk plays an important role in child development, being used to help learn new tasks or for problem-solving. Self-talk becomes internalised with age but persists in some adults with LD where it seems to serve a similar purpose, particularly during periods of anxiety (McGuire 1997). From time to time people may also present with *imaginary friends*, and *vivid internal auditory or visual imagery*.

Mood disorders

As elsewhere in psychiatry, anxiety and depression are the commonest clinical problems in people with LD and, as far as is known, bear similar relationships to genetic and social influences. Nonetheless, some specific points can be made. Diagnosis can be delayed because affective problems may initially present as behavioural problems, which may dominate the clinical picture. Except for people at the mild-to-borderline level of LD, typical depressive thinking and suicidal ideation are unusual. Greater reliance is placed on anhedonia (presenting as loss of interest in usual activities), changes in activity level and other biological symptoms in making the diagnosis (e.g. Collacott *et al.* 1992).

Mania, both in isolation and as part of bipolar disorder, also occurs. Although elation is sometimes seen, clinical experience suggests that irritability and dysphoria may be more common presentations.

Personality disorders

Although generally considered inappropriate as a diagnosis in people with severe LD, personality disorder can still be diagnosed using conventional criteria in those with mild LD. In a recent survey of patients in low- and medium-secure inpatient facilities specialising in LD (Flynn *et al.* 2002), the prevalence of severe personality disorder (defined as subjects meeting ICD-10 criteria for four or more personality disorder diagnoses concurrently) was found to be 39%. Almost all of these patients had emotional instability or severe antisocial behaviour as prominent clinical problems. Importantly, there was a strong association with severe psychosocial adversity (including abuse) in early life helping to confirm the validity of the diagnosis in this patient group. This relationship held even for patients with co-morbid psychosis.

The treatment of cluster B personality disorders in specialist LD services is generally empirical and pragmatic in the same way as for the majority of general psychiatric patients with similar clinical presentations. Because LD is generally an exclusion criterion for most mainstream personality disorder research there has been no formal evaluation of the effectiveness of important treatment settings such as therapeutic community or psychotherapeutic day hospitals, or therapeutic modalities such as dialectical behaviour therapy.

Then again, this difficult-to-manage group of patients can benefit from the general approach to case management that LD services traditionally adopt. Learning disability services take a long-term disability-orientated view of need, usually operate within a framework of mental health needs (rather than severe and enduring mental illness) and also patients can secure services due to the LD itself. Because of these factors there is a tendency for professionals to invest more heavily in engaging and working flexibly and creatively with such patients over protracted periods. For example, Esbensen and Benson (2003) describe a coordinated psychosocial and pharmacological approach to treating a young woman with borderline personality disorder and mild LD. This illustrates well the style of approach used by well-functioning LD services.

Autistic spectrum disorders

Autism was the term first used to describe a case series of children with poor social interaction, anxiety about change, hypersensitivity to sound and apparent good memory skills and who, in addition, seemed to come from families with highly achieving parents (mainly fathers). Although first described in 1943, it was not until the early 1980s that its use as a diagnosis became widespread. Autism has a strong association with LD: 80% of autistic people have LD and, conversely, 17% of those with LD have autism (rising to 27% in those with an IQ below 50).

The core features of autism constitute a triad of impairments:

1. **Disturbed mutual contact:** showing itself as aloofness or sometimes clumsy and indiscriminate 'overfriendliness', betraying a lack of interest

in social interaction or lack of understanding of how to approach others appropriately.

2. **Communication difficulties:** described above.
3. **Limited imagination, insistence on routine and repetitive or stereotyped behaviour:** an early developmental feature of autism involves problems with imaginative or pretend play, with toys used in unusual ways dictated more by their physical or local features than what they represent. Obsessions, routines and rituals are extremely common and are one of the most readily recognisable and disabling features of autism.

Classical autism is an uncommon disorder with a prevalence of about 1 in 2000, with males affected four times as often as females. However, since the early description it has become clear that the disorder lies at one end of a spectrum of pervasive developmental disorders, including Asperger syndrome, but also a variety of other interforms such as semantic-pragmatic disorder and disorders of attention, motor control and perception (DAMP) with different balances of the triad and stronger associations with normal intelligence (see Fitzgerald and Corvin 2001, for a summary).

Family and twin studies show that autistic disorders have a strong genetic component. The parents of autistic children differ from comparison groups with an excess of speech and pragmatic language deficits, problems with friendships, aloofness, rigid thinking and hypersensitivity to criticism (Piven and Palmer 1997; Graham *et al.* 1999). Autism is also associated with specific (and uncommon) medical conditions such as tuberous sclerosis, phenylketonuria, fetal alcohol syndrome and congenital rubella.

People with autistic spectrum disorders are especially prone to suffer anxiety and mood disorders (Sovner 1995), sometimes due to the demands of social interaction and also because of the distress associated with the disruption of routines. Depression in autistic disorders becomes prominent in adolescence, a time when young people begin to become exposed to increased levels of social expectation and responsibility, with pressures to settle on a stable identity. Adolescents with high-functioning autism

can be acutely aware of their difference and inability to fit in during this time.

Aggressive behaviour may result from the sort of personal struggles outlined above, but it perhaps more typically results from attempts to regain control in situations of unanticipated novelty or the removal of obstacles to the completion of routines. The ritualistic behaviours of autism can be phenomenologically distinguished from those in obsessive-compulsive disorder (OCD) by not being experienced as excessive or senseless or as an attempt to ward off a feared consequence. However, they share important biological similarities with, for example, OCD, which is over-represented in the relatives of people with autism; selective serotonin re-uptake inhibitor (SSRI) medications are effective for obsessional behaviour in both autism and OCD; and a significant number of autistic people independently meet diagnostic criteria for OCD (Russell *et al.* 2005).

The relationship between autism and psychotic illness continues to be a matter of debate (Berney 2000). Historically, Bleuler's (1911) use of the term autism as part of the syndrome of schizophrenia preceded its appropriation by Kanner (1943) by almost 50 years. Although transient psychotic symptoms are common in autistic spectrum disorders, there appears to be no major relationship between autism and schizophrenia, at least when the two syndromes are narrowly defined. However, alongside the appreciation that both disorders are dimensional in nature has been the realisation that schizophrenia has important developmental precursors, the disorder arising against a background of abnormal social and emotional development in childhood (e.g. Cannon *et al.* 2001), itself reminiscent of autism-like disorders. More recently, revised diagnostic criteria for schizotypal disorder (Shedler and Westen 2004) overlap considerably with many of the features otherwise attributed to high-functioning autism, notably eccentricity, social anxiety and preoccupation with odd ideas.

Perhaps more interesting than the classificatory issues has been the wider impact of the body of psychological theory that has been developed to explain autism. Most prominent and influential amongst these is the theory that autistic individuals are specifically unable to understand the actions of others in terms of belief, desire and other mental state constructs, a so-called Theory of Mind (ToM) deficit leading to what has been termed mind blindness (Baron-Cohen *et al.* 1985). This inability to adopt the intentional stance (Dennett 1991) towards human behaviour leaves the autistic person relying on more basic types of explanation to work out why other people do the things they do and to plan a response. Not surprisingly, social interactions can become overwhelming and unpredictable, with the result that autistic people prefer to avoid people in favour of, for instance, mechanical objects and computers.

It has long been noted that autistic people may process sensory information in fundamentally different ways, typically focusing on specific details rather than the whole picture. This can be likened to being unable to see the wood for the trees and may account for some difficulties with social understanding, with failures to grasp the gist of what people say or to read the information conveyed by overall facial expression in what has been termed a lack of central coherence. Then again, people with autism can have remarkable abilities to persist with repetitive tasks requiring sustained and accurate attention to small details and can be impervious to visual illusions. The extent to which this fits in with the ToM is unclear, but it has great practical significance because it emphasises that autistic disorders are associated with important potential *strengths* as well as weaknesses (Happé 1999).

Special aspects of clinical management

Pharmacological treatments

Approaches to the use of medication in adults with LD are dictated by the extent to which clinical problems are associated with a psychiatric diagnosis for which pharmacological treatments are well established. However, regardless of diagnosis, some general points can be made about using psychotropic drugs in the presence of LD. Firstly, it is common clinical experience that medications (particularly neuroleptics) may be efficacious at lower doses than generally used in general psychiatry. Secondly, adults with LD can be particularly sensitive to developing side-effects, especially sedative and extrapyramidal side-effects (although this is not invariably the case). The latter may present as a general worsening in posture or mobility in someone with other neurological disabilities, which become more common with more severe cognitive impairment. Anticholinergic drugs may also affect cognitive function through their impact on cholinergic activity in pathways subserving memory. Thirdly, it is common for people with LD to have other important health conditions, epilepsy being especially over-represented. Many psychiatric drugs need to be used with a degree of caution not only because of their propensity to reduce seizure thresholds, but also because of the potential significant drug interactions (e.g. carbamazepine can reduce the bioavailability of clonazepam by up to 50%). It is common practice for LD psychiatrists to start medications at lower than usual doses and titrate upwards relatively slowly. Sometimes a degree of creative thinking is required, for example starting with liquid fluoxetine so that patients can build up from starting doses of 5 or 10 mg daily to avoid nausea and agitation, before transferring to capsules for continuation. Arguably the most important impact of these complications is to alter considerations of the balance between risks and benefits, thus raising the bar for pharmacological intervention.

Where a diagnosis of mental illness can be made, the indications for and uses of psychotropic medication are similar for people with LD to those for anyone else with the same diagnosis. This includes, for example, clozapine for treatment-resistant psychosis (e.g. Antonacci and de Groot 2000, who showed it to be a highly effective and generally well-tolerated drug) and SSRIs in various specific and well-recognised indications including depression, OCD (in high doses) and borderline personality disorder. However, practice largely continues to be based on inferences drawn from evidence in general psychiatric patients and small case series, there being no well-conducted randomised controlled trials (RCTs) of medication for schizophrenia, affective disorders and other mental illnesses that specifically address the issue of LD.

An exception to this are recent RCTs which suggest that a case can be made for the disorder-specific use of low-dose risperidone (McDougle *et al.* 1998) and fluvoxamine (McDougle *et al.* 1996) in adults with autism and LD with significant behavioural problems. However, the relative efficacy of these drugs awaits formal evaluation. One important observation from these studies was that whilst risperidone was helpful in adults and children, fluvoxamine was associated with severe behavioural toxicity (agitation and aggression) in children.

It is common for medication to be used to help manage behavioural problems in situations where no diagnosis can be made. Frequently when this is the case drugs are used outside their licence, a situation that can feel uncomfortable for general psychiatrists and GPs without specialist advice and support. This has, and continues to be, an area of controversy in specialist LD services where there continue to be concerns amongst many patients, carers and some professionals about using drugs as general suppressants of behaviour to the detriment of social and psychological approaches. Nonetheless, used judiciously and as part of a comprehensive care plan, psychotropics play a valuable (and often essential) role.

The drugs most commonly used outside their normal licensed indications are *neuroleptics, lithium and the anticonvulsants*, and, occasionally, *opioid antagonists*.

Neuroleptics are the most researched medications in LD psychiatry (Einfeld 2001). However, a systematic review by Brylewski and Duggan (1999) surprisingly found only three adequate RCTs and these were inconclusive about the benefits. However, there remains considerable lower-level evidence and a strong professional consensus supporting the effectiveness of these drugs across a broad spectrum of behavioural disturbance including aggression and self-injurious behaviour. Nonetheless, because of

the high frequency of adverse effects in LD patients, the older neuroleptics have largely given way to the atypical antipsychotics. Risperidone has been the subject of a small number of RCTs and has found widespread clinical usage for behavioural indications, generally at low doses (less than 2 mg daily) for aggression in LD patients in the absence of autism or psychosis. For example, it has recently been shown to be effective compared with placebo for treating aggression in children with mild LD (Aman *et al.* 2002). A major multi-centre trial to assess its comparative effectiveness compared with haloperidol in adults with LD and aggression (NACHBID) is currently underway.

Carbamazepine and sodium valproate are often employed as alternatives to neuroleptics in the treatment of severe aggression, largely based on trial data in patients without LD. There is no strong consensus at this point on their effectiveness in LD patients and their use is subject to considerable variations in individual practice. Lithium continues to find occasional use as a third-line treatment for severe impulsive aggression and self-injurious behaviour and can be effective where other treatments have failed. In fact, and in contrast to the others, lithium retains behaviour disorder as a licensed indication for its use. Although the evidence base for lithium and aggression is small, it remains more extensive than for the anticonvulsants in LD (e.g. Langee 1990). When effective, it seems to produce a reflective delay that gives the patient the opportunity to put the brakes on impulsive acts.

The opioid antagonist naltrexone is sometimes used to treat severe intractable self-injurious behaviour in adults and children with severe LD. Its use in mild LD is currently rare. It is very unlikely to be used by general psychiatrists.

If a drug treatment seems effective for a behavioural problem, there is still the difficult matter of how long to persist with it. There are no studies looking at long-term recurrence rates during continuation treatment, but the chronic nature of much challenging behaviour prior to treatment biases practice towards carrying on with drugs in the long term. However, most clinicians will consider a careful trial of withdrawal if the problems arose in the context of adverse social circumstances that have since been satisfactorily remedied. A study by Ahmed and colleagues (2000) involving a randomised controlled discontinuation of antipsychotic medication in LD patients where it was used for a behavioural indication found that one-third could achieve full withdrawal and a further 19% could sustain a 50% reduction without recurrence of disturbed behaviour.

Psychological treatments

Psychosocial interventions for people with LD range from social casework, through the various psychotherapies, to approaches involving behavioural and environmental modification. Which approach is used in any one case depends on intellectual and communicative capacities, as well as resource availability. As with pharmacological treatments, there is little systematic evidence from clinical trials for the effectiveness of all forms of psychological intervention in LD, most studies being single cases or small case series from which large bodies of theory and practice have been developed. However, as with drugs, in clinical practice these approaches form an essential part of treatment planning.

Behavioural approaches within LD services are based on contemporary interpretations of operant learning theory, incorporating ideas of positive and negative reinforcement into a framework that also considers the social and physical environment. These methods have generally been developed with the needs of people with severe LD in mind, but their principles have wider application. Emerson (1995) provides a comprehensive and authoritative overview of the field but two key principles can be highlighted.

The first is that behavioural problems have a *social context* and interventions need to be *socially valid*. Behavioural problems may result from impoverished or frankly abusive environments, or lead the individual to descend into such environments with carers resorting to inappropriate (and sometimes retaliatory) interventions. Difficult-to-manage behaviour has an important effect on staff morale in care homes

and on wards that may need to be addressed through additional forms of support such as support groups, training and improved supervision.

These aspects need attention as much as behaviour itself, with outcomes planned and assessed in terms of their value for the individual (perhaps allowing return to a day centre or other increase in opportunities). This is sometimes referred to as the *constructional* approach to behavioural management, in contrast to the more traditional (and perhaps medically orientated) *pathological* approach, which attempts to minimise behaviour in its own right. Although constructional interventions are generally preferred, pathological approaches become necessary, and even essential, in acute and emergency settings where control of a difficult or dangerous situation is paramount (e.g. control and restraint, continuous observation, as-required medication use), or where the behaviour is resistant to functional analysis, outlined below (and techniques such as incentive programmes or differential reinforcement are sometimes necessary). The balance between pathological and constructional approaches changes as patients move towards rehabilitation from acute care.

The second principle is that wherever possible behaviour is seen as *purposive*. That is, it is associated with (and may be an expression of) personal meaning even in the absence of language. Assessing the motivation for behaviour forms part of the so-called *functional analysis of behaviour*, which sees behaviour as an attempt (albeit maladaptive in some instances) at communication. This may be communication of an unpleasant physiological state such as pain (perhaps leading to repetitive head-banging in the case of, say, toothache), a need for food or a desire for social contact and attention. Treatment involves educating carers about what is being communicated, thinking through how best to meet those needs and helping the person learn better ways of getting their point across (where possible through the development of some vocabulary, spoken or signed, or by using systems of tokens or pictures). Although the validity of viewing behaviour as communication may be a philosophical point, functional analysis provides a powerful way of reframing behaviour for carers (including ward staff) who may have become emotionally blunted in the face of recurrent aggression (perhaps directed at them) or self-injury and who may have taken to responding in stereotyped and unhelpful ways.

As cognitive level increases, it becomes appropriate to use language-based psychological interventions, and there is growing interest in psychodynamic and cognitive-behavioural therapies (CBT) for people with LD. In fact, although the functional analysis model outlined above is intended for severe LD, it resonates strongly with aspects of psychodynamic theory, where acting out behaviours are seen as non-verbal expressions of unconscious impulses that have bypassed the scrutiny of an ego deficient in language to frame and manage them. Again, there is as yet no strong body of evidence to support the use of these psychotherapies, the literature at this point being mainly concerned with how methods can be modified for this group of patients. In the case of CBT, a manual has been published (Stenfert Kroese *et al.* 1997) but formal clinical trials are likely to wait on wider clinical experience within services.

The principal modifications for CBT lie in the balance between the cognitive and behavioural components, with an emphasis on self-monitoring, self-control, coping and problem-solving. Most patients with LD lack the ability to adequately describe and differentiate emotional states (which often need to be reduced to 'good' and 'bad' moods). They are unable to write well enough to keep the detailed diaries of distorted thinking that are usually associated with CBT in adults without LD. It is more realistic to use simple recording methods which the person can use with a carer to help them keep track of particular behaviours, perhaps employing a simple pictorial scale for mood ratings, which can be used to foster a habit of personal reflection and inform discussion in therapy sessions. Cognitive restructuring most often takes the form of practising alternative behaviours or self-instructional statements for use in situations where a problem behaviour is likely to appear (e.g. educating patients to use procedures such as 'counting to ten' or saying to themselves 'just walk away' when feeling provoked).

For many LD patients concerns about the technical specifics of different verbal psychotherapies may be less important than their ability to act as vehicles for therapeutic relationships. People with LD, and particularly *milder* LD, frequently have low expectations of themselves and others, have trouble making and sustaining adaptive friendships and often feel marginalised and undervalued by society and even their own families. The evidence base for the effectiveness of psychodynamic therapies in LD is small. However, psychodynamic theory (and especially attachment theory) plays an essential role in informing general approaches to understanding and supporting people with LD as well as helping professional teams with the sorts of diverse theoretical orientations and priorities that LD work engenders to maintain a coherent outlook.

Mental health and mental capacity legislation

Patients with LD may, of course, be liable to detention in hospital if they satisfy the criteria and standards set out in the 1983 Mental Health Act in England and Wales, and its counterparts in Scotland and Northern Ireland. It is not known whether people with LD are over-represented amongst detention orders, but it is common for LD services (for various reasons, including philosophies of care and difficulties with access to acute beds) to resort to hospital admission only in extreme circumstances, when the need to use the Mental Health Act becomes more likely. On the whole, admissions of LD patients *by LD services* are uncommon events (in many districts amounting to only a handful each year), with Mental Health Act assessments less common still. This low incidence creates special challenges. Lack of practice inevitably leads to some atrophy of processes and relationships, especially between LD services on the one hand and admission wards and Approved Social Workers (who, with occasional exceptions, reside in the general adult service and whose area of expertise lies with severe and enduring mental illness) on the other.

Patients with LD only need show evidence of mental disorder (with concomitant risk and necessity for hospitalisation) for detention for *assessment*; difficulties arise when a decision has to be made about *continued* detention for *treatment* and it becomes necessary to specify a legal diagnostic category. The legal categories of mental illness and the troublesome psychopathic disorder apply to patients with LD, but there are also options to use mental impairment or severe mental impairment (differing from each other only in the substitution of 'severe impairment of intelligence' for 'significant impairment of intelligence' in their legal descriptions).

These legal categories are generally reserved for individuals with serious challenging (including offending) behaviour. Mental impairment carries a similar burden to psychopathic disorder in that a case for treatability needs to be made, a hurdle absent for severe mental impairment.

For professionals working in the UK, the final implications of the Bournewood Judgement remain uncertain for non-detained LD patients in hospital. The case, involving a man with severe LD admitted informally as an emergency to a psychiatric unit because of disturbed behaviour, achieved notoriety because the man's (adoptive) family had fundamental objections to his admission, which they saw as undermining their commitment to caring for him, objections they have pursued vigorously since, principally on the grounds that his admission amounted to illegal detention.

A recent review of the case in the European Court of Human Rights (*H.L.* v. the *United Kingdom* 2004) appears to reverse the judgement of the Law Lords that patients may be regarded as informal patients in the absence of their informed consent to remain in hospital provided they do not show or declare a clear intention to leave and acquiesce to their treatment. The European Court has ruled that H.L.'s detention in hospital as an informal patient contravened Section 5(1) of the European Convention on Human Rights. However, because the so-called Bournewood gap is principally an issue for patients with *severe* LD (who

are almost never in a position to give or withhold consent) rather than mild LD (where it is generally easier to be sure that compliance with care is with consent rather than the product of passive acquiescence), it is not a situation the general psychiatrist will encounter often. Interim NHS guidance following Bournewood pending further consultation is available through the Department of Health website.

In English law, capacity is always assumed for adults unless there is evidence to the contrary, a position that is independent of the diagnosis of LD or mental disorder. However, the presence of LD invariably has an impact on someone's ability to take complex decisions with the result that the assessment of mental capacity is something that regularly exercises specialist LD services. Nonetheless, the considerations are identical to those for patients with other mental disorders. For any decision to be the result of informed consent it must be expressed in the context of capacity (or competence) and without coercion. Capacity itself rests on an individual having access to appropriate information and being able to weigh that information in the balance. It is a fluid construction, influenced by a balance between personal characteristics (such as cognitive abilities), quality of information (including how that information is conveyed) and also the seriousness of the decision being made (bigger decisions needing correspondingly greater capacity), so that a person's capacity is enhanced or undermined according to circumstance.

The Mental Capacity Act 2005 (which came into force in April 2007) is an attempt to render into UK statute Common Law principles of good practice (in particular best interests, least restrictive intervention, presumption of capacity and the right to make eccentric or unwise decisions) in the assessment of capacity. It provides new mechanisms for proxy decision-making in those deemed to lack capacity in a particular area and applies to all areas not covered by Part IV of the Mental Health Act 1983. Perhaps the most significant development within the Act is a new power for courts to appoint deputies who may give consent on behalf of an incapacitated person on health and social welfare matters. This is a major departure from the longstanding doctrine that no one can give consent on behalf of any adult, and its operation will be the subject of much scrutiny. A draft code of practice has been published, but it remains to be seen how the new Act will operate in practice.

Generic or specialist inpatient services?

The UK has a unique tradition of recognising the psychiatric care of people with LD as a specialist area of training and practice, with its own certification process for psychiatrists completing higher professional training. Whilst most specialist LD psychiatrists opt to complete higher training solely in the specialist psychiatry of LD, a growing number are additionally training in general, forensic or child psychiatry, in part as an acknowledgement of the difficulties that exist at the interfaces between services. People with *mild* LD are a group particularly at risk of falling into gaps.

In the wake of deinstitutionalisation, the development of specialist psychiatric services for people with LD has become a difficult and contentious area. UK public policy actively supports the principle of mainstream access to services for people with LD, whether that be education, leisure or work opportunities or health (including mental health) care. The recent UK Government White Paper Valuing People (Department of Health 2001) sets out the role for LD services in meeting this goal and forms the framework for assessing their performance and allocating resources. There has been no formal attempt to reconcile Valuing People with the template outlined in the National Service Framework for Mental Health but there is now the expectation that people with mild LD will receive their mental health care through generic services, with the support of specialist LD services, unless there is a clear need for a more specialist (and, by implication, separate) service. The question arises, for the purposes of this discussion, as to when it becomes appropriate for someone with LD to be admitted to a *specialist LD-orientated* psychiatric unit.

In a recent systematic review, Chaplin (2004) highlighted a worrying paucity of research to help decide the issue or inform the development of services. Furthermore, the nature of acute admission wards has changed in recent years, with an increasing emphasis on their use for severe and enduring mental illness, short duration of stay, and pressures on staff to respond to crises. Patients with LD can pose considerable difficulties for units with rapid patient turnover and hard-pressed staff, who may find that they now have less time to devote to patients with communication impairments and who do not fit easily with contemporary general psychiatric models. Learning difficulty patients can also find it hard to participate in ward-based group activities. Finally, patients with LD can form a particularly vulnerable group on a busy ward, and are often victims of assault or exploitation by other patients.

For acute or emergency psychiatric admissions, there is little alternative to the acute psychiatric ward in almost all districts. Nonetheless, with appropriate support arrangements most admissions of people with LD to such wards are successful (Chaplin and Flynn 2000).

In some cases the LD component is a minor part of the overall clinical picture and patients can fit into the usual ward routine in a reasonably straightforward way. These patients are often looked after entirely within generic psychiatric services with little recourse to specialist advice or support.

Where LD is a *significant* complicating issue some sort of additional consideration is needed, and these patients will often have involvement from the multidisciplinary community learning disability team (CLDT). The CLDT provides a range of health and social care support, of which mental health is only one (and not necessarily the major) component. Apart from the consultant psychiatrist and psychologist, most CLDT staff do not have *specific* training in mental health care, although some will have developed a degree of expertise in this area. For example, LD nursing has a separate qualification to mental health nursing with only a small degree of overlap, and it is unusual for the LD social worker to be additionally trained as an Approved Social Worker or 'ASW' and so able to make applications under the Mental Health Act. Successful admission in this case relies on good working relationships between the ward and the LD service, including agreements about admission protocols.

Good working relationships in this context require a commitment by psychiatric staff on general wards, PICU and LSUs to work positively with LD patients and by the CLDT to actively (and visibly) support the ward in this effort. Sometimes this need only be advice and participation in discharge planning, but the CLDT can also often provide additional hands-on individual support for patients to help maintain or develop skills, become engaged with activities and reduce vulnerability. It is essential to have clarity about Resident Medical Officer ('RMO') responsibility, with different arrangements existing in different districts. In some, the LD consultants retain responsibility for their own inpatients throughout the admission episode whilst in others this role passes to the catchment area general psychiatrist until discharge. Issues of joint working and clinical responsibility may need to be supported by local agreed protocols. This becomes necessary where acute LD admissions are infrequent (probably the majority of inpatient units) and care arrangements are inevitably under-rehearsed.

There are times, however, when a patient with LD requires continuing care in a specialist LD unit able to provide a more appropriate therapeutic environment. In these cases, the patient's route to specialist care is often necessarily via the acute ward. This is because the need for specialist care may only become apparent during the course of an acute admission or because a patient needs initial local admission so that a safe transfer can subsequently be effected. There are relatively few such units in the NHS, a deficiency that has represented a significant business opportunity for the private sector. Specialist units are frequently geographically distant from the patient's area of residence, are geared towards long-term work (6–24 months), are rehabilitative in outlook and vary in their level of security and requirements for patients to be detained under the Mental Health Act.

Reasonable indications for transfer to a specialist unit include:

1. The patient needs *continued* detention for mental impairment or severe mental impairment, with or without psychopathic disorder. This will generally equate with severe challenging behaviour not secondary to major mental illness, including much offending behaviour such as serious recurrent violence, fire-setting or sex offending.

2. Patients with a significant degree of autism tend to have considerable difficulties on acute general wards because of the social intensity of the environment and insistence on routines (which may appear odd or idiosyncratic) that can be disruptive for general ward management. Active consideration should be given to transfer unless it is clear that admission will only be for a short period and the patient can be safely supported.

3. Patients with *severe* LD are rarely admitted to hospital and fit especially uncomfortably with acute wards. Brief admission may be necessary and appropriate for stabilisation of a pharmacological regime or, very rarely, interventions such as electroconvulsive therapy. These patients will almost always require one-to-one support on the ward and *prolonged* admission episodes should prompt consideration for referral.

4. Where PICU-type care is needed this should also initially be to the local generic service. This is as much a matter of necessity as of principle, with LD-specific PICUs being very rare. The PICU's role in such situations will be to help stabilise severely disturbed behaviour so that a decision about continuing care can be made. This may involve admission to a specialist bed if, say, the patient has a clear diagnosis of psychosis.

Conclusion

Recommendations like the ones above are inevitably impressionistic and their operation depends heavily on the configuration of mental health and LD services in a local area, the level of harmony between services and the attitudes of purchasers towards the mental health needs of people with LD. Unfortunately, they are not able to rely on much in the way of objective evidence. The development of specialist LD mental health services is hampered by a small evidence base and the low profile of LD patients with psychiatric disorders in national and local service priorities. Fascinating though it is as a specialism, LD psychiatry is perceived as neither fashionable nor, despite the ideological drive towards inclusiveness behind documents such as Valuing People, truly part of the mainstream.

In the absence of alternatives, patients with LD will continue to be admitted and maintained on acute psychiatric wards/PICUs and, in many cases, it is quite appropriate that this should be the case. Many of the skills needed to support people with mild LD, such as good communication skills, are indeed *generic*, and form part of the clinical competencies of all mental health professionals. It is however understandable that growing pressures on general psychiatrists and their colleagues to spend less and less time with more and more patients should result in disputes about where patients with mild LD ought to belong.

Generic services should seek help and advice from their local LD service, which should be prepared to provide active support if mainstream access is to be any more than a politically correct catchphrase. CLDTs have a responsibility to keep up to date on important mental health issues that may affect their work and to develop an understanding of the culture of, and pressures on, their local general psychiatric service. Arrangements to maintain these links when there are no LD patients on the ward should be considered, perhaps through training arrangements, shared posts and joint project work.

Then again, no matter how well set up a generic ward is, there will remain a subgroup of LD patients who need and deserve to have their care within a dedicated and specialist service and who should not have to endure their 'round pegs' being bashed into 'square holes'.

REFERENCES

Ahmed Z, Fraser W, Kerr MP *et al*. 2000 Reducing antipsychotic medication in people with a learning disability. Br J Psychiatry 176: 42–46

Aman MG, De Smedt G, Derivan A *et al*. 2002 Double-blind, placebo-controlled study of risperidone for the treatment of disruptive behaviours in children with sub-average intelligence. Am J Psychiatry 159: 1337–1346

Antonacci DJ, de Groot CM. 2000 Clozapine treatment in a population of adults with mental retardation. J Clin Psychiatry 61: 22–25

Baron-Cohen S, Leslie AM, Frith U. 1985 Does the autistic child have a 'theory of mind'? Cognition 21: 27–43

Bernal J, Hollins S. 1995 Psychiatric illness and learning disability: a dual diagnosis. Adv Psychiatr Treat 1: 138–145

Berney TP. 2000 Autism – an evolving concept. Br J Psychiatry 176: 20–25

Bleuler E. 1911 Dementia praecox or the group of schizophrenias (translated 1950 by J. Zinkin). New York: International Universities Press

Brylewski J, Duggan L. 1999 Antipsychotic medication for challenging behaviour in people with intellectual disability: a systematic review of randomised control trials. J Intellect Disabil Res 43: 360–371

Cannon M, Walsh E, Hollis C *et al*. 2001 Predictors of later schizophrenia and affective psychosis among attendees at a child psychiatry department. Br J Psychiatry 178: 420–426

Carpenter PK. 2002 Should there be a faculty of learning disability psychiatry? Psychiatr Bull 26: 83–84

Chaplin R. 2004 General psychiatric services for adults with learning disability and mental illness. J Intellect Disabil Res 48: 1–10

Chaplin R, Flynn A. 2000 Adults with learning disability admitted to psychiatric wards. Adv Psychiatr Treat 6: 128–134

Collacott R, Cooper SA, McGrother C. 1992 Differential rates of psychiatric disorders in adults with Down's syndrome compared with other mentally handicapped adults. Br J Psychiatry 161: 671–674

Dacey CM, Nelson WM 3rd, Stoeckel J. 1999 Reliability, criterion-related validity and qualitative comments of the fourth Edition of the Stanford-Binet Intelligence Scale with a young adult population with intellectual disability. J Intellect Disabil Res 43: 179–184

Dennett D. 1991 Consciousness Explained. Boston, MA: Little Brown

Department of Health. 2001 Valuing People: A New Strategy for Learning Disability for the 21st Century. London: HMSO

Einfeld SL. 2001 Systematic management approach to pharmacotherapy for people with learning disabilities. Adv Psychiatr Treat 7: 43–49

Emerson E. 1995 *Challenging Behaviour: Analysis and Intervention in People with Learning Disabilities.* Cambridge: Cambridge University Press

Emerson E. 1998 People with challenging behaviour. In: Emerson E, Hatton C, Bromley J, Caine A (eds.) Clinical Psychology and People with Intellectual Disabilities. Chichester: Wiley

Esbensen AJ, Benson BA. 2003 Integrating behavioural, psychological and pharmacological treatment: a case study of an individual with borderline personality disorder and mental retardation. Mental Health Aspects Dev Disabil 6: 107–113

Fitzgerald M, Corvin A. 2001 Diagnosis and differential diagnosis of Asperger syndrome. Adv Psychiatr Treat 7: 310–318

Flynn A, Matthews H, Hollins S. 2002 Validity of the diagnosis of personality disorder in adults with learning disability and severe behavioural problems. Br J Psychiatry 180: 543–546

Fryers T. 1997 Impairment, disability and handicap: categories and classifications. In: Russell O (ed) *Seminars in the Psychiatry of Learning Disabilities.* London: Gaskell, pp. 16–30

Graham P, Turk J, Verhulst FC. 1999 Neurodevelopmental and neuropsychiatric disorders: pervasive developmental disorders. In: Child Psychiatry: A Developmental Approach. Oxford: Oxford University Press, pp. 120–131

Gudjonsson GH, Clare I. 1986 Suggestibility in police interrogation: a social psychology model. Soc Behav 1: 83–104

Happé F. 1999 Understanding assets and deficits in autism: why success is more interesting than failure. Psychologist 12: 540–547

Kanner L. 1943 Autistic disturbances of affective contact. Nervous Child 2: 217–250

Langee HR. 1990 Retrospective study of lithium use for institutionalised mentally retarded individuals with behaviour disorders. Am J Mental Retard 94(4): 448–452

McDougle CJ, Naylor ST, Cohen DJ, Volkmar FR, Heninger GR, Price LH. 1996 A double-blind, placebo-controlled study of fluvoxamine in adults with autistic disorder. Arch Gen Psychiatry 53: 1001–1008

McDougle CJ, Holmes JP, Carlson DC, Pelton GH, Cohen DJ, Price LH. 1998 A double-blind, placebo-controlled study of risperidone in adults with autistic disorder and other pervasive developmental disorders. Arch Gen Psychiatry 55: 633–641

McGuire DE. 1997 'Self-Talk' in adults with Down syndrome. Disabil Solut 2 [Issue 2] [http://www.altonweb.com/cs/downsyndrome/agetalk.html]

O'Brien G, Yule W. 1995 *Behavioural Phenotypes.* Cambridge: McKeith Press

Piven J, Palmer P. 1997 Cognitive deficits in parents from multiple-incidence autism families. J Child Psychol Psychiatry 38: 1011–1021

Russell AJ, Mataix-Cols D, Anson M, Murphy D. 2005 Obsessions and compulsions in Asperger syndrome and high-functioning autism. Br J Psychiatry 186: 525–528

Shedler J, Westen D. 2004 Refining personality disorder diagnosis: integrating science and practice. Am J Psychiatry 161: 1350–1365

Sovner R. 1995 Autism spectrum disorder and affective illness. Habilitative Healthcare Newsletter 14: 53–55

Stenfert Kroese B, Dagnan D, Loumidis K. (eds). 1997 Cognitive-Behavioural Therapy for People with Learning Disabilities. London: Routledge

Turner T. 1989 Schizophrenia and mental handicap: an historical overview, with implications for further research. Psychol Med 19: 301–314

Whitaker S. 2003 Should we abandon the concept of mild learning disability? Clin Psychol 29: 16–19

16

The interface with general psychiatric services

Trevor Turner

Introduction

The development of Psychiatric Intensive Care Units (PICUs) as originally outlined some years ago (Beer, *et al.* 1997) has very much followed an ad hoc pattern, depending on local demand and local champions. Likewise, the way in which individual PICUs have become embedded in the provision of general psychiatric services, to a defined catchment area or district, has not been systematically studied. The location of units varies, from being part of an acute general hospital with other wards on site, to stand-alone buildings, within or outside a general or mental hospital area. A further problem is that there has been no established consensus as to the siting or size of adult psychiatric inpatient units, although the Royal College of Psychiatrists' Report, Not Just Bricks and Mortar (Royal College of Psychiatrists, 1998), attempted to look at these issues in the context of new developments and their appropriate conformation, staffing and setting. Of course, general psychiatric services are much more than just 'bricks and mortar', their components being a comprehensive provision of care for individuals with a wide range of disorders, and thus requiring a combination of diagnostic and treatment skills, with multidisciplinary staffing, for both inpatient and community-based services. It is now generally accepted that a pragmatic balance of both community and hospital services is necessary in all areas (Thornicroft and Tansella

2004), and that general adult psychiatry must integrate care, as seamlessly as possible, from the GP surgery to the inpatient unit, and back out into the community.

The Royal College of Psychiatrists' recommendations (1998) can be summarised as follows with regard to psychiatric inpatient units in general.

1. Clinicians, users, other local stakeholders (e.g. relevant voluntary groups) and carers should all be involved in developing the project and drawing up operational policies.

2. Ideal ward sizes, whether PICU or general acute, are between ten and fifteen beds. Stand-alone units should be between three and five wards in size, with the design standards of a comfortable modern hotel, not exceeding two storeys, and with an associated landscape area. Single bedrooms should be the norm.

3. Units are best sited on a district general hospital (DGH) campus, with their own entrance, with security an integral factor in all aspects of design, and with appropriate staffing (e.g. nurses, doctors, therapists), suitable for safety and therapy.

4. Appropriate policies in terms of single-sex accommodation (the disadvantages of purely single sex-wards are emphasised), air conditioning and cigarette smoking, and intensive care provision, need to be in place. In the latter regard 'intensive care provision should be designed into all new units'.

Psychiatric Intensive Care, 2nd edn., eds. M. Dominic Beer, Stephen M. Pereira and Carol Paton.
Published by Cambridge University Press. © Cambridge University Press 2008

5. Appropriate training, leave arrangements, liaison with local police and other agencies, and agreed protocols and guidelines should be part and parcel of the unit's organisation and development.

Alongside modern, safe and appropriately designed units, what else do general adult services provide? Again, there is no established consensus, but it is assumed that general adult psychiatrists will be part of multidisciplinary teams able to provide the following at least:

1. Assessment and treatment in primary care (e.g. GP liaison clinics), in community mental health teams (CMHTs), in outpatient clinics, and (if necessary) in the patient's home.

2. Provision of day hospital and day centre (continuing care) facilities, alongside a range of non-acute residential units, from the temporary 'halfway house', to medium and high dependence supported placements.

3. An active inpatient and community-orientated rehabilitation service, providing continuing care for those with chronic illnesses as well as acute-on-chronic relapses.

4. Team-based approaches, in particular local, comprehensive and multidisciplinary CMHTs, linking ward and community resources, applied to a specific catchment area and working with local GPs. Catchment area size will depend on location and socioeconomic indices, varying from 15 000 to 10 0000 in population, but increasingly tending towards the lower end.

5. The provision of crisis intervention, early intervention and assertive outreach teams, integrated (depending on local variety and need) with the CMHTs and acute wards, usually via agreed interface arrangements.

6. An associated psychotherapy/psychological treatments service, operating either via secondary or tertiary referral processes, again depending on local agreement.

7. A number of areas will have more specialist units, often providing treatment resources for a number of districts, for example mother and baby (perinatal) units, eating disorders units, specialist psychotherapeutic day hospitals, and alcohol and/or drug rehabilitation units. The latter are now increasingly located in the private sector.

Interface issues

Given the comprehensive nature of modern general services, and their ever-changing configuration, it has not been easy to research or clarify the integration of a PICU service. What follows therefore is a personal overview of current problems and practice based on over 20 years of working within an inner city, community-focused service. This analysis has been made more difficult by the vexed interface between general adult and forensic services, there being considerable overlap between patients found in general adult wards and Medium Secure Units (MSUs). This is partly due to the differing attitudes of local courts, partly due to bed availability, but certainly related to the rising tide of more complex patients detained under the Mental Health Act, especially in urban areas (Fitzpatrick *et al.* 2003). The apparent reluctance of police and courts to prosecute those with mental illness, not least because of the rising burden of mentally ill prisoners (Birmingham 2003), has exacerbated this problem. With plans afoot to enhance inreach by CMHTs into local prisons (Department of Health 2001), it is likely that these dilemmas will be exacerbated.

As a result in some areas the local PICU may even be managed by the forensic directorate rather than the local general adult directorate, and even within a given trust (particularly the larger mental health trusts that have emerged over the last 4 years) there may be differing policies. An internal survey in East London revealed significantly different lengths of stay, depending on whether or not the PICU was used for true 'intensive care' or as an available locked unit for forensic assessments. There has been a persistent view, from the forensic perspective, that a PICU bed can be seen as a form of low secure provision, and thus mentally disturbed prisoners may be transferred for assessment, usually via court orders. The Department of Health (2002) Policy Guidance did in fact implicitly link the two approaches, but defined low secure as for those patients requiring 'the provision of security' and 'needing rehabilitation usually for up to 2 years'.

Such usage does not fit with the perception amongst general psychiatrists that PICU should be primarily for true intensive care (i.e. extra nursing in a specifically designed environment), rather than merely for security to suit legal requirements. From the general adult perspective therefore, PICU is considered as an integrated part of a flexible range of inpatient resources designed to look after all types and phases of mental illness. Whether perceived as a pyramidal structure, with a broad range of outreach, home-based and primary care services at the base, moving on to day hospital and day patient care, then to acute general wards and then to the 'pinnacle' of PICU, or whether a PICU is seen as an associated resource of an effective acute psychiatric hospital, the essence of PICU/adult general ward arrangements should be *interface invisibility*. That is to say, assuming a patient-centred model, and an approach as classically outlined in the archetypal Reed Report (Department of Health and Home Office 1992), patients should be cared for as near to home as possible and in the least restrictive environment. Likewise the National Service Framework (Department of Health 1999) notes under Standard Five that patients shall have 'timely access to an appropriate hospital bed . . . in the least restrictive environment consistent with the need to protect them and the public – as close to home as possible'.

It follows from this that all PICU services should be part and parcel of general adult provision, with the PICU consultant (and it is accepted by most general adult consultants that each PICU should have an independent lead consultant) working with his/her colleagues in as flexible a way as possible. The more the formalities for admission and discharge from PICU, the less the patients' needs can be quickly dealt with. Certain basic principles emerge from this approach in terms of what general adult psychiatric consultants and services should reasonably expect from their PICU colleagues.

1. A bed should always be available for acutely disturbed patients, because, by definition, the most acutely ill patients in any unit should, in essence, be cared for in the local PICU.

2. Such availability demands that every patient on PICU should have an agreed, updated care plan and contingency transfer plan, enabling the least disturbed quickly to be taken back to their locality ward without disruption to their treatment.

3. This responsive availability also requires close and constant cooperation between senior medical and nursing staff, all being prepared to accept that there is a quid pro quo that enables urgent transfer of a severely ill patient with (often) reciprocal transfer back of a less unwell patient. In my view such transfers are best nurse-led rather than consultant-led, nurses being in the front line of day-to-day care, and consultants not necessarily being available.[1]

4. This flexibility of transfer requires absolute trust between colleagues, and this can be reinforced by intermittently joining in ward rounds across the general ward/PICU boundary, regular joint discussions on management of patients (e.g. via case conferences) and acceptance that the PICU consultant is only Resident Medical Officer for all aspects of a patient's care while they are in PICU. This will include medication, Care Programme Approach (CPA) meetings, Mental Health Act assessments, and tribunals, and even early leave arrangements, by agreement with the CMHT, who must be prepared to attend PICU-based CPA meetings. Once transferred out of PICU the locality CMHT and consultant should take on all of these tasks.

5. Direct admission to PICU, and even direct discharge, should be available, again by agreed arrangements with the CMHT and relevant consultant. Again, the principle of such arrangements should always be the answer to the question, 'where will this patient best be cared for in our unit?'.

---

[1] This acceptance of nursing responsibility reflects both the traditional role of the consultant as treatment adviser to a ward (not manager or 'in charge of') and the modern partnership of true multidisciplinary working.

6. The role of the PICU consultant in terms of relating to his/her general colleagues will vary. Some will take on an attached Emergency Clinic, with an outpatient role, but it is generally accepted that they should not be responsible for a catchment area, GP liaison clinics or regular outreach services. Specific expertise in modern therapeutics, as well as skills in acute tranquillisation, will be assumed, but some individuals may take on additional roles.

7. Managing the flexibility of PICU/ward interface issues probably requires daily PICU ward rounds and multidisciplinary reviews if joint assessments are required. Likewise, the provision of reports, initial discharge summaries, and information to carers/relatives should be the role of PICU staff until transfer has taken place.

8. To ensure that the processes of admission and transfer do not lead to arguments or concerns about 'cherry-picking' or inappropriate practice, regular review by all ward managers, ideally led by an experienced nurse consultant and involving the Clinical Director, will be required so as to work through individual patient problems and general guideline issues.

9. Reconciliation procedures in cases of dispute, especially if an untoward incident occurs (e.g. injury to a nurse or an at-risk patient going absent without leave) should be established and given an agreed priority and supervisor. In modern clinical governance terms, the results of any serious untoward incident (SUI) should be used to inform and educate all those involved.

Protocols and guidelines

It has been generally accepted that all wards, whether general or specialist, should have documented and established policy guidelines, and this is now extended to the more general area of National Institute for Health and Clinical Excellence (NICE) guidelines for a range of conditions. The evidence for the effectiveness of guidelines, unfortunately, remains rather thin, and 'what passes today for the standards of clinical care – thousands of practice guidelines, often conflicting sometimes disreputable . . . is a mess' (Reilly 2004). Nevertheless, it is generally accepted that some form of written contract, agreeing the principles of interface arrangements between wards and CMHTs, wards and specialist teams, or different areas of the service does provide some useful ground rules. The most basic of these within psychiatry currently is the 'catchment area', a unique division of responsibility that does not apply to any other specialities in the NHS.

The reason for establishing separate catchment areas has not been widely explored in the public debate about protocols and guidelines, but is usefully indicative of the dilemmas faced by general adult psychiatric teams. In particular, although not uniquely, psychiatric patients can be very difficult to deal with both physically and emotionally, especially mentally disordered offenders (Birmingham 2003). By agreeing on a particular (geographical) area of responsibility, it has been possible to ensure that locality teams deal with their own 'local' problem patients, rather than shift them off via nefarious transfers to someone else. This of course still happens, given the increased transiency of some patients (Fitzpatrick *et al.* 2003), but defined and continuing financial and care responsibility are documented. The role of the Care Programme Approach (CPA) has been part of the ongoing attempt to stabilise this area of practice. This agreement on borders and responsibilities has generally been effective (although often misunderstood by non-psychiatrists and GPs), even though the more mobile population of the inner city tends to create considerable difficulties for hard-pressed urban acute psychiatric units. It is in this context that the relationship between the general psychiatry side, in particular the acute wards, and PICU becomes extremely sensitive.

The dilemma around protocols and/or guidelines, if used religiously to decide who should go to a PICU, who should be transferred and so forth, is that they may not allow for the individual variations in patients, ward teams (whose competence may vary, particularly if there are bank staff working) and the capacity of a given PICU. While it is reasonable to have a broad outline of the kind of patient who should be transferred to a PICU, this should, generally, be a flexible guideline rather than something set in stone. For example, key features, from the general perspective, of the kind of patient who would probably require transfer to a PICU would include the following.

1. Threatening or assaultative behaviours that cannot be contained by the staff on a general ward, either because of limited staff numbers or limited staff experience.

2. The need for additional nursing staff to observe and/or manage and/or interact with a given patient, whether for mental health, physical health or security needs.

3. Substantial risk of absconding from the open ward, leading to at-risk behaviours, either in terms of self-harm or harm to others.

4. In association with all of the above the presence of a severe mental illness, usually requiring detention and treatment under the Mental Health Act (but not necessarily so), that is likely to be treatable within a psychiatric ward.

5. The acceptance that there should be no absolute exclusions, since a PICU should be prepared to accept any patient that has been admitted to a general psychiatric ward.

Given that a patient fits such criteria, who should decide on the transfer? While some consultants insist on reviewing all admissions, it is increasingly being accepted that senior and front-line nurses have a much more nuanced understanding of patients' needs within the ward context. They will know if their team can handle a particular patient, and constant liaison between acute wards and the PICU team (on a daily basis if necessary, or even more frequently) will be required to ensure the right balance of transfer and continuing care. As outlined above, the key to a positive relationship between acute general wards and PICU will be the acceptance that transfer of a 'difficult' or 'unmanageable' patient will often be met by the equivalent transfer back of another patient, who may still be exhibiting some problems in terms of management, but who will be, by definition, less in need of PICU and its specific staffing and security environment. Furthermore many patients are well known to hospitals and it may need merely the mention of a given name to set in train an agreed transfer.

There will of course always be disputes. An effective acute psychiatric unit (i.e. the combination of a PICU and the surrounding acute wards and related CMHTs and other teams) will have a dispute-resolution system set up. This may involve a nurse consultant, the senior duty nurse, the clinical director or duty consultant, or even the medical director. Again, laying down the rules as to who should be involved is much less important than having a local and agreed system of avoiding, working through, and continuing to monitor any disputed care arrangements. In fact, it is probably worth considering a disputed care arrangement between a PICU and a general ward as a form of near-miss SUI. Investigation, discussion, audit if necessary and regular review of such incidents should be used as a means of minimising their occurrence, ongoing training and enhancing the quality of patient care.

PICU and special problems (rehabilitation, personality disorder and substance misuse)

The relationship between general adult psychiatry and other specialities, for example substance misuse services, forensic services, learning difficulties and rehabilitation, has been carefully reviewed via a series of Interface documents prepared by the Royal College of Psychiatrists. These are not meant to be prescriptive, but do try to lay down practical ground rules as to how such services should interact. This has been a particularly problematic factor for general psychiatry, which has tended to be left holding the baby as specialist services have drawn up clear limits as to who they will and will not see. In addition forensic services have been severely restricted by financial considerations and the limited number of beds available in expensive MSUs. This tendency for difficult and multiply diagnosed patients (e.g. those with psychosis, substance misuse *and* a degree of personality disorder) to be left in the hands of general adult services, and particularly general adult wards, has been cited as a key factor in the comparative unpopularity of general psychiatry within the profession. Depending on area, some 10%–15% of consultant jobs are unfilled, and the role of the consultant is being closely reviewed, particularly by the General Adult Faculty of the College.

Given that patients have a range of illness levels and chronicity of impairment, rehabilitation and management of substance misuse and personality disorder tend to be part and parcel of routine general adult psychiatry. It should not therefore be seen as surprising that a PICU may be involved. While it is clear that such patients do have special needs, in many areas specific resources are simply not available, despite the established National Service Framework (NSF), outlined after much debate and fanfare (Department of Health 1999). A basic rule should be that if an acute ward is involved in the care of a patient, then a PICU may also have to be involved, again depending on the patient's needs. As outlined above, exclusion clauses should be as few as possible, if PICUs are to work effectively in partnership with general adult psychiatry, to which they are ineluctably bound as part of a mesh of services.

A specific dilemma arises, of course, when a particular patient stays on a PICU beyond his or her PICU needs. That is to say, there is nowhere to move them on to, in terms of an appropriately supportive, usually high dependency, residence, and/or no one is prepared to continue their care in the community. In this regard, what specific arrangements should be put in hand for these patients?

Rehabilitation

By definition, patients being treated by rehabilitation teams will have long-standing and relatively severe forms of mental illness, usually schizophrenia. One in ten of these can be expected to relapse at any one time, and every psychiatric unit should have a facility for dealing with such relapses. This may be based in the rehabilitation unit itself, having perhaps two or three respite beds, or versions of these on the acute wards, or via special outreach measures, for example from a branch of the Assertive Outreach Team. Nevertheless, some patients will sometimes require a PICU environment, because of the nature of their relapse.

Fears of difficulty in discharging will need to be dealt with via clear-cut agreements that (1) any admission of a rehabilitation patient is based upon the assumption that they will accepted back to their previous place of residence, once the need for an acute or PICU place no longer pertains, and (2) that the care coordinators (who will often know such patients very well) regularly attend the inpatient unit (e.g. PICU) to maintain contact and support during the relapse admission. If a patient cannot continue in his/her previous living environment (because of higher needs), there should be an agreement that the original place of residence will provide interim care rather than PICU. If this involves employing temporary additional staff then so be it. Such arrangements clearly need to be established by agreed and written protocols, within a locality, and involving NHS, social services and voluntary bodies. They should be regularly reviewed, with audit used to refine their effectiveness and acceptability.

Personality disorder

Many patients admitted to acute psychiatric units have both psychotic symptoms and elements of a personality disorder (PD). Use of PICUs should be confined to managing treatable 'mental illness' symptoms rather than criminality or socially unacceptable behaviour per se. Use of PICUs as an alternative to a police cell, or merely due to persisting offending behaviour should never be accepted. Certain patients will require special leadership skills from senior nursing, consultant or management staff, and at present a 'treatability' clause is still part of the Mental Health Act. This treatability should remain the criterion for any ongoing inpatient stay. Close liaison with the police with regard to prosecuting those patients who are assaultative, and an agreed trust policy around supporting staff in this area are mandatory requirements. Clearly this is an area where PICU and forensic services interface, and policies for PICUs should be similar to those on acute general wards. Exceptions may occasionally be necessary, on a temporary basis, for example to clarify the basis of an episode of disturbed behaviour, but should never be the rule.

Substance misuse and dual diagnosis

It is more likely than not that up to 50% of patients on a PICU will have a significant substance dependence problem, given the relationship of chronic psychotic disorders such as schizophrenia with substance misuse. This will usually be abuse of alcohol, cannabis or (especially in the inner city) cocaine or crack cocaine. The assumption should be made (unlike modern prisons!) that drugs or alcohol *can* be excluded from a typical PICU, so that treatment of severe mental illness can take place alongside appropriate management and/or withdrawal from, for example, alcohol dependence. In fact, from a general perspective, the placing of a dual diagnosis patient on a PICU can be especially helpful, in a diagnostic sense, in clarifying whether a psychotic illness is *associated with or secondary to* drug/alcohol abuse.

Once a patient no longer requires the environment and staffing of a PICU, for example in managing a psychotic relapse, the fact that they have ongoing dependence needs and are likely to return to a pattern of alcohol or drug dependence should not be used as a means of keeping them on the PICU. There is no evidence that such an environment is required for the management of dependence, and in fact the modern approach, for example using motivational interviewing and/or other cognitive approaches, is based upon individuals making decisions (without coercion) to deal with their dependence. Given the prevalence of such dual diagnosis conditions, it would seem reasonable that a number of staff members of a PICU should have training in dual diagnosis, and should be able to initiate approaches to helping patients withdraw from their dependence. Whether or not a specific, separate, dual diagnosis worker, employed across the PICU and for example a CMHT or substance misuse service, should be employed will depend on local arrangements and resources.

Acute wards and PICUs

The rise of the PICU movement, in terms of resources, specialisation and staffing, has led to a number of concerns as to the role of general acute wards. Are PICUs really necessary, or could their approaches be integrated into general acute wards, which may be seen as at-risk of being de-skilled by the presence of a PICU? While these concerns have been expressed, the evidence for this happening remains unclear. Although there certainly have been a number of reports looking critically at the current state of acute psychiatric wards (e.g. Haigh 2002; Rethink 2004), these seem usually to have led to increasing demands to enhance crisis intervention and assertive outreach teams, on the assumption that such teams will mean that admission should no longer be required. While certainly enhancing the quality of care available to patients out of hospital (by the simple fact of additional staffing), the end result has been the increasingly severe nature of the illnesses affecting patients on the wards (Haigh 2002). That is to say, anyone manageable outside of hospital, in terms of behaviour or insight and in terms of appropriate family support, is kept out. Those with no family support, suffering from more severe illnesses, lacking insight and requiring treatment under the Mental Health Act (by definition needing 'treatment in hospital') tend to gather in the acute wards, thus the increasing tension and disruption found in such units.

The rising Mental Health Act (MHA) section rates in the UK during the 1990s, which seem to have stabilised now, have quite clearly created a different atmosphere on acute wards and PICUs (Thompson *et al.* 2004). Some have very much become intensive, psychosis-only (almost) units. They are faced with the paradox of trying to keep out patients who seem to want admission (i.e. those with borderline disorders, threatening self-harm and drinking excessively), while trying to keep in and treat patients who have no insight into their illnesses and who want to leave. Three separate cycles of stay tend to occur: those in for a few days, those in for a few weeks and those in for a number of months. Often it is the latter, whose discharge is difficult to plan and whose needs are complex, who create the worst management problems. Experienced nursing and consultant leadership, being prepared to move on patients who cannot benefit from acute ward admission, is vital in this regard. Consultants returning to being just ward based (Dratcu *et al.* 2003) may create ward/community interface difficulties.

However, having a separate PICU can be seen as a positive asset (Haigh 2002), given the complex nature of the patients that acute general wards have to manage. For example, general wards are unlikely to become de-skilled in managing acute crises, since it is usually they who have to initiate treatment before transfer to a PICU. Likewise, they will often have to manage patients with a range of behavioural disorders, given the variation in the demands on beds (and PICUs) that naturally occurs. Finally, the presence of an active PICU can significantly enhance the responses available for acutely disturbed patients, in terms of providing a psychiatric 'crash' team, a centre for training for control and restraint techniques, the ability to maintain treatment of patients who otherwise would lead to significant injuries to staff (and other patients), and (in some units) the ability to provide a time out resource. It is generally accepted that having more than two behaviourally disturbed patients on an average-size acute ward is about the limit, given staffing levels (for example four nurses to fifteen to twenty patients), the vulnerability of the other patients and the emergency resources available. Separating out the functions of acute wards and PICUs in this sense can be seen as helpful from the following perspectives:

1. Staff have to regularly make assessments as to the environmental needs of individual patients, thus regularly having to review rather than accept an unchanging environment.

2. Other patients can have a more beneficial and therapeutic inpatient experience, since disruptive, noisy, or otherwise behaviourally disturbed individuals can be appropriately dealt with in another environment.

3. Staff on acute wards can develop skills in terms of regular assessment, insight work and even cog-nitive approaches, rather than continuing de-escalation, restraint, high-dose medication and behavioural control.

4. Providing different levels of ward environment can produce useful different training resources for nurses, doctors and other mental health specialists.

5. Research into the role, practices and organisation of PICUs versus acute wards can lead to a better understanding of the training and resources required for managing patients on acute inpatient wards in general.

While it is accepted that most patients who go onto an acute psychiatric ward, whether a general ward or a PICU, come out better, there is remarkably little research showing the positive benefits of such treatment. By contrast, there are a number of critical commentaries (e.g. Muijen 1999), and acute wards (as well as PICUs) regularly come in for negative comments, attributing to the ward itself the difficulties engendered by the nature of the illnesses they manage. This is akin to blaming the messenger for bad news, and it has taken a long time for management to grasp the importance of understanding the role of the acute ward. Not only should it be regularly refurbished and maintained (just like, for example, an operating theatre), but it should be understood as a vital diagnostic, assessment, therapeutic and rehabilitative environment. The unique skills of acute psychiatric ward nurses enable a whole-person understanding of a patient's illness, how it affects their behaviour in social interactions, and their biological and interpersonal functioning. In this sense acute general wards and PICUs should stand side by side, essentially providing similar services, but agreeing on the particular priorities of the different stages of a patient's journey through illness.

Conclusions

There is little formal research into the interface between general psychiatric units and PICUs. This chapter therefore has been derived from known reports and guidelines as well as personal experience. The history of inpatient care for psychiatric patients has varied enormously over time, but even in the largest forms of institution (the asylums) it was accepted that specialist wards for more demanding patients should be established. Whether these were called 'refractory' wards or 'Psychiatric Intensive Care Units' reflects the particular nature of the underlying institution, and the available treatment resources. From a historical perspective, we are relatively lucky in the modern age, in being able to provide intensive forms of treatment in highly structured environments, that can substantially alter the course of serious illnesses and bring patients back to health. The essence of an effective psychiatric hospital lies in its ability to provide a range of treatment environments for all patients, and in this sense the jewel in the crown of any such unit will be its PICU. If a PICU is working appropriately, then the acute wards can do so as well, and the establishment and maintenance of a flexible, nurse-led and consultant-supported interface between such units seems of the essence. This requires regular monitoring and review, at senior nursing, consultant and management levels, and an agreed philosophy of care that will involve guidelines but will also centre itself upon putting the patient's needs first in every dilemma.

REFERENCES

Beer D, Paton C, Pereira S. 1997 Hot beds of general psychiatry. A national survey of psychiatric intensive care units. Psychiatr Bull 21: 142–144

Birmingham L. 2003 The mental health of prisoners. Adv Psychiatr Treat 9: 191–199

Department of Health. 1999 National Service Framework for Mental Health. Modern Standards and Service Model. London: Department of Health

Department of Health. 2001 Changing the Outlook. A Strategy for Developing and Modernising Mental Health Services in Prisons. London: Department of Health

Department of Health. 2002 Mental Health Policy Implementation Guide. National Minimum Standards for General Adult Services in Psychiatric Intensive Care Units (PICUs) and Low Secure Environments. London: Department of Health

Department of Health and Home Office. 1992 Review of Health and Social Services for Mentally Disordered Offenders and Others Requiring Similar Services. The Reed Report. Final Summary Report. Cm 2088. London: HMSO

Dratcu L, Grandison A, Adkin A. 2003 Acute hospital care in inner London: splitting from mental health services in the community. Psychiatr Bull 27: 83–86

Fitzpatrick NK, Thompson CJ, Hemingway H et al. 2003 Acute in-patient admissions in inner London: changes in patient characteristics and clinical admission thresholds between 1988 and 1998. Psychiatr Bull 27: 7–11

Haigh R. 2002 Acute wards: problems and solutions. Modern milieux, therapeutic community solutions to acute ward problems. Psychiatr Bull 26: 380–382

Muijen M. 1999 Acute hospital care: ineffective, inefficient and poorly organised. Psychiatr Bull 23: 257–259

Reilly BM. 2004 The essence of EBM. Br Med J 329: 991–992

Rethink. 2004 Behind Closed Doors. Acute Mental Health Care in the UK. London: Rethink

Royal College of Psychiatrists. 1998 Not Just Bricks and Mortar. Council Report CR62. Report of the Royal College of Psychiatrists' Working Party on the Size, Staffing, Structure, Siting and Security of New Acute Adult Psychiatric In-Patient Units. London: Royal College of Psychiatrists

Thompson A, Shaw M, Harrison G, Verne J, Ho D, Gunnell D. 2004 Patterns of hospital admission for adult psychiatric illness in England and Wales: analysis of Hospital Episode Statistics data. Br J Psychiatry 185: 334–341

Thornicroft G, Tansella M. 2004 Components of a modern mental health service: a pragmatic balance of community and hospital care. Br J Psychiatry 185: 283–290

17

The interface with the Child and Adolescent Mental Health Services

Gordana Milavić

Introduction

There are many similarities between the psychiatric intensive care of adults and the management of children and young people who present with serious mental health problems. However, there are equally a number of differences stemming from the biological, developmental and social aspects pertinent to childhood and adolescence.

In everyday clinical practice young people presenting with severe and complex psychiatric disorders requiring inpatient treatment receive that treatment in a variety of settings. At best they are treated in adolescent inpatient units or the few adolescent intensive care or forensic units, but an increasing number of young people go on to receive treatment in adult mental health units including Psychiatric Intensive Care Units (PICUs). This happens mainly because of a lack of specialist inpatient resources in the Child and Adolescent Mental Health Service (CAMHS) sector.

This chapter will focus on the key components and functions of CAMHS with particular reference to the group of young people with serious psychiatric and/or behavioural disorders who pose a high risk to themselves or others and are likely to require admission to adult PICUs.

CAMHS service structure

Child and Adolescent Mental Health Services can be managed by Primary Care Trusts, Mental Health Trusts or in some cases acute hospital services as part of paediatric services. Children's Trusts are a more recent development in which social services, education and health come together jointly to commission and to provide comprehensive children's services including CAMHS. The tiered approach to the provision of services spans the range from primary mental health to specialist inpatient services (see Appendix 17.1; NHS Health Advisory Service 1995).

Inpatient provision

The Royal College of Psychiatrists' Research Unit was commissioned by the Department of Health to assess the level of inpatient provision for children and adolescents in England and Wales. The National Inpatient Child and Adolescent Psychiatry Study (NICAPS) (O'Herlihy et al. 2001) established that there was a lack of emergency beds, an insufficient number of beds, poor provision for severe and high-risk cases and poor liaison with other services.

The study (O'Herlihy et al. 2001) found that most of the specialist and forensic inpatient provision was provided by the private sector. There were only three NHS units in England and Wales providing forensic adolescent care and no intensive care beds for this age group.

A large number of children and young people were placed on paediatric and adult mental health wards. The rate of 'inappropriate' admissions to adult services was estimated to be 4.6 per 100 000

Psychiatric Intensive Care, 2nd edn., eds. M. Dominic Beer, Stephen M. Pereira and Carol Paton.
Published by Cambridge University Press. © Cambridge University Press 2008

of 18-year-olds and under per year, and to paediatric services the rate was 1.4 per 100 000 of 18-year-olds and under per year (O'Herlihy *et al.* 2001).

Generic and even more so specialist and forensic inpatient provision in the country remains highly inadequate. Many adolescents with mental disorders continue to be inappropriately placed in Social Services Secure Units, HM prisons and Young Offenders Institutions.

Equally general adult wards and PICUs remain under pressure to admit adolescents with severe mental illness. Factors that determine admission to these inpatient services include the severity and complexity of the psychiatric condition, safety issues, family circumstances, and a number of less directly related factors such as the experience and knowledge of the referring clinician, the nature and structure of the referring organisation and the availability of funding.

Caring for children and young people in general adult wards and PICUs raises a number of concerns about the quality of care provided. These include a lack of understanding of child and adolescent mental health practice, issues of consent and confidentiality; unavailability of access to legal advice; and differences in approaches to risk assessments. There may also be a paucity of trained specialist staff; unfamiliarity with child protection procedures and an absence of links with social services and education.

Whereas increased investment for provision of specialist inpatient services for young people with severe mental illness remains a priority it may still be necessary to admit young people to adult PICUs. The quality of care can be improved and the clinical risks reduced by increasing the awareness of CAMH services and specialist practice and ensuring basic levels of safety and security.

Policy initiatives with specific reference to inpatient provision

The National Service Framework for Mental Health (Department of Health 1999a) makes specific reference to the use of adult wards 'for a short period' when an adolescent bed cannot be found, in order to ensure the safety and welfare of the young person or others. The report states that NHS Trusts should identify wards or settings that would suit the needs of young people with agreed protocols between adult and CAMH services (Department of Health 1999a).

The Health Advisory Service Report on Child and Adolescent Mental Health set the basis for inpatient CAMHS standards stressing the need for privacy and dignity of patients, age-appropriate security and maintenance of liaison with other agencies including social services and education (Health Advisory Service 1995).

Standard 9 (The Mental Health Wellbeing of Children and Young People) of the National Service Framework for Children, Young People and Maternity Services (Department of Health 2004) establishes that, although relatively rarely, a number of young people will develop psychotic disorders or present with complex, persistent and severe behavioural disorders requiring treatment in specialist adolescent inpatient units for young people.

The Report on the implementation of Standard 9 (Department of Health 2006) established that although progress has been made in the commissioning and provision of CAMHS, gaps in the provision of services persist with almost a quarter of children and young people diagnosed with psychiatric disorder not being able to access appropriate mental health services over a three-year period.

Mental health problems in children and adolescents

Prevalence

Mental health problems are relatively common in children and young people. The Audit Commission Report, Children in Mind (1999) stated that 20% of children and young people suffer with mental health problems at some time in their life. Indeed 10% – 15% of 5- to 15-year-olds have a diagnosable mental health disorder and it is estimated that 1.1 million

Table 17.1. Factors determining the significance of a mental health problem or disorder

Severity	The level of distress or concern it is causing to the child, family or agency and hence the amount of care the child may require
Complexity	The number of incapacitating features or symptoms present and the presence or otherwise of another disorder or complex family and social situations
Persistence	The length of time the problem has been present or is likely to last
The risk of secondary handicap	For example, the possibility of specific learning difficulties contributing to the development of a conduct disorder
State of child's development	Whether the problem is considered to be 'normal' for the age and stage of development of the child, e.g. nocturnal enuresis, fear of the dark
Presence or absence of protective factors	For example, good-quality early attachment relationships
Presence or absence of risk factors	Marital disharmony or parental separation with persisting conflict
Presence or absence of stressful social and cultural factors	For example, family under stress from social or economic disadvantage

Adapted from Street (2000).

Table 17.2. Multi-axial diagnostic model

Axes	Multiaxial framework categories	Examples
I	Clinical psychiatric syndromes	Conduct disorder
II	Specific disorders of psychological development	Of speech and language, of scholastic skills
III	Intellectual level	Normal range, mild, moderate, severe mental retardation
IV	Medical conditions	Severe, chronic or life-threatening illness, such as diabetes, epilepsy, hearing impairment
V	Associated abnormal psychosocial situations	Parental mental disorder, sexual abuse, bullying
VI	Global assessment of psychosocial disability	Ranging from superior social functioning to gross social disability

World Health Organization 1996.

children and young people under 18 in Great Britain would benefit from specialist services, with 45 000 having a severe mental health disorder (ONS 2000; Department of Health 2004).

Factors determining the significance of mental health problems or disorders

The prevalence of any particular problem or disorder will be determined by a number of factors (Table 17.1). Some disorders such as conduct disorders and substance misuse or emotional difficulties, related to quality of parenting or child abuse, will be more sensitive to socioeconomic influences than others. Other disorders, such as those related to brain damage, other neurological disorders, genetically transmitted conditions or chronic physical illness, will be less so.

Multi-axial classification of child and adolescent psychiatric disorders

The multi-axial diagnostic model (Table 17.2) used in everyday clinical practice reflects the complexity of the multi-factorial nature of the aetiology of disorders of childhood and adolescence.

Common serious mental health problems of childhood and adolescence

Severe mental illness in adolescence is rare but often has its onset in adolescence.

Conditions that are most likely to require treatment in specialist inpatient settings include:

- Psychoses, mood disorders including depressive disorders and bipolar disorders, schizophrenia and severe eating disorders, mental disorders arising from substance abuse.
- Serious risk of self-harm or suicide.
- Conduct disorders and challenging behaviour.
- Complex mental conditions linked to learning disability and neurodevelopmental disorders.

Substance abuse

It is difficult to establish the prevalence of substance abuse in the young population as it often goes unreported and effects upon physical and mental health are not as prominent as in the adult population. In a survey of 15- and 16-year-olds (Miller and Plant 1966) three-quarters of young people had been drunk at least once, and an equal number had smoked. Half the sample had tried illicit drugs. Drug experimentation has shown a surprising course more recently. In the late 1980s and early 1990s drug experimentation increased to reach a peak in the mid-nineties (Balding 1999). But there appears to have been a levelling off more recently; for instance, Ramsey *et al.* (2001) found that the use of any drugs by 16- to 19-year-olds in the previous year fell from approximately one-third to just above a quarter between 1994 and 2000. However, early smoking and alcohol consumption appear to have increased in young people and the correlation between an early start in drug use and drinking and illicit substance misuse is high (Health Advisory Service 1996).

Cannabis is the most widely used drug (Institute for the Study of Drug Dependence 1993) but alcohol, tobacco and solvents are also used by young people. It is estimated that about 1% of British secondary school pupils inhale organic solvents (Goodman and Scott 1997).

The association between psychiatric disorder and substance misuse is well documented in terms of both aetiology and co-morbidity (Zeitlin 1999).

Conduct-disordered children and young people and those who continue to suffer from attention deficit hyperactivity disorder (ADHD) are particularly at risk of developing substance misuse although peer influences and availability are important aetiological factors. It should be noted that stimulant treatment of ADHD is associated with reduced illicit drug misuse (Biederman *et al.* 1999) and that it is usually the group of young people who have both conduct disorder and untreated ADHD who are most likely to end up misusing drugs.

There is evidence of an association between substance abuse and a number of psychiatric disorders. Affective disorders, personality disorders and eating disorders, are correlated with substance misuse. Suicide is much more common in this group. Psychiatric disorders with an onset in childhood have a poorer prognosis and are likely to continue into adult life particularly if complicated by substance misuse.

In everyday clinical practice it is accepted that psychosis can be precipitated by drug misuse. Psychotic symptoms are most common following the use of amphetamine and cocaine, hallucinogenic drugs such as lysergic acid diethylamide (LSD) and ecstasy. Psychosis can also develop in association with cannabis use and, given the wide use of cannabis by young people, it is not surprising that the role of cannabis in the aetiology of psychotic disorders has been the subject of renewed interest. Cannabis use can be linked to increased risk, increased relapse rate and poor oucome (Martinez-Arevalo *et al.* 1994; Linszen *et al.* 1994). Alternatively cannabis has been seen as a form of self-medication in the prodromal stages of psychotic disorders.

The pharmacological management of young people is complicated by the fact that medications used for detoxification, substitution and relapse prevention are not licensed for people under 18.

Nevertheless in emergency situations naloxone and flumazenil are useful since both have specific pharmacological antagonistic effects, in being an opiate and a benzodiazepine. Detoxification is not necessary in the majority of adolescent substance misusers who have as yet not developed dependence. However, on the rare occasions when opiate detoxification is necessary, methadone, lofexidine, clonidine, buprenorphine and dihydrocodeine can be used. In alcohol withdrawal chlordiazepoxide can be used on a short-term basis (Crome *et al.* 2004). The recently published public health intervention guidance on Community based Interventions to Reduce Substance Misuse among Vulnerable and Disadvantaged Children and Young People recommend early intervention, multi-agency involvement including parents and the provision of motivational interviewing, family based programmes and structured support over periods as long as two years or more (NICE 2007).

Deliberate self-harm and suicide

Rates of deliberate self-harm (attempted suicide, parasuicide) are relatively low in childhood but much more common in adolescence and early adulthood. Suicidal preoccupations are not rare among community samples of adolescents but fewer young people go on to harm themselves. The rate of suicide in Britain is 5/1 000 000 children aged 10–14 per year and 30/1 000 000 in young people aged 15–19. Boys outnumber girls at all ages (McClure *et al.* 1966).

Self-poisoning or self-injury is common in adolescents, with an estimated 20 000 to 30 000 presentations to general hospitals annually to England and Wales with a life time prevalence of 13.2% (Hawton and Rodham 2006). Self-harm is strongly associated with suicide. Gaps in service provision may lead to repeated deliberate self-harm and life-threatening outcomes.

The assessment and management of deliberate self-harm are usually conducted through the rapid response by emergency CAMHS with follow-up in the community or in CAMHS outpatient services. Serious suicidal intent presents a psychiatric emer-

Table 17.3. Indications of serious suicidal intent

- Carried out in isolation
- Timed so that intervention is unlikely
- Precautions taken to avoid discovery
- Preparations made in anticipation of death
- Other people informed beforehand of the individual's intention
- Extensive premeditation
- Suicide note left
- Failure to alert other people following episode

Adapted from Goodman and Scott (1997).

gency, which is likely to result in an admission to inpatient services.

Completed suicides in young people bear some common characteristics: 90% had a history of psychiatric disorder including depressive illness, conduct disorder and substance abuse; a history of previous suicidal behaviour; adverse family circumstances including a history of mental illness, suicide, self-harm and substance abuse; and access to firearms or other lethal means.

The assessment should include an evaluation of the circumstances of the suicidal intent (Table 17.3), the identification of precipitating and predisposing risk factors, a mental state examination and an assessment of the capacity to engage in treatment.

All children and young people who have self harmed should normally be admitted overnight to a paediatric or medical ward and assessed fully the following day by the CAMHS services prior to their discharge. Further treatment and care should be unitiated at this point (NICE 2004).

Should it be established that a young person is at risk of further serious deliberate self-harm or suicide, psychiatric inpatient care is indicated. Issues related to consent to treatment and capacity become even more pertinent in these situations. Treatment on a PICU will need to be considered in those situations where the further management on open specialist psychiatric wards becomes untenable usually due to the intensity of the level of care required and the young person's non-compliance with treatment.

Major psychotic disorders

Major psychotic disorders in childhood and adolescence follow a similar pattern to that manifested in adulthood although there are a number of differences stemming from factors pertinent to the period of adolescence and from differences in the manifestation of the psychotic disorder. Swedish studies using case register data from Goteberg established a prevalence for all psychotic disorders at age 13 to be 0.9 per 10 000 increasing steadily to reach a prevalence of 17.6 per 10 000 at the age of 18 (Hollis 2000).

The main conditions include: schizophrenia, schizoaffective disorder, affective psychosis and mania, psychotic depression and mixed affective psychosis and drug-induced psychosis.

First episodes of psychosis in young people are often undifferentiated, not fitting easily into schizophrenic or affective type syndromes. Although it is important to identify the driving symptomatology, particularly when suspecting drug-induced psychosis, if there are no clear indicators to suggest a specific category it is often more accurate to refer to these episodes as 'psychotic disorders'.

Schizophrenia

Schizophrenia is one of the most devastating psychiatric disorders to affect children and adolescents. It is rare before the age of 10 years. The incidence rises steadily to reach its peak between the ages of 20–25 years.

The childhood onset has a poorer prognosis and there is evidence of greater neurodevelopmental impairment than in adult-onset schizophrenia. The diagnostic criteria applied to schizophrenia arising in childhood or adolescence are, however, the same as those in adults (World Health Organization 1992; American Psychiatric Association 1994).

Premorbid impairments in child- and adolescent-onset schizophrenia (CAOS) include poor premorbid functioning, early developmental delays, and lower premorbid IQs than in adult-onset schizophrenia, suggesting a strong neurodevelopmental aspect of CAOS (Hollis 2000).

Box 17.1. Clinical features of schizophrenia in childhood

- Poor premorbid functioning
- Below-average IQ
- Insidious onset
- Deterioration of scholastic and social skills
- Strong family history of psychosis/schizophrenia
- Predominantly negative symptoms
- Severe and unremitting course

Adapted from Hollis (2000)

A clear prodromal phase is more common in childhood-onset schizophrenia. Children and young people begin to show a decline in educational and social functioning before the onset of active psychotic symptoms. Rarer prodromal behavioural characteristics include obsessional symptoms and social disinhibition.

Box 17.2. Psychotic symptoms of child-onset in contrast to adult-onset schizophrenia (Hollis 2000)

- More prominent negative symptoms, including flattened and inappropriate affect, and bizarre and manneristic behaviour
- Disorganised behaviour
- Hallucinations in different modalities
- Relatively few well-formed systematised or persecutory delusions

---

The differential diagnosis includes a number of neurological, neurodevelopmental and drug-related conditions.

Schizophrenia in young people requires early identification and treatment. Atypical antipsychotics are the first-line treatment. Side-effects in young people are particularly concerning and include extrapyramidal side-effects (EPSE), weight gain, hyperprolactinaemia, sedation and seizures. Side-effect profiles differ between the atypicals. Children and young people appear to be more prone than adults to developing side-effects. Other treatments include family and individual work and psychological and psycho-educational measures (NICE Guidelines for Schizophrenia 2002).

Depressive disorders

Children and adolescents suffer with depressive disorders that resemble adult depressive disorders (American Academy of Child and Adolescent Psychiatry 1998). However, there are important developmental differences (Goodyer and Coopes 1983; NICE 2005). As in adults the main symptom clusters of depression include mood changes, cognitive impairments and altered activity levels sufficiently severe to cause impairments in day-to-day functioning. It is estimated that the point prevalence rates of depression and dysthymia in prepubertal children are 1%–2% and 2%–5% in the older age group (Fonagy *et al.* 2002). The sex ratio is approximately 1:1 before puberty and rises with age, with a preponderance in girls in adolescence. Suicidal intentions occur as in adults and are often present, particularly in the older age adolescents. Comorbidity is high, with anxiety disorders and conduct disorders being present in more than half of children and young people who suffer with depression.

The course and prognosis of depression occurring in childhood and adolescence can be concerning: 10% of children recover spontaneously within 3 months and a further 40% go on to recover within the first year. However 50% remain depressed at 1 year and around 20%–30% of young people do not recover after 2 years (Harrington and Dubicka 2001; Goodyer *et al.* 2003; Dunn and Goodyer 2006). The most serious consequence of persisting depression is suicide with a rate of about 3% in the next 10 years (Harrington 2001).

The severely depressed young people with suicidal symptoms who have failed to respond to treatment in the community and at Tier 3 are likely to be admitted for inpatient treatment and are likely to require admission to adult PICUs.

There is increasing evidence that severe depressive disorders in children and adolescents are most likely to respond to medication as the first line of treatment (TADS study 2004; March and Silva *et al.* 2006) in emergencies.

Fluoxetine is the only selective serotonin reuptake inhibitor (SSRI) recommended for use in depressive disorders in young people under 18. It should be started in low doses of 5–10 mg daily and increased to at least 20 mg daily. Young people prescribed SSRIs are at increased risk of emergent suicidal thoughts and acts requiring vigilance (NICE 2005). The recommended length of treatment is the same as in adults (6 months after recovery for a single episode). Psychological treatments should always be used first line.

Bipolar disorders

Mania, hypomania and bipolar disorders are rare in young children (Harrington 1994). In adolescence, both mania and depression are more common, with the first episode usually occurring after the age of 15. Each episode can be primarily manic or depressive, or a mixture of the two with rapid mood changes. One-year prevalence rates vary between 0.2% and 0.3%. A positive family history and previous episodes of depression are risk factors and contribute to accurate diagnosis.

The diagnosis and management of bipolar disorder in children and adolescents is similar to that in adults except that when diagnosing Bipolar Disorder I mania should be present and 'euphoria must be present most day, most of the time for a period of seven days' (British Psychological Society and the Royal College of Psychiatrists 2006). Irritability in this context is not a pathognomonic symptom and Bipolar Disorder II should not normally be diagnosed in children and adolescents as the diagnostic criteria are not well established. The differential diagnosis includes ADHD (attention deficit hyperactivity disorder), schizophrenia, abuse and neglect, substance misuse, learning difficulties and organic disorders. Inpatient treatment will be considered for those who are severely behaviourally distressed and at risk of suicide. Mixed episodes of mania and depression carry additional risks of self-harm and suicide. Atypical antipsychotics, lithium for females and males and sodium valproate for male patients are the first line of treatment. In more severe cases rapid tranquilisation with haloperidol should be avoided because of the increased risk of side-effects in this young population (British Psychological Society and the Royal College of Psychiatrists).

Seriously challenging behaviour and conduct disorders

Conduct disorders are characterised by repetitive and persistent dissocial, aggressive and defiant behaviour. They represent the commonest childhood psychiatric disorder ranging from 5% to 10% of non-clinical samples. Boys are affected more than girls in a ratio of 3:1. It is argued sometimes that such behaviour, by definition, is merely a contravention of socially accepted rules and norms, and should not merit psychiatric classification or treatment. Nevertheless a number of young people with serious forms of disordered behaviour will at some point warrant intensive psychiatric treatment and require admission to an adult PICU. Hyperactivity and depression are associated conditions. Long-term outcome is linked to educational and job difficulties and delinquency.

In the community early intervention is recommended and psychosocial interventions are the first line of treatment. Parent training programmes are based on helping parents to promote prosocial behaviours in their children and eliminate problem behaviour. Webster Stratton and Oregon social learning centre programmes are some of the best well known parenting interventions. Child-orientated interventions include social skills and anger-coping skills. Psychodynamic therapies have not been shown to be of value.

In inpatient settings one is more likely to resort to pharmacotherapy, including the use of stimulants. Drug approaches to the treatment of conduct disorders include the use of stimulants (methylphenidate and dexamphetamine), particularly given the coexistence of ADHD. Lithium can be used for the treatment of explosive and severely aggressive manifestations of conduct disorder. Antipsychotics, particularly the atypicals, may have a place in reducing aggressiveness.

Complex mental conditions linked to learning disability and neurodevelopmental disorders including autistic disorders

Although children and young people affected by these conditions will present to CAMHS from an early age, once they reach adolescence they may require treatment in acute inpatient and residential settings. A number of young adolescents will develop epileptic seizures. Some will become prone to periods of agitation and may develop extreme forms of challenging behaviour. Disinhibited and inappropriate sexualised behaviour is also common and some may develop psychosis.

Treatment includes a combination of behavioural, pharmacological and educational measures including anticonvulsants, stimulants and antipsychotics.

The rights of the child and adolescent

Issues of competence and consent

Assessment and treatment can be perceived by the patient as an assault. Consent issues in relation to children and young people are different to those in adults. Young people aged 16 and 17 are in most circumstances deemed competent to provide consent to treatment. The Gillick 'test' of competence (*Gillick v Norfolk and Wisbech Area Health Authority* 1985) needs to be applied to all children under 16 years old. Treatment can be given without consent where the Mental Health Act 1983 applies (White *et al.* 2004).

Case study

- A 15-year-old girl is brought into A& E by two policemen after hours
- She is drunk and violent and has slashed her wrists with a razor
- She is refusing medical attention for her cuts
- She has already tried to abscond and is threatening to do so again

- She is known to social services but still lives with her parents
- There is no out-of-hours child psychiatrist
- The parents cannot be contacted
- The Duty Social Worker is in another hospital

Consent and treatment considerations

- Is the young person Gillick competent?[a] The patient is under 16 years; she may have a right to consent to treatment but she cannot refuse
- Can she hold in mind implications of treatment and no treatment and the consequences of each?
- Mental, physical and social assessment should precede any emergency intervention

Clinical management

- Assess competence to consent or refuse treatment
- Prevent the patient from leaving the A & E Department
- Common law can be used (doctrine of necessity) as it is an emergency and the patient's life is at risk
- Administer medical treatment
- Assess the patient's competence bearing in mind Gillick competence; don't forget refusal of treatment can be over-ruled by a parent/guardian
- Duty Social Worker or Manager would have to act in loco parentis
- Consider admission to specialist adolescent unit particularly if patient is suicidal
- If no specialist beds, admit to adult ward

---

[a] Following a case concerning a young person's right to consent to medical treatment without the parents' knowledge The House of Lords ruled that the degree of parental control varied according to the child's understanding and intelligence (*Gillick* v *Norfolk and Wisbech Area Health Authority* 1986). Subsequently developed case law held that 'Gillick competence' related to the particular child and the particular treatment. The parental right to determine whether or not their child below the age of 16 will have medical treatment no longer held once the child achieved sufficient understanding and intelligence to enable him or her to understand fully what was being proposed. The courts have in the past over-ruled refusal of potentially life-saving treatment by patients under 16 years, even if they are Gillick competent. The courts can over-ride the wishes of both parents and children where treatment is vital to the child's welfare.

- If patient still refusing admission and risk of suicide high invoke the Mental Health Act 1983
- If the patient continues to try to abscond or cause significant self-harm on adolescent/adult ward, discuss with the PICU
- Consider tranquillisation and watch out for continuing effects of drug/alcohol intoxication

The law

- If it is established that the patient lacks capacity to make the necessary decisions due to immaturity or alcohol intoxication, the Law allows the administration of immediate treatment necessary to preserve life or prevent serious deterioration in health
- Consider use of the Mental Health Act 1983 if the patient is assessed to be suicidal or a danger to others or themselves – but this would enable treatment of mental health issues and not immediate physical issues
- A restriction of liberty under Section 25 of the Children Act may be considered after the patient receives emergency medical treatment if the risk of absconding and the danger to self and others persists
- Involve Trust/hospital solicitor early – emergency rulings can be obtained even out of hours
- These are not decisions that should be taken on your own. Consult managers, Trust/hospital solicitors, medical defence body and keep good notes

Management of serious psychiatric disorders in young people: models of care

Community-based outreach adolescent teams

The HAS report, Bridge over Troubled Waters (Health Advisory Service 1986), argued for dedicated, accessible community adolescent mental health services.

More recently a number of CAMHS have developed local multidisciplinary teams whose main objective is the provision of early assessment and treatment interventions with a broad range of therapeutic options including the management of referrals to Tier 4 (see Appendix Table 17.1) adolescent inpatient services. Criteria for referral are based on a need for rapid response and more intensive treatment than could be offered by generic Tier 3 CAMHS. Eligibility criteria include self-harm and acute depression and suicidal ideation, prodromal psychotic conditions, psychosis, acute post-traumatic stress disorder (PTSD) and severe eating disorders. The evaluation of one such community-based service demonstrated that most acute presentations could be managed locally within the context of the family, occasionally relying on short periods of inpatient treatment. The advantages of such an approach included the provision of continuous and consistent therapeutic programmes, as well as the support of family and social networks and rehabilitation (Kaplan *et al.* 2002).

Inpatient adolescent services

Inpatient adolescent units were described by the NICAPS (O'Herlihy *et al.* 2001) research team as those units that predominantly admitted young people between the ages of 12 and 18 years. These included eating disorder and forensic specialist units. The study identified 54 such units (668 available beds on the day of the census) in England and Wales with 30% of these units in the private sector.

Eligibility criteria for inpatient units are based on the need for a rapid response to serious mental health or complex and persisting behavioural problems covering the principal major psychiatric diagnostic groups. A higher percentage of the inpatient population is rated as having moderate to severe problems on the Health of the Nation Outcome Scale for Children and Adolescents (HoNOSCA) in comparison with the outpatient population (Audit Commission 1999). The main diagnostic categories of young people aged 13–18 years admitted to inpatient units were schizophrenia and other psychotic disorders, affective disorders, conduct disorders and eating disorders for boys, and eating disorders, affective disorders, schizophrenia and other psychotic conditions for girls.

The main treatments offered on adolescent wards are drug therapy, cognitive therapy, behavioural therapy, cognitive-behavioural therapy (CBT), group and family therapy, creative therapies and social skills training.

The NICAP Study looked at length of stay of discharged patients during the study period. It should be pointed out that these were aggregated results for both child and adolescent admissions. The mean length of stay was 3.7 months with a standard deviation of 181 days and a range of 0–2194 days.

Snowsfields

A new approach to CAMHS inpatient treatment is exemplified in a London-based adolescent unit (Street 2000). The unit opened in 1998 in the setting of a teaching general acute hospital and offers ten beds and four day places for young people aged between 13 and 18 years. The unit has attempted to improve the accessibility of inpatient care for young people with severe mental illness. Young people with learning difficulties, substance abuse problems and those who are homeless are considered for admission, departing from the usual practice in the more traditional models of inpatient adolescent care. Urgent cases are admitted on the day of referral, 24 h a day 7 days a week. The unit provides a wide range of treatments and educational provision on site. In the first 2 years of operation the bed occupancy was 88% with a median length of stay of 33 days.

Early intervention in psychosis units

Early intervention in psychosis models of service have developed against a backdrop of a growing body of evidence indicating that young people's first access to mental health services is delayed for up to 1–2 years even when there are clear indications of serious mental health disorder (Aitchison *et al.* 1999; Shiers *et al.* 2004).

An early example of one such unit set up in July 2000 is described in the Young Minds Study (Street 2000), which looked into the needs of young people with serious mental problems. The unit provides services for the age group 16–25 years and is a street-based agency alongside a range of different services for young people. Young people presenting to the service for the first time are engaged in an initial assessment leading to a Care Programme Approach care plan. Links with specialist inpatient services are routinely maintained.

Multi-agency provision model of services

The Southampton Behaviour Resource Service (Street 2000) opened in 2000. In this model, health, social services and education have come together to provide a resource for those children and young people who often fall between agency categories and their eligibility criteria but who are nevertheless seriously at risk and present with a combination of complex mental health and behavioural needs. The unit caters for children and young people aged 5–18 years with four inpatient beds for young people aged 13–18 years. The maximum length of stay is 4 weeks. Therapeutic and care programmes instituted alongside each other are based on close cooperation between the jointly staffed service and collaboration in planning and management.

PICU provision for severe and high-risk cases

It is accepted by both providers and commissioners of mental health services that the provision for severely ill young people who require intensive psychiatric care, containment and security remains inadequate. It is likely that a proportion of young people whose needs cannot be met on generic inpatient adolescent wards and where there is no access to specialist adolescent PICUs will continue to be admitted to adult PICUs. Young people presenting with severe psychiatric illness, including psychosis, dual diagnosis disorders, learning difficulties including those with pervasive developmental disorders and autistic spectrum disorders and conduct-disordered children with challenging behaviour are particularly difficult to place and may be admitted to adult wards and PICUs. In this instance, the need for joint protocols becomes that much greater.

A common scenario: the admission of a young person to a PICU

Patients requiring admission to PICU will usually already be known to CAMHS staff. Attempts will have been made to secure more appropriate provision but often the young person cannot be contained in the community or in the generic inpatient adolescent setting. The most common reasons for requiring an intensive care ward admission include serious and complex psychiatric presentations where patients are not responding to treatment or are refusing treatment, or where there is a high risk of absconding in the face of suicide and/or violence to others.

Case study

An example of a typical case requiring intensive psychiatric services is that of a 15-year-old adolescent who presented to CAMHS with psychotic symptoms in the setting of heavy and regular cannabis use since he was 11 years old. There was a history of several months duration and a history of deterioration of academic, social and personal functioning. He was started on olanzapine but refused to take the medication. His mental state deteriorated. He required an inpatient admission to a specialist adolescent unit and an informal admission was arranged. A diagnosis of a psychotic disorder was confirmed. The patient failed to cooperate with the assessment and treatment regime offered on the ward and he was placed on Section 2 of the Mental Health Act 1983. The patient continued to refuse his antipsychotic medication and started to abscond. He was subsequently prescribed oral risperidone and then quetiapine with continued non-compliance. The patient often ran back to his family home and smoked cannabis. He was repeatedly brought back to the ward and became violent to the nursing staff when they tried to administer his medication or detain him on the ward. Oral lorazepam and haloperidol IM were used when he became very aggressive. His aggression and violence deepened. Continued assessment and treatment were required to establish the exact nature of his mental health problems and to ensure his safety. He was transferred to the adult PICU. On admission he tested positive for cannabis and cocaine. A diagnosis of paranoid schizophrenia was established. He was started on depot medication.

He remained on the PICU for 8 weeks. A period of stability followed his discharge but further admissions have been necessary to date. The main problems are his non-compliance and continued drug misuse.

Procedures on admission

Box 17.3. Prior to admission of a young person to a PICU the following issues should be considered:

- Consider legal issues with reference to patient's and parental/carer's consent to admission
- Assess competence and capacity to consent
- There is no age limit restricting the use of mental health legislation. The Mental Health Act 1983 should be used whenever there is evidence of mental health disorder.
- Consideration may be given to the use of the Police Protection Order (Children Act 1989) although this is rarely the case. This would apply to a child under the age of 18 where the police have reasonable cause to believe that the child would otherwise be at risk of significant harm.
- Some young patients may be subject to mental health legislation via the police and courts
- The detention of a minor under the Mental Health Act in a facility other than a specialist adolescent unit must be reported to the Mental Health Act Commission by the CAMHS team. They will then make arrangements to visit the facility, interview the patient, carers and staff involved

---

Procedures during admission

- Consultant responsibility for psychiatric care will transfer to the PICU consultant
- Employ additional specialist nursing staff
- Safeguard the young person and ensure adherence to child protection policies
- Apply accepted standards and policies on safety and dignity
- Maintain vigilance with respect to bullying and violence by adult patients

- Set up care planning meeting as soon as possible after admission including adult and CAMHS staff
- Formulate the treatment plan including input of other therapists and professionals including specialist nursing
- Set clear and firm boundaries with respect to accepted norms of behaviour on the ward; discuss smoking, sexual behaviour and the use of alcohol and drugs in line with ward policy
- Ensure young person's needs for education are met by contacting school and hospital school services
- Involve social services and educational authorities at the outset
- Clear record keeping is essential particularly with respect to time out, the use of physical restraint and any critical incidents
- Seclusion and restraint, including pharmacological restraint, are interventions of last resort
- The decision to discharge from the ward will involve parents, carers and other agencies including the GP

Managing acute aggressive behaviour in children and adolescents

Approved physical restraint and the use of pharmacological agents in managing acute aggressive behaviour in inpatient settings are subject to codes of practice and clear ward protocols (Department of Health 1993, 1999b). Careful advance planning, adequate numbers of specialist and fully trained staff may preclude the use of extreme measures. Should restraint and rapid tranquillisation be necessary the young person's diagnostic profile should always inform the procedure. Previous successful strategies in managing a particular patient should be adhered to. Contributing factors should be considered including acute stressors, current medication, side-effects and any contributing physical state factors. Feedback should regularly be offered to both the patient and their family.

In practice, atypical antipsychotic medication is used in addressing acute aggressive behaviour even though these medications are not licensed for such use in children and adolescents. Equally the use of

Table 17.4. The therapeutic process for managing acute aggressive behaviour of children and adolescents

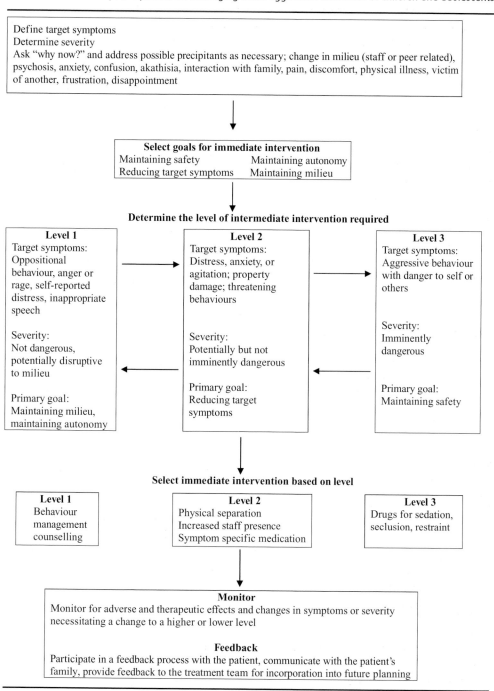

Define target symptoms
Determine severity
Ask "why now?" and address possible precipitants as necessary; change in milieu (staff or peer related), psychosis, anxiety, confusion, akathisia, interaction with family, pain, discomfort, physical illness, victim of another, frustration, disappointment

Select goals for immediate intervention
Maintaining safety   Maintaining autonomy
Reducing target symptoms   Maintaining milieu

Determine the level of intermediate intervention required

Level 1	**Level 2**	**Level 3**
Target symptoms: Oppositional behaviour, anger or rage, self-reported distress, inappropriate speech	Target symptoms: Distress, anxiety, or agitation; property damage; threatening behaviours	Target symptoms: Aggressive behaviour with danger to self or others
Severity: Not dangerous, potentially disruptive to milieu	Severity: Potentially but not imminently dangerous	Severity: Imminently dangerous
Primary goal: Maintaining milieu, maintaining autonomy	Primary goal: Reducing target symptoms	Primary goal: Maintaining safety

Select immediate intervention based on level

Level 1	**Level 2**	**Level 3**
Behaviour management counselling	Physical separation Increased staff presence Symptom specific medication	Drugs for sedation, seclusion, restraint

Monitor
Monitor for adverse and therapeutic effects and changes in symptoms or severity necessitating a change to a higher or lower level

Feedback
Participate in a feedback process with the patient, communicate with the patient's family, provide feedback to the treatment team for incorporation into future planning

Adapted from dosReis *et al.* (2003).

Table 17.5. Common child and adolescent psychiatric conditions and evidence-based preferred treatments[a]

Condition	Preferred pharmacotherapy	Main psychotherapeutic and psychosocial intervention
Anxiety disorders	• SSRIs[b] • Efficacy of benzodiazepines and beta-blockers not confirmed	• CBT • Behavioural therapy
Depressive disorders	• SSRIs[b]	• CBT • Social skills training • Family therapy • Interpersonal therapy for adolescents
Conduct disorders	• Atypical antipsychotics, e.g. risperidone for aggressive outbursts • Stimulants when there is an ADHD component	• Parent training: Webster Stratton, the Oregon Social Learning Center Programs, Parent and Child programmes • Family therapy • Social and anger management skills • Classroom management
ADHD	• Methylphenidate • Dexamphetamine • Atomoxetine • Clonidine as second-line treatment	• Behavioural therapies • Parent training • Social skills training
Tourette's disorder	• Antipsychotic drugs	• Anxiety management • Psycho-education • Family interventions
Schizophrenia	• Risperidone • Olanzapine • Clozapine	• Psycho-education • Psychosocial treatments; social skills training and family interventions
Bipolar disorders	• Lithium • Antipsychotic drugs • Valproate	• Family and individual work • Psycho-education
Pervasive developmental disorder such as autism and Asperger's syndrome	• Risperidone • SSRIs[b] may be useful in some patients	• Intensive behavioural programmes in home and school settings
Eating disorders: • Anorexia nervosa	• No drug treatment is of proven benefit • Appropriate nutritional and other supplements	• Weight restoration through gradual refeeding as part of a behavioural programme • Family therapy for onset < 19
• Bulimia nervosa	• SSRIs	• CBT • Behavioural therapy

[a] Fonagy *et al.* (2002) and Wolpert *et al.* (2006).
[b] Care should be taken when prescribing SSRIs for young people. Only fluoxetine can be prescribed for the treatment of depression in children and adolescents <18 years of age.
There is no evidence that tricyclic antidepressants are effective in young people; they are also poorly tolerated and very cardiotoxic.
ADHD, Attention deficit hyperactivity disorder; CBT, cognitive-behavioural therapy; SSRIs, selective serotonin reuptake inhibitors.

intramuscular formulations such as olanzapine in the treatment of acute agitation are not licensed for use in children although they are regularly used particularly for rapid tranquillisation (Table 17.4).

An overview of therapies

Treating children and young people will involve the family and immediate social environment, the school and often social services. Frequently acute or community paediatric services are also involved in the care of the child or young person. In the case of some parents there may be important links with adult mental health services. The engagement and appropriate sharing of information with all agencies will form the basis of any successful intervention. With increasing emphasis on evidence-based practice, a range of pharmacological and psychotherapeutic approaches are being established in everyday child and adolescent practice (Table 17.5; Fonagy *et al.* 2002). Overall there are changes towards specific focused treatment methods such as behavioural and cognitive therapies.

These therapeutic principles also apply to the treatment of severe disorders of childhood and adolescence in adult PICUs. Antipsychotic drugs, psycho-education, family and individual counselling, CBT and attention to continuation of education are the main components of a multimodal treatment approach. In young people with first-onset psychotic disorders, atypical antipsychotics should be the first line of treatment. Early treatment with antipsychotics may improve outcome. Treatment resistance is established after a lack of response to at least two atypical antipsychotics, each from a different chemical class, used for at least 4–6 weeks and/or when severe side-effects occur in response to atypical antipsychotics. Clozapine may be effective in these cases.

Conclusions

Young people with serious psychiatric and/or behavioural disorders who pose a high risk to themselves or to others are at some point during their treatment likely to require admission to an adult ward or to an adult PICU, given the persisting lack of specialist inpatient provision for young people. Awareness of CAMHS issues and the legal framework are essential. Issues include access to specialist nursing and appropriate therapeutic interventions. The early involvement of family, establishment of links with education and social services and an increased vigilance with respect to safety and protection will ensure better outcomes for young people.

APPENDIX 17.1
Key components, professionals and functions of tiered CAMHS

Tier 1

A primary level which includes interventions by:
• GPs
• Health visitors
• School nurses
• Social services
• Voluntary agencies
• Teachers
• Residential social workers
• Juvenile justice workers
CAMHS at this level are provided by non-specialists who are in a position to:
• Identify mental health problems early in their development
• Offer general advice – and in certain cases treatment for less severe mental health problems
• Pursue opportunities for promoting mental health and preventing mental health problems

Tier 2

A level of service provided by uni-professional groups which relate to others through a network rather than within a team. These include:
• Clinical child psychologists
• Paediatricians, especially community
• Educational psychologists
• Child psychiatrists

- Community child psychiatric nurses/nurse specialists

CAMHS professionals should be able to offer:
- Training and consultation to other professionals (who might be within Tier 1)
- Consultation for professionals and families
- Assessment which may trigger treatment at a different tier
- Outreach to identify severe or complex needs which require more specialist interventions but where the children or families are unwilling to use specialist services

Most children or adolescents with mental health problems will be seen at Tiers 1 and 2. All agencies should have structures in place to facilitate the referral of clients between tiers, and to maximise the contribution of CAMH specialists at each tier.

Tier 3

A specialist service for the more severe, complex and persistent disorders. This is usually a multidisciplinary team or service working in a community child mental health clinic or child psychiatry outpatient service, including:
- Child and adolescent psychiatrists
- Social workers
- Clinical psychologists
- Community psychiatric nurses
- Child psychotherapists
- Occupational therapists
- Art, music and drama therapists

The core CAMHS in each district should be able to offer:
- Assessment and treatment of child mental health disorders
- Assessment for referrals to Tier 4
- Contributions to the service, consultation and training at Tiers 1 and 2
- Participation in R & D projects

Tier 4

Services at this level include specialised outpatient teams, such as forensic teams or teams for sexually abused children, specialist day provision, inpatient adolescent units, eating disorder services, learning disability, forensic and secure treatment units. Adolescent PICUs which did not exist at the time of writing not exist in the NHS sector would fall under Tier 4 services. Tier 4 services are geared towards children and adolescents who are severely mentally ill and who pose suicidal risks. These services are provided on a supra-district and regional level as not all services can be expected to offer the level of expertise. Examples include:
- Adolescent inpatient units
- Secure forensic adolescent units
- Eating disorder units
- Specialist teams for sexual abuse
- Specialist teams for neuropsychiatric problems

This appendix is adapted from NHS Health Advisory Service (1995) and Street (2000).

REFERENCES

Aitchison JK, Meehan K, Murray RM. 1999 First Episode Psychosis. London: Martin Dunitz, pp. 16–27

American Academy of Child and Adolescent Psychiatry. 1998 Practice parameters for the assessment and treatment of children and adolescents with depressive disorders. J Am Aca Child Adolesc Psychiatry 37 [Suppl. 10]: 63S–83S

American Psychiatric Association. 1994 Diagnostic and Statistical Manual of Mental Disorders, 4th edn. Washington, DC: American Psychiatric Association

Audit Commission. 1999 National Report (1999). Children in Mind: Child and Adolescent Mental Health Services. London: Audit Commission

Balding JW. 1999 Young People in 1998. With a Look Back as Far as 1983. Exeter: Schools Health Education

Biederman J, Wilens T, Mick E et al. 1999 Pharmacotherapy of attention deficit/hyperactivity disorders reduces risk of substance use disorder. Paediatrics 104: e20

British Psychological Society and the Royal College of Psychiatrists. 2006 The Management of Bipolar Disorder in Adults, Children and Adolescents in Primary and Secondary Care. National Clinical Practice Guideline Number 38. London: British Psychological Society and Royal College of Psychiatrist

Crome BI, McArdle P, Gilvarry E, Bailey S. 2004 Treatment. In: Crome I, Ghodse H, Gilvarry E, McArdle P (eds) Young

People and Substance Misuse. London: The Royal College of Psychiatrists

Department of Health. 1999a NHS National Service Framework for Mental Health. London: HMSO

Department of Health. 1999b Code of Practice to the Mental Health Act 1983 (revised 1999). London: The Stationery Office

Department of Health. 2003 NHS Confidentiality Code of Practice. London: Department of Health

Department of Health. 2004 Standard 9. The Mental Health and Psychological Wellbeing of Children and Young People. London: Department of Health

Department of Health. 2004 National Service Framework for Children, Young People and Maternity Services: Executive Summary. London: The Stationary Office

Department of Health. 2006 Report on the Implementation of Standard 9 of the National Service Framework for Children, Young People and Maternity Services. London: Department of Health

dosReis S, Barnett S, Love RC, Riddle MA, Maryland Youth Practice Committee. 2003 A guide for managing acute aggressive behavior of youths in residential and inpatient treatment facilities. Psychiatric Serv 54(10): 1357–1363

Dunn V, Goodyer IM. 2006 Longitudinal investigation into childhood and adolescence-onset depression: psychiatric outcome in early adulthood. Br J Psychiatry 188: 216–222

Fonagy P, Target M, Cottrell D, Phillips J, Kurtz Z. 2002 What Works for Whom? A Critical Review of Treatments for Children and Adolescents. New York: Guilford Press

Gillick v West Norfolk and Wisbech Area Health Authority. 1986 AC 112

Goodman R, Scott S. 1997 Child Psychiatry. Oxford: Blackwell Science

Goodyer IM, Cooper PJ. 1993 A community study of depression in adolescent girls. II: the clinical features of identified disorder. Br J Psychiatry 163: 374–380

Goodyer IM, Herbert J, Tamplin A. 2003 Psychoendocrine antecedents of persistent first-episode major depression in adolescents: a community-based longitudinal enquiry. Psychol Med 33: 601–610

Harrington R. 1994 Affective disorders. In: Rutter M, Taylor E, Hersov L (eds) Child and Adolescent Psychiatry: Modern Approaches, 3rd edn. Oxford: Blackwell Science, p. 330–350

Harrington R. 2001 Depression, suicide and deliberate self harm in adolescence. Br Med Bull 57: 47–60

Harrington R, Dubicka B. 2001 Natural history of mood disorders in children and adolescents. In: Goodyer IM (ed) The Depressed Child and Adolescent. Cambridge Child and Adolescent Psychiatry Series. Cambridge: Cambridge University Press, pp. 311–343

Hawton K, Rodham K. 2006 By their Own Young Hand, Deliberate Self Harm and Suicidal Ideas in Adolescents. London: Jessica Kinglsey

Health Advisory Service. 1986 Bridge over Troubled Waters: A Report on Services for Adolescents. London: HMSO

Health Advisory Service. 1995 A Handbook on Children and Adolescent Mental Health. London: HMSO

Health Advisory Service. 1996 Children and Young people: Substance Misuse Services: The Substance of Young Needs. London: HMSO

Hollis C. 2000 Adolescent Schizophrenia: Advances in Psychiatric Treatment. London: Royal College of Psychiatrists

Institute for the Study of Drug Dependence. 1993 National Audit of Drug Misuse in Britain. London: Institute for the Study of Drug Dependence

Kaplan, T et al. 2002. From a short life project to a mainstream service: convincing commissioners to fund a community adolescent mental health team. Child Adolesc Mental Health 7 (3): 114–120

Linszen D et al. 1994 Cannabis abuse and the course of schizophrenic disorder. Arc Gen Psychiatry 51: 273–279

March J, Silva S et al. 2006 The Treatment for Adolescents with Depression Study (TADS): methods and message at 12 weeks. J Am Acad Child Adolesc Psychiatry 45(12): 1393–1403

Martinez-Arevalo MJ, Calcedo-Ordonez A, Varo Prieto JR. 1994 Cannabis consumption as a prognostic factor in schizophrenia. Br J Psychiatry 164(50): 679–681

McClure W, Schaffer D et al. 1966 Psychiatric diagnosis in child and adolescent suicide. Arch Gen Psychiatry 53: 339–348

Mears A, White R, Banerjee S et al. 2001 An Evaluation of the Use of the Children Act 1989 and the Mental Health Act 1983 in Children and Adolescents in Psychiatric Settings (CAMHA –CAPS). College Research Unit Report. London: Royal College of Psychiatrists

Miller P, Plant M. 1966 Drinking, smoking and illicit drug use among 15 and 16 year olds in the United Kingdom. Br Med J 313: 394–397

NHS Health Advisory Service. 1995 Together We Stand: Thematic review of the Commissioning, Role and Management of Child and Adolescent Mental Health Services. London: The Stationery Office

NICE 2002 Schizophrenia: Core Interventions in the Treatment and Management of Schizophrenia in Primary and Secondary Care. Clinical Guideline 1. London: NICE

NICE 2004 Self Harm Clinical Guideline 16. The Short Term Physical and Psychological Management and Secondary Prevention of Self Harm in Primary and Secondary Care. London: NICE

NICE 2005 Depression in Children and Young People. Identification and Management in Primary, Community and Secondary Care. Clinical Guideline 28. London: NICE

NICE 2007 Community Based Interventions to Reduce Substance Misuse Among Vulnerable and Disadvantaged Children and Young People. NICE public Health Intervention Guidance 4. London: NICE

O'Herlihy A, Worrall A, Banerjee S, Jaffa A *et al.* 2001 National In-patient Child and Adolescent Psychiatry Study. College Research Unit Report submitted to Department of Health, May 2001

Ramsey M, Baker P, Goulden G *et al.* 2001 Drug Misuse Declared in 2000: Results from the British Crime Survey. Home Office Research Study 224. London: Home Office

Royal College of Nursing. 2003 Restraining, Holding Still and Containing Children and Young People. Guidance for Nursing Staff (1999 updated 2003). London: Royal College of Nursing

Secretary of State for Health. 1999 Saving Lives: Our Healthies Nation. London: The Stationery Office

Shiers D, Lester H. 2004 Early intervention for first episode psychosis: needs greater involvement of primary care professionals for its success. Br Med J 328: 1451–1452

Street C. 2000 Whose Crisis? Meeting the Needs of Children and Young People with Serious Mental Health Problems. A Young Minds Study. Ward Guidelines. Guy's Hospital, South London and Maudsley Trust: Snowsfields Adolescent Unit

Treatment for Adolescents With Depression Study (TADS) Team. 2004 Fluoxetine, cognitive-behavioral therapy, and their combination for adolescents with depression: Treatment for Adolescents with Depression Study (TADS) randomized controlled trial. J Am Med Assoc 292: 807–820

UK Government. 2000 The Mental Health of Children and Adolescents in Great Britain. London: Office of National Statistis

White R, Harbour A, Williams R. 2004 London: The Royal College of Psychiatrists

Wolpert L. *et al.* 2006 Drawing on Evidence. Advice for Mental Health Professionals Working with Children and Adolescents, 2nd edn. London: CAMHS Publications

World Health Organization. 1992 The ICD-10 Classification of Mental and Behavioural Disorders: Clinical Descriptions and Diagnostic Guidelines. Geneva: World Health Organization

World Health Organization. 1996 Multiaxial Classification of Child and Adolescent Psychiatric Disorders. Cambridge: Cambridge University Press

Zeitlin H. 1999 Psychiatric comorbidity with substance misuse in children and teenagers. Drug Alcohol Depend 55: 225–234

18

Severe mental illness and substance abuse

Zerrin Atakan

Introduction

There has been a growing and justified interest in co-morbid severe mental illness and substance abuse over recent years, due to its high prevalence and significant impact on clinical and social problems, as well as the heavy burden laid on the health services. The annual health and social costs of misuse of alcohol and illegal substances in England and Wales are each estimated to be nearly £20 billion amongst people aged under 45 (Williams *et al.* 2005). The great majority of such patients are admitted to Psychiatric Intensive Care Unit (PICU) settings and their management can cause considerable difficulties, especially where there are no adequate evidence-based treatment models designed for inpatients.

The interaction between a psychotic illness and the use of substances is complex and is known to have major detrimental effects on the course of the illness, risk of violence, outcome, physical health complications and even possibly aetiology. In this chapter, these complex interactions will be examined and some management strategies will be discussed.

As mentioned in Chapter 10 on complex needs patients, substance use is one of the main characteristics of this group. Even though most of the studies in this area originate from the USA, the prevalance of substance abuse amongst the severely mentally ill is also known to be high in the UK where the estimated prevalence ranges between 20% and 60% (Miles *et al.*

2003). In PICU settings the average prevalence can be as high as 85% percent (Isaac *et al.* 2005). Polydrug abuse is common and under-detection of substance use can be as high as 50% (Kavanagh *et al.* 2002). Frequently the use of one substance leads to the use of another.

It is important to point out that mentally ill patients have a higher prevalence of substance misuse compared to the general population, even though the figures vary according to the country and over time. The most frequently used substances amongst patients with severe mental illness are: nicotine, alcohol, cannabis, crack cocaine and amphetamines. In Australia a population survey found that among those who had a psychotic illness regular nicotine, alcohol and cannabis use were much more common and they were more likely to be dependent compared to the general population (Degenhardt and Hall 2001).

Several studies have found that there is a high correlation between alcoholism and anxiety disorders, affective disorders and antisocial personality disorder. Drug abuse has been shown to be high in patients with major depression, bipolar disorder, antisocial personality disorder and schizophrenia. Table 18.1 shows the prevalence rates of the Epidemiological Catchment Area (ECA) Study (Regier *et al.* 1990). Both alcohol and drug abuse amongst the mentally ill are highly co-morbid, irrespective of gender (Kessler *et al.* 1994).

Psychiatric Intensive Care, 2nd edn., eds. M. Dominic Beer, Stephen M. Pereira and Carol Paton.
Published by Cambridge University Press. © Cambridge University Press 2008.

Table 18.1. Co-morbidity of substance abuse and other psychiatric disorders: prevalence ratios from the Epidemiological Catchment Area study

	Females		Males	
	Alcohol abuse/Dependence	Other drug abuse/Dependence	Alcohol abuse/Dependence	Other drug abuse/Dependence
Antisocial	29.6	26.6	12.0	7.3
Alcoholism	—	9.0	—	2.9
Other drug abuse	8.8	—	4.8	—
Major depression	2.7	3.6	2.4	4.9
Mania	9.3	11.1	6.5	11.3
Panic	4.4	2.9	4.2	4.1
Phobias	2.1	1.9	1.8	2.4
OCD	2.1	3.5	3.0	3.6
Schizophrenia	5.6	6.4	4.6	6.2

OCD, Obsessive-compulsive disorder.

Interaction between substance use and severe mental illness

Before examining the effects of substances on severe mental illness, it is important to make a distinction between a substance-induced psychosis and a newly developing primary psychotic disorder that co-occurs with the use of alcohol or substances. This is especially significant in understanding the illness course and planning of the appropriate management. There is limited research making the distinction between the two categories and one recent study shows that there are significant differences between the two groups (Caton *et al.* 2005). Parental substance abuse is more common among the substance-induced psychosis group, whilst those with a primary diagnosis of a psychotic illness are less likely to be dependent on any substance and have higher positive and negative symptom scores. Substance-induced psychosis usually resolves more quickly compared to primary psychosis. Patients in PICUs are mostly those who belong to the second group, but on occasions patients can acutely present with a substance-induced illness. In this chapter we deal mainly with patients who have more enduring conditions and abuse substances.

Substance use amongst first-onset psychosis patients

There are numerous studies showing the detrimental effects of substances on severe mental illness. The complex interaction between the two varies from aetiology to the progress of the illness itself. As seen in the general population, substance misuse is especially common amongst those who are young, male, unemployed and have a lower level of education, a history of family adversity and conduct disorder. Early-onset psychosis services report significantly high rates of substance misuse, in particular cannabis, in newly diagnosed patients (van Mastrigt *et al.* 2004; Wade *et al.* 2006). Adolescence is a period when biological, psychological and social factors have a significant impact on the formation of the adult self and experimentation, together with high-risk-taking behaviour, can be common. Use of a substance, such as cannabis, appears to be an aetiological factor in the development of an enduring psychotic illness, especially in those who are predisposed to developing it (Henquet *et al.* 2005). In a recent study examining the course of substance misuse and daily tobacco use in first-episode psychosis patients, it was found that about three-quarters of patients had a lifetime substance misuse and half of all patients had current use of mainly cannabis during the initial 15-month treatment period (Wade *et al.* 2006). They found that despite receiving at least basic counselling regarding the potential risks of substance use on recovery from psychosis, three in every four patients maintained daily tobacco use. However, it was also found that patients who continued substance misuse were likely to reduce the severity and/or frequency of their substance use during the study period.

Substance misuse predicts a poor clinical outcome in patients with early psychosis and its negative impact on the course of the illness can be independent from medication adherence, diagnosis and potential confounding factors (Sorbara *et al.* 2003). Medication non-adherence, however, can also be related to the underlying depressive symptomatology and unstable living circumstances, rather than the substance misuse per se, as suggested in a recent study (Elbogen *et al.* 2005). In this study 528 patients with schizophrenia were examined in order to study the relationship between substance abuse and medication non-adherence, and multivariate analyses showed that factors such as substance abuse, depressive symptoms and living stability each contributed to medication non-adherence. The authors emphasise the importance of the utility of assessment of depression and living circumstances when evaluating adherence among people with psychosis.

Effects of substance use on the course of the illness

There is ample evidence in the literature showing that substance misuse can have a detrimental effect on the course of the illness, especially when patients with already established severe mental illness continue using substances or alcohol. The effects vary from medication compliance to increased hospi-

talisation. Medication non-compliance is found to be strongly associated with substance abuse among patients with schizophrenia (Owen *et al.* 1996). Persistent substance use after first admission for psychosis has a deleterious impact on clinical outcome, such as increased risk of readmission, of presenting with psychotic symptoms and with developing a more continuous course of illness (Sorbara *et al.* 2003). In another outcome study comparing adolescent and adult first episode patients, it was shown that the adolescents used more cannabis and had an increased number of relapses (Pencer *et al.* 2005).

Substance use and risk of violence

When taken during a psychotic state, substances can increase the risk of a patient's wanting to act on his or her delusions and display violence. Symptoms such as hostility, paranoid ideation and substance abuse are the most significant short-term predictors of violent behaviour. Furthermore, substances such as alcohol can cause disinhibition, which again increases the risk of violence and impulsive behaviour.

There is ample research evidence showing the association between violence and substance abuse, but little is available regarding the specific links between psychiatric disorder, violence and substance misuse (Phillips 2000). However, over the last 10 years there have been some important studies shedding light on the complex interactions between the three entities. One such study is the MacArthur Violence Risk Assessment Study, which involved comprehensive follow-up of 1000 patients who were discharged from acute care settings (Dyer 1996). It was found that the risk of violence in patients with substance use and psychotic disorder was increased fourfold. The same study also suggests that violent behaviour is mediated by sociological, pharmacological and psychological factors within the individual. Another key study is the Epidemiological Catchment Area Survey Study in the USA, in which 10 000 people were surveyed (Swanson *et al.* 1996). In this study severely mentally ill patients were four times more likely to have been violent by 1 year and this figure was 17-fold when the patients abused substances.

In a national survey of 3142 prisoners in the UK, severe dependence on cannabis and psychostimulants was found to be associated with a higher risk of psychosis and was in contrast to severe dependence on heroin (Farrell *et al.* 2002). They also found that those who started abusing cannabis, amphetamine, cocaine or opiates before the age of 16 years were at greater risk of psychosis. The same group of researchers also found that one in four prisoners with a psychotic disorder had psychotic symptoms attributed to toxic or withdrawal effects of psychoactive substances (Brugha *et al.* 2005). These studies emphasise how a combination of mental illness and substance misuse can lead to an increased risk of criminal behaviour.

Substance use and victimisation

Even though much attention is given to violent behaviour perpetrated by patients with severe mental illness, they are often the victims of violence themselves (Table 18.2). Results of an Australian National Survey show that the odds of being a victim were increased in those who were female, homeless and had a lifetime history of substance abuse (Chapple *et al.* 2004).

Table 18.2. The co-occurrence of severe mental illness and use of drugs and/or alcohol is associated with the following

- Early psychotic breakdown
- Poor compliance with treatment
- Increased rates of hospitalisation
- Increased rates of violence
- Increased rates of suicide
- Increased rates of victimisation
- Criminal behaviour
- Homelessness

Menezes *et al.* 1996; Swanson *et al.* 1996; Kovasznay *et al.* 1997; Chapple *et al.* 2004.

Most commonly used substances

Most studies treat patients as a homogenous population, grouping together different substances, and there appears to be less substance-specific research (Crawford *et al.* 2003). A study carried out in the UK by Miles *et al.* (2003) investigated whether patients could be defined according to the main substance they misused. They found that there was a significant difference in the lifetime history of violence, which was more frequent among stimulant users. Alcohol users were older and more likely to be white. Currently there are no research data available on whether the management of such patients should vary according to the substance they primarily use. Substances such as heroin and opiates are not commonly used by this group of patients. We will now look at the substances most commonly used by severely mentally ill patients.

Nicotine

Even though more and more people are quitting smoking in the general population, patients with severe mental illness still have extremely high rates of smoking ranging from 58% to 90%, and they are therefore at greater risk for smoking-related illnesses (McCreadie 2002). Because nicotine induces the metabolism of some antipsychotic medications, smokers with schizophrenia require higher doses of medications such as clozapine, which in turn increase their risk of experiencing side-effects. Smoking behaviour has also been found to be significantly related to an enhanced risk for alcohol abuse (Margolese *et al.* 2004).

Despite the size of the problem, there are only a few studies looking at the success rate of cessation programmes. It is difficult to design cessation programmes for people with schizophrenia that take into account their various cognitive and social deficits. Some of these programmes focus on nicotine replacement (NRT) methods only (Chou *et al.* 2004), whilst others use atypical antipsychotics in addition to NRT (George *et al.* 2000). Such methods have been found to be successful but additional behavioural cessation programmes are thought to be needed to accompany these methods. More recently there have been a few programmes which use a combination of motivational enhancement, relapse prevention, social skills training and supportive therapy with promising results, especially when used in conjunction with NRT (Evins *et al.* 2004). Another recent study applied the Transtheoretical Model which focuses on listing the pros and cons of smoking and beliefs and attitudes about smoking to patients with schizophrenia-spectrum disorders who were either chronic or first-episode patients (Esterberg and Compton 2005). They found significant differences between the new and chronically ill patients in the areas of readiness to quit and beliefs about smoking cessation and an overall negative attitude toward NRT. Esterberg and Compton (2005) make a specific comment about the difficulty in applying this method due to impaired cognitive functioning and lack of motivation frequently found, especially in those with chronic forms of the illness. Most of these intervention studies for cessation of smoking take place in the USA and there are as yet no known programmes designed for people with severe mental illness established in the UK.

Conclusions

- Compared to the general population, the smoking rate amongst patients with severe mental illness is extremely high
- Patients who smoke carry significant physical health care risks
- There are as yet no established treatment programmes for smoking cessation for this group, but nicotine replacement therapies along with education on health risks should be actively introduced

Alcohol

Alcohol dependence is more common amongst those who have bipolar disorder, schizophrenia, schizoaffective disorder and antisocial personality disorder than in the general population (Schuckit *et al.* 1997; Etter and Etter 2004). It is also known that a great majority of those who are dependent on alcohol suffer from anxiety states prior to their dependence. It is suggested that patients use alcohol to relieve anxiety, but in fact alcohol adds to their problems by worsening psychotic symptoms, as well as increasing risks for poor physical health. Due to its disinhibiting effect alcohol use is significantly linked with increased risk for violent behaviour and also with victimisation. However, the risk is not only high during intoxication states but also during withdrawal from alcohol.

Alcohol use usually co-exists with the use of other substances and is especially prevalent in non-affective and affective psychoses. Interestingly, alcohol use can be seen in any age group, whilst the use of other substances is seen in younger age groups (Kavanagh *et al.* 2004). Under-reporting of alcohol consumption amongst patients with severe mental illness is significant and therefore careful and detailed assessment of current alcohol use, as well as other substance use, is crucial when taking histories from patients and their carers.

Conclusions

- Alcohol dependence is high amongst those with severe mental illness compared to the general population and carries serious health risks
- Alcohol is frequently linked with the use of other substances
- Under-reporting of alcohol use is common and a detailed assessment of current use is important

Cannabis

Cannabis is used by people with severe mental illness significantly more than is found in the general population. On a recent review of cannabis use and misuse prevalence among people with psychosis, when the findings of fifty-three treatment samples and five epidemiological studies were analysed, it was found that lifetime use is 42% and lifetime misuse is 22.5% (Green *et al.* 2005). Current use was reported to be 23%, whilst current misuse was 11.3%. In a recent UK study which took place in a PICU setting, where

115 patients were studied, 71.3% of patients were abusing cannabis (Isaac *et al.* 2005). These patients were found to be more severely ill and spent longer periods in PICU care. Furthermore, they had greater weight increase and higher blood glucose levels on admission as compared to those who did not use cannabis.

With the relaxation of the law and growing views that cannabis is a 'harmless' drug, its use has been increasing steeply in many countries, whilst the age of initial use has been decreasing (Johns 2001; Degenhardt *et al.* 2003). Especially among young people, cannabis use is increasing (Rey and Tennant 2002).

More recently there has been some significant research emerging in relation to the association between use of cannabis amongst young people and the subsequent risk of developing a psychotic illness. The first significant research on this is the Swedish conscript study, in which over 50 000 subjects were studied and heavy cannabis use at age 18 years was found to increase the risk of later schizophrenia six-fold (Andreasson *et al.* 1987). This study was later criticised for its methodology and more recently Zammit and colleagues have re-evaluated the data taking into account these criticisms. They found that the findings were still consistent with a causal relation (Zammit *et al.* 2002).

The Dunedin study is the first prospective longitudinal study of adolescent cannabis use as a risk factor for adult schizophreniform disorder, taking into account childhood psychotic symptoms ante-dating cannabis use (Arseneault *et al.* 2002). A birth cohort of 1037 individuals was followed up until age 26 years. As well as agreeing with the causal link, the researchers report that cannabis use is not secondary to a pre-existing psychosis, that early cannabis use carries a greater risk for schizophrenia than later cannabis use (by age 18 years) and the risk is specific to cannabis use as opposed to the use of other drugs.

Another recent longitudinal study which involved a population survey examining the mechanisms between cannabis use and psychosis was carried out by van Os and colleagues (2002). A 3-year follow-up of over 4000 individuals showed that cannabis use increases the risk of both the incidence of psychosis in previously non-psychotic persons and a poor prognosis in those with psychotic disorder.

Henquet and colleagues (2005) followed up 2437 young people (14–24 years), with and without predisposition for psychosis, for 4 years and after adjustment for other factors they found that the effect of cannabis use was much stronger in those with predisposition for psychosis (23.8%) than in those without (5.6%), and that there is a dose–response relation with increasing frequency of cannabis use (Henquet *et al.* 2005).

There has been a considerable interest in whether or not there is a causal relationship between cannabis use and the development of a psychotic illness. To examine this Moore *et al.* (2007) carried out a systematic review of longitudinal and population-based studies. They found that there is sufficient evidence that cannabis use increased the risk of psychosis outcome by 1.4 times. Furthermore they found a dose-dependent link, with greater risk in those who used it more frequently. They also reviewed studies looking into the association between cannabis use and affective disorders but found that the available evidence for this was less consistent.

Even though the verdict on the causal relationship is not yet finalised, there is ample evidence that ongoing use of cannabis by those with established severe mental illness can worsen the course of the disorder (Mueser *et al.* 2000; Arseneault *et al.* 2002; Degenhardt and Hall 2002). As well as affecting the outcome and leading to the exacerbation of symptoms, cannabis use amongst patients with psychosis can also lead to behavioural disturbances, such as increased risk of violence and criminal activity (Miles *et al.* 2003). After smoking cannabis, the worsening of symptoms, especially suspiciousness and subsequent hostility, is a frequently observed phenomenon in PICU and acute admission ward settings.

Even though there are a few treatment programmes developed for outpatients with 'dual diagnosis' and some for cannabis use for healthy people, there are no programmes designed for inpatients who predominantly use cannabis. Most treatment programmes use a combination of motivational enhancement and cognitive behaviour techniques for harm reduction or cessation.

Conclusions

- People with psychosis use cannabis more compared to the general population
- There is epidemiological evidence that cannabis use at early ages (below 18 years) may increase the risk of development of psychosis, especially in those who are genetically vulnerable or predisposed to developing it
- Regular cannabis use negatively affects the course of psychosis by leading to:
  - Exacerbation or precipitation of symptoms
  - Higher risk of relapse and increased hospitalisation
  - Longer duration of psychotic episode
  - Poor social functioning
  - Increased risk of behavioural problems, violence, criminal activity
- There are as yet no specific treatment models designed for inpatients who use cannabis.

Crack cocaine

The use of cocaine, especially in the form of crack cocaine, by those with severe mental illness has increased worryingly over the last decade due to its easy availability and cheap price. Crack cocaine is obtained by heating the ordinary cocaine hydrochloride in a solution of baking soda until the water evaporates. This type of cocaine makes a cracking sound when heated; hence, the name 'crack'. Crack vaporises at a low temperature, so it can be easily inhaled via a heated pipe. The initial short-lived euphoria is followed by a 'crash' when the person experiences anxiety, depression, irritability, extreme fatigue and paranoia. Some may have tactile hallucinations of insects crawling underneath the skin, known as formication. Cocaine-induced paranoia is well known and is especially

seen in those who use it on a regular and heavy basis (Floyd *et al.* 2006).

Cocaine when taken with alcohol forms a metabolite called cocethylene, which has a significantly long half-life and is more potent than cocaine (Crawford *et al.* 2003). Alcohol dependence is linked with cocaine use and puts alcohol-dependent patients at greater risk of violence and unsafe sexual encounters (Heil *et al.* 2001). In PICU and acute admission settings, some patients with severe mental illness report that their current use of crack cocaine has a negative impact, due to their acute awareness of it making them 'paranoid'. The withdrawal from crack cocaine can be very fast and is then followed by intense craving and withdrawal symptoms. During such states violent and impulsive behaviour is frequently observed and this creates further challenges in the management of patients with severe mental illness.

Conclusions

- The use of crack cocaine by patients with severe mental illness is increasing because of its easy availability and cheap price
- Mixing cocaine and alcohol is specifically dangerous due to the release of a potent metabolite
- Cocaine withdrawal happens quite intensely and consequent craving can lead to violent and impulsive behaviour and increased risk of offending

Benzodiazepines

Benzodiazepine use is high among people who abuse substances. Patients with severe mental illness who use substances are often prescribed benzodiazepines, not only for their anxiety symptoms, but also for sedation purposes and to combat medication side-effects. In a 5-year prevalence of benzodiazepine study, patients with schizophrenia and substance misuse were found to have 63% prevalence rate. This rate was even higher (75%) for patients with bipolar disorder. The rates were significantly high compared to patients who did not have a co-occurring substance misuse disorder (Clark *et al.* 2004).

Even though it can be possible to use benzodiazepines safely under close supervision, more often patients are allowed to just continue using benzodiazepines, which in turn leads to their being addicted to yet another drug. There is very limited research evidence on the use of benzodiazepines in this specific group of patients. One prospective longitudinal 6-year follow-up study examined 203 outpatients with severe mental illness and co-occurring substance abuse (Brunette *et al.* 2003). A high rate of use of prescribed benzodiazepines (43%) was found in this group and 15% of them were abusing it 6 years later. Benzodiazepine abuse rate was 6% amongst those who were not prescribed benzodiazepines at the outset. Authors suggest that clinicians should consider other treatments for anxiety in this population. If benzodiazepines have to be prescribed however, they need to be carefully monitored and stopped at the earliest opportunity. It is highly recommended that cessation occurs well before the patient is discharged.

Conclusions

- Benzodiazepine abuse is high amongst patients with severe mental illness who also abuse substances
- Benzodiazepines are widely prescribed to this group of patients
- Benzodiazepine prescription should be avoided, as far as possible, as those who are prescribed it are more likely to continue to abuse it
- If a benzodiazepine has to be prescribed, close monitoring is essential and it should be stopped before the patient is discharged to the community

Managing severe mental illness and substance abuse

Effective management of patients with severe mental illness and substance abuse is at an early stage in its development and there is limited research evidence for successful models. However, some strategies can be developed for better management and treatment,

which are based on existing research, and these are discussed here.

Assessment

Comprehensive assessment is the first step towards effective management and treatment of a patient with a co-morbid condition. It is not enough to make a brief comment on whether or not he/she uses or has used certain substances. A thorough assessment will provide a better understanding of the interactions between the two conditions. Even though there are some valid assessment scales available for this purpose, and these will be discussed, their use may not always be possible for practical reasons. In any case, a comprehensive substance history needs to be taken to include systematic information such as length of abuse, types of preferred substances, reasons for substance taking, method of use, subjective experience, what the patient gains or loses from it, how it affects his or her mental and physical health, social life, medication, compliance and finances. Whilst making an assessment it is important to maintain a non-judgemental manner, remembering that under-reporting is very common. Further information can be gathered from carers and friends, whenever possible.

The use of substances and alcohol can continue in acute care and PICU/LSU settings, despite efforts to prevent it, and can have detrimental effects on the progress made in the treatment of the patient. The deterioration of the clinical state can demoralise not only the patient but also the staff. However, it is important to acknowledge the possibility of such occurrences without losing the determination to assist them in changing their drug-taking behaviour. Having an open and honest communication about these matters will encourage the patient to be more open about his or her reasons for drug use. It is crucial to engage the patient in all steps of care by ensuring their active involvement in their treatment and management. This includes drawing up care plans with the patient, which may include preventative measures such as agreeing to talk about their craving behaviour and to accept randomised urine drug analyses.

Attention to stage of use

During the assessment special attention should be given to the stage patients are at in relation to their substance use behaviour, as the effect and impact can vary according to the stage of use. For instance, during the intoxication state, patients become more vulnerable to victimisation, accidental injuries and expression of violence to others and themselves. They are also more likely to have unprotected sex and increase the risk of sexually transmitted diseases, including positive-HIV status. These risks occur due to increased impulsivity, impaired cognition and disinhibition during intoxication. When a patient is withdrawing from a substance, craving behaviour can lead to increased criminal behaviour and violence, as well as confusion and extreme discomfort. Ongoing use of substances can lead to cognitive impairment, changes in personality traits, criminal behaviour and the impact of the habit on their economic state. Physical health care needs are usually multiple and special attention should be paid to assessing these, whilst carrying out relevant investigations, with a view to providing medical care when required.

Assessment tools

Even though there are numerous valid and reliable scales available to assess and measure substance use for substance abusers in the normal population, it is only over the last decade that some scales have been developed specifically for those with a severe mental illness (Table 18.3). Such tools can be used for a more thorough assessment to ensure the collection of good quality data. In the literature there are numerous scales which have established reliability and validity. For instance, Psychiatric Research Interview for Substance and Mental Disorders (PRISM) has been shown to be reliable with enhanced diagnostic accuracy (Hasin *et al.* 1996). However, this scale can take time to complete. The Chemical Use, Abuse and Dependence (CUAD) scale, on the other hand, is shorter but valid and reliable at the same time (Appleby *et al.* 1996). Some other scales provide information on the motivational level

Table 18.3. Some useful assessment of substance misuse scales for patients with severe mental illness

- PRISM: Psychiatric Research Interview for Substance and Mental Disorders Scale
- CUAD: Chemical Use, Abuse and Dependence Scale
- SOCRATES: Stages of Change Readiness and Treatment Eagerness Scale
- SATS: Substance Abuse Treatment Scale
- ASI: Addiction Severity Index

for change, such as the Stages of Change Readiness and Treatment Eagerness Scale (SOCRATES), which is a self-report nineteen-item measure. In a study which compared various similar scales Carey and colleagues found that such scales had validity and were stable over time. They also suggest that self-report scales support efforts to quantify readiness to change substance misuse in those who have severe mental illness, but they should not be used exclusively (Carey *et al.* 2001). There is also a scale which evaluates treatment progress and outcome called the Substance Abuse Treatment Scale (SATS). Based on its use in a community-based sample of persons with co-morbid disorder, it is reported to be valid and reliable by McHugo *et al.* (1995).

Some of the assessment tools which are normally used for non-psychotic populations have also been tried on patients with severe mental illness and substance use problems. For instance, Addiction Severity Index, which has a well established reliability and validity (McLellan *et al.* 1980), has been revised to include new sections, including psychiatric problems (McLellan *et al.* 1992) and more recently has been found to be a reliable method of assessing drug and alcohol use amongst patients with a psychotic disorder (Helseth *et al.* 2005).

Psycho-education on the effects of substances

The impact of promoting healthy choices and early education on the effects of tobacco smoking has led to a steady decrease of use in the UK (Henry *et al.* 2003). However, the number of cannabis smokers, especially among young people, has been increasing.

According to a survey of students in Exeter, the number of 14 to 15-year-olds who tried cannabis increased from 19% to 29% in boys and 18% to 25% in girls in one year (Schools Health Education Unit 2002). There has not yet been a successful campaign in schools on the health effects of cannabis smoking. Education, especially as a preventative measure, is particularly crucial given the available evidence on the harmful effects of cannabis in triggerring an enduring psychotic illness, especially in those who have a predisposition to it.

There is limited evidence-based data on the effects of psycho-education on substance use by patients with severe mental illness. However, a review of studies over a 10-year period on smoking cessation programmes for people with mental illness concludes that the majority of interventions combined psycho-education and medication (El-Guebaly *et al.* 2002). Providing information to patients on the effects of substance use and how it interacts with their treatment and the outcome of their illness can be a daunting task, as it is frequently seen that most patients cannot easily retain this information. This information needs to be provided without taking a judgemental tone, bearing in mind that under-reporting of use and misuse is quite common. There is some evidence, however, that well-structured educational sessions can have some impact on the patient's insight into their mental health problems (Macpherson *et al.* 1996). Authors suggest that a series of patient education sessions is needed to consolidate learning and a single session will not be sufficient. In addition, carers involvement is crucial and they too require information on all aspects of mental illness and the impact of substance use. Further work needs to be done in this area to provide evidence of the impact of psycho-education on harm reduction or cessation of substance use.

Treatment models

Despite the size of the problem, there are not yet any established and effective treatment methods available. However, a variety of treatment models have been proposed. These will be discussed here.

Specially designed services for severe mental illness and substance misuse or use

Over the last decade, with increasing concern at the impact of dual diagnosis patients on existing resources, there has been a movement to create specially designed services and treatment programmes. However, in the USA, the creation of services which integrate substance misuse and adult mental health services has not been easy, due to separate funding sources or different administrative divisions. In the UK, although the substance misuse service is part of the mental health service, the day-to-day functioning of services and personnel are also known to be separate. There are some significant differences between these services, especially in relation to their philosophies and treatment approaches. Mental health services have specially trained clinical staff and favour assertive efforts to maintain people in treatment, medication and psychosocial approaches. Then again substance misuse staff can be people who have been drug abusers themselves and the patients are not treated in an assertive manner, but are encouraged to take responsibility and use voluntary organisations. These major differences of approach need to be taken into consideration when a special programme to treat dual-diagnosis patients is being planned (Table 18.4).

One treatment model is that following the treatment of psychiatric illness, the substance abuse is treated. The other method involves concurrent but separate treatment of both psychiatric and substance misuse disorders, when different teams from each service treat patients. Both of these models can be applied when there are no integrated services available, but they require seamless planning and time management, with special care not to overload the patient. The third method is the integrated model, where both disorders are treated concurrently by the same clinical team. This model requires the presence of well-integrated inpatient care, assertive community services and supportive living environments. Treatment methods vary within this model. Motivation-based treatments and engagement with services and psychosocial methods have

Table 18.4. Three treatment models

- **Serial treatment:** one treatment is followed by the other
- **Parallel treatment:** the concurrent but separate treatments delivered by two teams.
  Both serial and parallel treatment programmes require:
    - Seamless planning
    - Time management
    - Special care not to overload the patient
- **Integrated treatment**: both treatments are delivered by the same team and this model requires:
    - Well-integrated inpatient and substance misuse treatments and assertive community services
    - Assertive styles of engagement
    - Supportive living environments

both been advocated. This model can be costly and requires careful planning of existing resources or the creation of new ones.

Although there are some studies showing that the third model, with integrated case management services, can lead to a better outcome in dual diagnosis patients (Rosenthal *et al.* 1992; Ries and Comtois 1997), there does not appear to be any clear evidence that one model is superior to another or that these models produce a better outcome compared to traditional services. A recent systematic Cochrane review aimed to evaluate the effectiveness of treatment programmes for people with dual diagnosis identified six studies which met their selection criteria (Jeffery *et al.* 2000). However, most of these studies were either small in size or did not report important clinical outcome measures. The reviewers concluded that there is no clear evidence supporting an advantage of any one type of substance misuse programme over another. They add that the current momentum for integrated services is not based on good evidence and suggest that the implementation of new specialist services should be within the context of simple, well-designed controlled trials.

It can be suggested that within the PICU/LSU setting, where there is a high staff-to-patient ratio, training staff in substance abuse issues may have beneficial effects, at least for a proportion of dual-diagnosis patients. Indeed in our clinical experience,

providing regular information on the adverse effects of substances and rewarding abstinence by leaves from the unit, combined with the use of atypical antipsychotics, have been beneficial in increasing the motivation to stop abusing drugs in a number of patients.

Motivation to stop abusing substances can be very low in dual diagnosis patients and may vary according to the substance abused. In a study of outpatients, the percentage of low motivational level (precontemplation and contemplation) was 41% for opiates and 60% for cocaine (Ziedonis and Trudeau 1997). The same authors used a motivation-based treatment to increase the level of motivation for change. In addition, they advocate the following to achieve extended abstinence: the use of community reinforcement approaches (i.e. treatments focusing on engagement with treatment), external and internal levers to increase motivation, case management and blending traditional substance abuse psychotherapy approaches with mental health treatment with atypical antipsychotics.

Psychological interventions

Over recent years some psychological intervention methods have been developed to provide patient-tailored treatment programmes to tackle substance misuse problems for patients with severe mental illness. Such methods match treatment to the individual according to their motivational level. In a study where motivational level was assessed, it was shown that low motivation to quit substances varied according to the substance used. For instance, the cessation figures were 41% for opiates, 48% for alcohol, 51% for cannabis and 60% for cocaine (Ziedonis and Trudeau 1997). In other words, quitting substances such as opiates and alcohol required higher motivational levels.

Motivational interviewing therapies are based on a five-stage scale which determines the motivational level of the individual in terms of readiness to change. These are defined as follows:

1. **Precontemplation:** continuous use with no interest to quit in the previous 6 months

2. **Contemplation:** continuous use with ambivalent interest to quit
3. **Preparation:** continuous use with interest to quit in the subsequent 30 days
4. **Action:** active attempt to stop
5. **Maintenance:** abstinent for more than 3 months but less than 5 years

Motivational interviewing or enhancement therapy aims to build patient's motivation for change by increasing awareness of the impact of the substance use, whilst taking an empathic approach to encourage responsibility, according to the patient's motivational stage. The interaction between the therapist and the patient is based on being open, non-judgemental and realistic about what can be achieved. Giving advice or immediate problem solving is usually avoided. The interview is strategically directed towards the patient's use of substances and related life events. In some patients the aim may be harm reduction, in others it can be cessation or maintenance.

The efficacy of motivational interviewing has been well established, especially in the non-psychotic populations, and most recently it has also been applied to patients with severe mental illness. In a recent multi-site cluster randomised trial, when a single session of motivational interview was applied to non-psychotic young people, it was found that those who were randomised to motivational interview sessions reduced their use of cigarettes, alcohol and cannabis, mainly through moderation of ongoing substance use, rather than cessation at 3 months follow-up (McCambridge and Strang 2004). However, studies carried out on patients with severe mental illness indicate that a single session would not be sufficient in this group. The reasons for this are that patients with severe mental illness may have hindering cognitive deficits and disordered thinking. A recent study applied motivational interviewing principles to patients with severe mental illness, taking into account their deficits by simplifying open-ended questions, refining reflective thinking skills, heightening emphasis on affirmations and integrating psychiatric issues into personalised feedback (Martino *et al.* 2002). They also highlighted the importance of taking clinical considerations, such as crisis events and handling psychotic exacerbations, into account when treating this group of patients.

Some psychosocial treatment programmes combine various therapy models. For instance, relapse prevention treatment may involve a hybrid behavioural therapy approach that integrates prevention of substance abuse relapse and social skills training in a patient who is in the action stage. The needs of the patient would be expected to be different at each stage. For instance, if a patient is moving from the action stage to the maintenance stage, special attention would be given to the restoration of relationships, seeking employment or meaningful activities, especially in social settings with non-drug users.

Recently there have been a number of studies published solely carried out on outpatients. There are, as yet, no valid treatment models applied to inpatients. There are only a few validated models for outpatients and one of these is a manualised group-based intervention which aims to help patients to reduce their substance use. The actual intervention is based on motivational enhancement and cognitive-behaviour therapy principles and is tailored to patient's stage of change and motivational level. The intervention consists of weekly 90-min sessions over 6 weeks. In a randomised control study which involved sixty-three patients, 92% completed a 3-month follow-up assessment of psychopathology, antipsychotic medicine dose, alcohol and substance use, severity of dependence and hospitalisation. Significant improvements were found in most outcome measures in the treatment group in comparison to the control, following the described intervention (James *et al.* 2004). However, this study is limited in that it only indicates benefit in short-term follow-up.

In the UK, a randomised controlled study evaluated the efficacy of individual- and family-orientated cognitive-behaviour therapy for treatment resistant psychosis combined with motivational intervention for substance use problems over an 18-month follow-up period, when the treatment group patients received approximately twenty-nine sessions of combined therapy (Haddock *et al.* 2003). Significant improvements in patient functioning were found in the treatment group, compared to standard care patients, over 18 months. The cost was comparable to the control treatment.

In addition to the motivational enhancement therapies, recently some other psychological intervention models have been proposed. For instance, the Insight-Adherence-Abstinence triad is introduced as an integrated treatment focus for patients with first-episode schizophrenia who also use cannabis. This model focuses on building adherence to medication treatment, abstinence from substances and insight building during the first year of treatment, in order to prevent further relapses, and specifically targets the unique characteristics of the first-episode patients. It provides supportive, cognitive-behavioural, behavioural and motivational therapies as well as skill building and psycho-education. In a recent study which involved sixty-eight patients, thirty of whom were abusing cannabis, this form of intervention was applied and significant improvements in the treatment group were observed (Miller *et al.* 2005).

There is a need to have psychological intervention programmes applicable to inpatient groups. In PICU/LSU and acute care settings, substance use can unfortunately continue and as a consequence create further treatment and management problems. Interestingly some patients, especially at the beginning of their admission, can admit to the deleterious effect of their substance use, as it may still be fresh in their memory that, for instance, cannabis or crack cocaine use has made them suspicious and led to their admission to hospital. This level of motivation can be facilitated into harm reduction or cessation, if there is a valid treatment model available. Studies examining effective treatment models are needed for this group.

Conclusion

- There is some evidence, based on a few randomised controlled trials on outpatient groups, that cognitive-behaviour therapy and motivational intervention methods can be superior to routine care
- There are as yet no treatment models developed for inpatient groups

Pharmacotherapy of severe mental illness and substance abuse

The pharmacotherapy of dual-diagnosis patients is a recently developing area. It studies both the pharmacokinetics of the substance and the psychotropics and their interactions. Animal studies show that cocaine seeking behaviour may be diminished by administering dopamine-like agonists to rats who have been primed with cocaine previously (Self *et al.* 1996). Deriving from this premise, amantadine, a dopamine agonist that is normally used to alleviate extrapyramidal side-effects, may have a desired effect when used for prevention of a stimulant relapse. Some tricyclic antidepressants, such as desipramine (a dopamine re-uptake inhibitor), have also been suggested to prevent cocaine relapse. In an open, double-blind, placebo-controlled study, desipramine was given to cocaine abusing patients with schizophrenia and the preliminary results suggest that cocaine-abusing schizophrenic patients who received desipramine for 12 weeks used less cocaine in a 15-month follow-up period, compared to those who received the placebo (Wilkins 1997). Wilkins, in his review article, concludes that the treatment of cocaine-abusing schizophrenic patients may be enhanced by the addition of desipramine to the treatment regime and that cocaine-induced depression is alleviated by desipramine. He also adds that cannabis, when taken concomitantly with cocaine, may also reduce the depressive symptomatology, whilst increasing hostility and suspiciousness.

It is suggested by research that one of the major reasons why schizophrenic patients take substances is to 'self-treat' the negative symptoms or to reduce the side-effects of neuroleptics. For instance, cannabis has been shown to reduce negative symptoms, whilst increasing the positive symptoms of schizophrenia (Peralta and Cuesta 1995). Hence, targeting the treatment of negative and affective symptoms of schizophrenia may have beneficial effects on reducing the drive or the need to take substances.

As mentioned previously, an ideal medicine for a stimulant-abusing schizophrenic patient should target the reduction of negative and positive symptoms and the drive to take stimulants. Clozapine has been shown to alleviate negative symptoms and in principle should have some effects on the drive to take drugs. In a study comparing substance-abusing schizophrenics with non-abusing ones, clozapine produced similar improvements in symptoms and psychosocial functioning levels and the history of substance abuse did not appear to negatively influence response to clozapine (Buckley *et al.* 1994). In a recent review article Buckley advocates the use of clozapine as the therapeutic option for patients with dual diagnosis as it has been shown to reduce alcohol, tobacco and cocaine use (Buckley 1998). In another study of patients with severe mental illness who also abuse alcohol and/or cannabis, the effects of clozapine has been compared with risperidone in forty-one patients (Green *et al.* 2003). It is suggested that co-morbid patients treated with clozapine are more likely to abstain from alcohol and cannabis use than are those treated with risperidone. Furthermore, it is suggested that clozapine may also have antiaggressive effects (Buckley *et al.* 1995). A retrospective analysis of 331 patients with schizophrenia showed that at baseline 31.4% displayed overt physical aggression and this rate fell to 1.1% after an average 47-week period on clozapine (Volavka 1999). The author adds that this finding cannot be explained by sedation or antipsychotic effects alone, as the effect on aggression was more pronounced than the effects on other symptoms.

In a recent systematic review article a total of fifty-four experimental or observational studies were identified to examine the evidence on the interactions between the stimulant use and psychotic reactions, as well as looking at the impact of the antipsychotic medications on those who already had a psychotic illness (Curran *et al.* 2004). The authors say that the use of stimulants leads to the exacerbation of psychotic symptoms which are unaffected by use of antipsychotic medication in this group. In other words, antipsychotic medication does not block the action of stimulants and prevent deterioration.

Recently there have been a few studies looking at the effect of other atypical antipsychotic medications in this group, but most of these were carried out using a small number of patients. For instance, the effect of quetiapine was studied in nine inpatients and benefits were observed in terms of reduced substance use (Sattar *et al.* 2004). In another study, three patients with treatment-resistant psychosis and alcohol abuse were reported to have reduced alcohol use and craving following clozapine augmentation with lamotrigine (Kalyoncu *et al.* 2005). In a first-episode patient study, the effect of olanzapine was compared to haloperidol on 262 patients (Green *et al.* 2004). The 12-week response data indicated that 27% of patients with substance use disorder responded to either medication, compared to 35% of those who did not use substances. Patients with alcohol use disorder were less likely to respond to olanzapine than those without. It is suggested that the use of substances or alcohol by first-episode patients may negatively affect the response to both typical and atypical antipsychotics.

Amidst newly emerging information regarding the reasons why patients with schizophrenia turn toward substances and that atypical neuroleptics may prove to be beneficial, it has to be remembered that substance abuse behaviour cannot be explained by pharmacology alone. Adding contingency management, psycho-education and social skills training may enhance the efficacy of pharmacotherapy (Table 18.5).

Summary

In this chapter we examine the scale of the substance use problem amongst people with severe mental illness as well as its detrimental effects on their condition, ranging from increased risk of violence to frequent hospitalisation. We also list the substances most commonly used by this group of patients by looking at the available evidence. This

Table 18.5. Studied medications used in substance use

Medication	Traditional use	Substance abuse mechanism	Pharmacological effect on substance abuse
Benzodiazepines	Anti-anxiety	GABA agonist	Alcohol, opioid detoxification
Carbamazepine	Bipolar illness	Anticonvulsant	Stimulant relapse prevention, alcohol detoxification
Desipramine	Antidepressant	Dopamine, noradrenaline reuptake inhibitor	Stimulant relapse prevention
Flupentixol	Antipsychotic	Dopamine antagonist	Cocaine relapse prevention
Clozapine Olanzapine Risperidone	Atypical antipsychotics	DA and serotonin antagonists	Stimulant relapse prevention

chapter also includes some useful assessment tools, as well as comparing different treatment models. Available psychological interventions and pharmacological treatments are also discussed. There is an urgent need to have effective intervention programmes applicable to patients who are in inpatient settings. Unfortunately the size of the problem does not yet match the available and effective treatment programmes and much work needs to be done in this area.

REFERENCES

Andreasson S, Allebeck P, Engstrom A, Rydberg U. 1987 Cannabis and schizophrenia. A longitudinal study of Swedish conscripts. Lancet 26: 2 (8574): 1483–1486

Appleby L, Dyson V, Altman E, McGovern MP, Luchins DJ. 1996 Utility of the chemical use, abuse and dependence scale in screening patients with severe mental illness. Psychiatr Serv 47(6): 647–649

Arseneault L, Cannon M, Murray R, Poulton R, Caspi A, Moffitt TE. 2002 Cannabis use in adolescence and risk for adult psychosis: longitudinal prospective study. Br Med J 325: 1212–1213

Brugha T, Singleton N, Meltzer H et al. 2005 Psychosis in the community and in prisons: a report from the British National Survey of psychiatric morbidity. Am J Psychiatry 162(4): 774–780

Brunette MF, Noordsy DL, Xie H, Drake RE. 2003 Benzodiazepine use and abuse among patients with severe mental illness and co-occurring substance use disorders. Psychiatric Serv 54: 1395–1401

Buckley PF. 1998. Substance abuse in schizophrenia: a review. J Clin Psychiatry 3 [Suppl. 59]: 26–30

Buckley PF, Thompson P, Way L, Meltzer HY. 1994 Substance abuse among patients with treatment-resistant schizophrenia: characteristics and implications for clozapine therapy. Am J Psychiatry 151(3): 385–389

Buckley PF, Bartell J, Donenwirth K, Lee S, Torigoe F, Schulz SC. 1995 Violence and schizophrenia: clozapine as a specific antiaggressive agent. Bull Am Acad Psychiatry Law 23(4): 607–611

Carey KB, Maisto SA, Cary MP, Purnine DM. 2001 Measuring readiness-to-change substance misuse among psychiatric outpatients: I. Reliability and validity of self-report measures. J Stud Alcohol 62(1): 79–88

Caton CL, Drake RE, Hasin DS et al. 2005 Differences between early-phase primary psychotic disorders with concurrent substance use and substance-induced psychoses. Arch of Gen Psychiatry 62(2): 137–145

Chapple B, Chant D, Nolan P, Cardy S, Whiteford H, McGrath J. 2004 Correlates of victimisation amongst people with psychosis. Soc Psychiatry Psychiatr Epidemiol 39 (10): 836–840

Chou KR, Chen R, Lee JF, Ku RB. 2004 The effectiveness of nicotine-patch therapy for smoking cessation in patients with schizophrenia. Int J Nurs Stud 41(3): 321–330

Clark RE, Xie H, Brunette MF. 2004 Benzodiazepine prescription practices and substance abuse in persons with severe mental illness. J Clin Psychiatry 65(2): 151–155

Crawford V, Crome IB, Clancy C. 2003 Co-existing problems of mental health and substance misuse (dual diagnosis): a literature review. Drugs Educ Prevent Policy Suppl 10: S1–S74

Curran C, Byrappa N, McBride A. 2004 Stimulant psychosis: systematic review. Br J Psychiatry 185: 196–204

Degenhardt L, Hall W. 2001 The association between psychosis and problematic drug use among Australian adults: findings from the National Survey of Mental Health and Well-Being. Psychol Med 31: 659–668

Degenhardt L, Hall W. 2002 Cannabis and psychosis. Curr Psychiatry Rep 4(3): 191–196

Degenhardt L, Hall W, Lynskey M. 2003 Testing hypotheses about the relationship between cannabis use and psychosis. Drug Alcohol Dep; 71(1): 37–48

Dyer C. 1996. Violence may be predicted among psychiatric patients. Br Med J 313: 318

Elbogen EB, Swanson JW, Swartz MS, Van Dorn R. 2005 Medication nonadherence and substance abuse in psychotic disorders: impact of depressive symptoms and social stability. J Nerv Mental Disord 193(10): 673–679

El-Guebaly N, Cathcart J, Currie S, Brown D, Gloster S. 2002 Smoking cessation approaches for persons with mental illness or addictive disorders. Psychiatr Serv 53(9): 1166–1170

Esterberg ML, Compton MT. 2005 Smoking behaviour in persons with a schizophrenia-spectrum disorder: a qualitative investigation of the transtheoretical model. Soc Sci Med 61(2): 293–303

Etter M, Etter JF. 2004 Alcohol consumption and the CAGE test in outpatients with schizophrenia or schizoaffective disorder and in the general population. Schizophr Bull 30(4): 947–956

Evins AE, Cather C, Rigotti NA et al. 2004 Two-year follow-up of a smoking cessation trial in patients with schizophrenia: increased rates of smoking cessation and reduction. J Clini Psychiatry 65(3): 307–403

Farrell M, Boys A, Bebbington P et al. 2002 Psychosis and drug dependence: results form a national survey of prisoners. Br J Psychiatry 181: 393–398

Floyd AG, Boutros NN, Struve FA, Wolf E, Oliwa GM. 2006 Risk factors for experiencing psychosis during cocaine use: a preliminary report. J Psychiatr Res 40(2): 178–182

George TP, Ziedonis DM, Feingold A et al. 2000 Nicotine transdermal patch and atypical antipsychotic medications for smoking cessation in patients with schizophrena. Am J Psychiatry 157(11): 1835–1842

Green AI, Burgess ES, Dawson R, Zimmet SV, Strous RD. 2003 Alcohol and cannabis use in schizophrenia: effects of clozapine vs. risperidone. Schizophr Rese. 60: 81–85

Green AI, Tohen MF, Hamer RM et al. 2004 First episode schizophrenia-related psychosis and substance use disorders: acute response to olanzapine and haloperidol. Schizophr Res 1;66(2–3): 125–135

Green B, Young R, Kavanagh D. 2005 Cannabis use and misuse prevalence among people with psychosis. Br J Psychiatry 187: 306–313

Haddock G, Barrowclough C, Tarrier N et al. 2003 Cognitive-behavioural therapy and motivational intervention for schizophrenia and substance misuse: 18 month outcomes of a randomised control trial. Br J Psychiatry 183: 418–426

Hasin DS, Trautman KD, Miele GM. 1996 Psychiatric Research Interview for Substance and Mental disorders (PRISM): reliability for substance abusers. Am J Psychiatry 153: 1195–1201

Heil SH, Badger G, Higgins ST. 2001 Alcohol dependence among cocaine-dependent outpatients: demographics, drug use, treatment outcome and other characteristics. J Stud Alcohol 62: 14–22

Helseth V, Lykke-Enger T, Aamo TO, Johnsen J. 2005 Drug screening among patients aged 17–40 admitted with psychosis. Tidsskr Nor Laegeforen 4;125(9): 1178–1180

Henquet C, Krabbendam L, Spauwen et al. 2005 Prospective cohort study of cannabis use, predisposition for psychosis and psychotic symptoms in young people. Br Med J 330(7481): 11

Henry JA, Oldfield WL, Kon OM. 2003 Comparing cannabis with tobacco. Br Med J 326: 942–943

Isaac M, Isaac M, Holloway F. 2005 Is cannabis an anti-antipsychotic? The experience in psychiatric intensive care. Hum Psychopharmacol 20(3): 207–210

James W, Preston NJ, Koh G, Spencer C, Kisely SR, Castle DJ. 2004 A group intervention which assists patients with dual diagnosis reduce their drug use; a randomized controlled trial. Psychol Med. 34(6): 983–990

Jeffery DP, Ley A, McLaren S, Siegfried N. 2000 Psychosocial treatment programmes for people with both severe mental illness and substance misuse. Cochrane Database Syst Rev. Issue 2. Art. No.: CD001088. DOI: 10. 1002/14651858. CD001088

Johns A. 2001 Psychiatric effects of cannabis. Br J Psychiatry 78: 116–122

Kalyoncu A, Mirsal H, Pektas O, Unsalan N, Tan D, Beyazyurek M. 2005 Use of lamotrigine to augment clozapine in patients with resistant schizophrenia and comorbid alcohol dependence: a potent anti-craving effect? J Psychopharmacol 19(3): 301–305

Kavanagh DJ, McGrath J, Saunders JB, Dore G, Clark D. 2002 Substance misuse in patients with schizophrenia, epidemiology and management. Drugs 65(5): 743–755

Kavanagh DJ, Waghorn G, Jenner L et al. 2004 Demographic and clinical correlates of comorbid substance use disorders in psychosis: multivariate analyses from an epidemiological sample. Schizophr Res 66(2–3): 115–124

Kessler RC, McGonagle KA, Zhao S *et al.* 1994 Lifetime and 12-month prevalence of DSM-III-R psychiatric disorders in the United States. Arch Gen Psychiatry 51: 8–19

Kovasznay B, Fleischer J, Tanenberg-Karant M, Jandorf L, Miller AD, Bromet E. 1997 Substance use disorder and the early course of illness in schizophrenia and affective psychosis. Schizophr Bull 23(2): 195–201

Macpherson R, Jerrom B, Hughes A. 1996 A controlled study of education about drug treatment in schizophrenia. Br J Psychiatry168: 709–717

Margolese HC, Malchy L, Negrete JC, Tempier R, Gill K. 2004 Drug and alcohol use among patients with schizophrenia and related psychoses: levels and consequences. Schizophr Res 67(2–3): 157–166

Martino S, Carroll K, Kostas D, Perkins J, Rounsaville B. 2002 Dual diagnosis motivational interviewing: a modification of Motivational Interviewing for substance-abusing patients with psychotic disorders. J Subst Abuse Treat 23: 297–308

McCambridge J, Strang J. 2004 The efficacy of single-session motivational interviewing in reducing drug consumption and perceptions of drug-related risk and harm among young people: results from a multi-site cluster randomized trial. Addiction 99: 39–52

McCreadie RG. 2002 Use of drugs, alcohol and tobacco by people with schizophrenia: case-control study. Br J Psychiatry 181: 321–325

McHugo GJ, Drake RE, Burton HL, Ackerson TH. 1995 A scale for assessing the stage of substance abuse treatment in persons with severe mental illness. J Ner Men Dis 183: 762–767

McLellan AT, Luborsky L, Woody GE, O'Brien CP. 1980 An improved diagnostic evaluation instrument for substance abuse patients. The Addiction Severity Index. J Nerv Ment Dis 168: 26–33

McLellan AT, Kushner H, Metzger, *et al.* 1992 The fifth edition of the addiction severity index. J Subs Abuse Treat 9(3): 199–213

Menezes PR, Johnson S, Thornicroft G *et al.* 1996 Drug and alcohol problems among individuals with severe mental illness in South London. Br J Psychiatry 168(5): 612–619

Miles H, Johnson S, Amponsah-Afuwape S, Finch E, Leese M, Thornicroft G. 2003 Characteristics of subgroups of individuals with psychotic illness and a comorbid substance use disorder. Psychiatr Serv 54: 554–561

Miller R, Caponi JM, Sevy S, Robinson D. 2005 The Insight–Adherence–Abstinence triad: an integrated treatment focus for cannabis-using first-episode schizophrenia patients. Bull Meninger Clin 69(3): 220–230

Moore THM, Zammit S, Lingford-Hughes A *et al.* 2007 Cannabis use and risk of psychotic or affective mental health outcomes: a systematic review. Lancet 370: 319–328

Mueser KT, Yarnold PR, Rosenberg SD, Swett C Jr, Miles KM, Hill D. 2000 Substance use disorder in hospitalized severely mentally ill psychiatric patients: prevalence, correlates and subgroups. Schizophr Bull 26(1): 179–192

Owen RR, Fischer EP, Booth BM, Cuffel BJ. 1996 Medication noncompliance and substance abuse among patients with schizophrenia. Psychiatr Serv 46(8): 853–858

Pencer A, Addington J, Addington D. 2005 Outcome of a first episode of psychosis in adolescence: a 2-year follow-up. Psychiatry Res 133(1): 35–43

Peralta V, Cuesta MJ. 1995 Negative symptoms in schizophrenia: a confirmatory factor analysis of competing models. Am J Psychiatry 152(10): 1450–1457

Phillips P. 2000 Substance misuse, offending and mental illness: a review. J Psychiatr Ment Health Nurs 7: 483–489

Regier DA, Burke JD, Burke KC. 1990 Comorbidity of affective and anxiety disorders in the NIMH epidemiologic catchment area (ECA) program. In: Maser JD, Cloninger CR (eds) Comorbidity of Mood and Anxiety Disorders. Washington, DC; American Psychiatric Press

Rey JM, Tennant CC. 2002 Cannabis and mental health. Br Med J 325: 1183–1184

Ries RK, Comtois KA. 1997 Illness severity and treatment services for dually diagnosed severely mentally ill outpatients. Schizophr Bull 23(2): 239–246

Rosenthal RN, Hellerstein DJ, Miner CR. 1992 A model of integrated services for outpatient treatment of patients with comorbid schizophrenia and addictive disorders. Am J Addic 1(4): 339–348

Sattar SP, Subhash CB, Petty F. 2004 Potential benefits of quetiapine in the treatment of substance dependence disorders. J Psychiatry Neurosci 29(6): 452–457

Schools Health Education Unit. 2002 Young people in 2001. University of Exeter: School of Education

Schuckit MA, Tipp JE, Bucholz KK *et al.* 1997 The life-time rates of three major mood disorders and hour major anxiety disorders in alcoholics and controls. Addiction 92(10): 1289–1304

Self DW, Barnhart WJ, Lehman DA, Nestler EJ. 1996 Opposite modulation of cocaine-seeking behaviour by D_1- and D_2-like dopamine receptor agonists. Science 271(5255): 1586–1589

Sorbara F, Liraud F, Assens F, Abalan F, Verdoux H. 2003 Substance use and the course of early psychosis: a 2-year follow-up of first-admitted subjects. Eur Psychiatry 18: 133–136

Swanson JW, Borum R, Swartz MS, Monahan J. 1996 Psychotic symptoms and disorders and the risk of violent behaviour in the community. Crim Behav Ment Health 6: 309–329

van Mastrigt S, Addington J, Addington D. 2004 Substance misuse at presentation to an early psychosis program. Soc Psychiatry Psychiatr Epidemiol 39 (1): 69–72

van Os J, Bak M, Hanssen M, Bijl RV, de Graaf R, Verdoux H. 2002 Cannabis use and psychosis: a longitudinal population-based study. Am J Epidemiol 156(4): 319–327

Volavka J. 1999 The effects of clozapine on aggression and substance abuse in schizophrenic patients. J Clin Psychiatry 60 [Suppl. 12]: 43–46

Wade D, Harrigan S, Edwards J, Burgess PM, Whelan G, McGorry PD. 2006 Course of substance misuse and daily tobacco use in first-episode psychosis. Schizophr Res 81(2–3): 145–150

Wilkins JN. 1997 Pharmacotherapy of schizophrenia patients with comorbid substance abuse. Schizophr Bull 23(2): 215–228

Williams S, Hickman M, Bottle A, Aylin P. 2005 Hospital admissions for drug and alcohol use in people aged under 45. Br Med J 330: 115

Zammit S, Allebeck P, Andreasson S, Lundberg I, Lewis G. 2002 Self reported cannabis use as a risk factor for schizophrenia in Swedish conscripts of 1969: historical cohort study. Br Med J 325: 1199–1201

Ziedonis DM, Trudeau K. 1997 Motivation to quit using substances among individuals with schizophrenia: implications for a motivation-based treatment model. Schizophr Bull 23(2): 229–238

19

Social work issues in PICUs and LSUs

David Buckle

Introduction

Mental health social work began in the 1920s and, traditionally, social workers have followed a psychosocial model of mental health which, whilst valuing the medical model, would argue for a more holistic approach (Ramon 2001). This approach concurs with the principle of multidisciplinary team working to provide comprehensive care within Psychiatric Intensive Care Units (PICUs) and Low Secure Units (LSUs). Many patients find themselves in a cycle of social exclusion which often leads to loss of social networks, debt, poor housing, rejection by society, unemployment and worsening mental health (Social Exclusion Unit 2004). A major policy direction to address this inequality is social inclusion which, undoubtedly, increases the importance of social care within mental health services. Consequently, it is argued that each multidisciplinary team should have a dedicated social worker, especially for long-stay low secure environments, to promote the social care agenda and bring about positive social change in what is, traditionally, a health care setting (Department of Health 2002a).

This chapter briefly defines social work, considers the social policy focus on social inclusion and identifies the need for social work within the multidisciplinary team in order to provide a holistic package of care. It then proceeds to propose a model of social work that focuses on the social causes of illness and the need for a social response to the problems people often experience. Four specific areas of social work are then discussed; namely, anti-discriminatory practice which permeates social work, child welfare, advocacy and the representation of people being questioned within the criminal justice system. Finally, the chapter considers the areas of social work in relation to the chronological phases of admission and assessment, continuing care and treatment, predischarge and community support.

Definition of social work

The International Federation of Social Workers claims that the social work profession promotes social change, problem-solving in human relationships and the empowerment and liberation of people to enhance wellbeing. Moreover, they say that the principles of human rights and social justice are fundamental to social work (Horner 2003). A more pragmatic definition of social work is described thus:

Social work is a very practical job. It is about protecting people and changing their lives, not about being able to give a fluent and theoretical explanation of why they got into difficulties in the first place. (Jacqui Smith, former Minister of Health, 2002) cited in Horner (2003)

Social workers utilise the social model of disability, which recognises that the symptoms of mental ill health often prevent people from engaging in

Psychiatric Intensive Care, 2nd edn., eds. M. Dominic Beer, Stephen M. Pereira and Carol Paton.
Published by Cambridge University Press. © Cambridge University Press 2008

their customary roles, relationships and activities – in much the same way as physical impairments (Oliver 1993). Therefore, the aim of service provision should be to help people overcome these socially constructed barriers.

Social inclusion

A major policy direction within the European Union and the UK's Department of Health is social inclusion with the aim of enabling people to participate in mainstream society (Social Exclusion Unit 2004). Indeed, Standard One of the Department of Health's National Service Framework requires action to reduce discrimination against individuals and groups and promote their social inclusion (Department of Health 1999).

It is widely accepted that people with mental ill health are amongst the most socially excluded in the UK (Sayce 2000) and that mental ill health is not distributed randomly in society. It may affect one in four people but not any one in four: it reflects the social divisions of class, age, gender, ethnicity and disability (Rogers and Pilgrim 2003). The Social Exclusion Unit (2004) identified five main reasons why mental ill health too often leads to and reinforces social exclusion:

- Stigma and discrimination is pervasive throughout society
- Professionals often have low expectations of what people can achieve
- There is a lack of clear responsibility for promoting vocational and social outcomes
- People can lack ongoing support to enable them to work
- People face barriers to engaging in the community and struggle to access the basic services they need, especially decent housing

The relationship between mental ill health and social exclusion is, undoubtedly, complex and many of the elements of social exclusion, such as low income, unemployment, lack of opportunities to establish a family, small or non-existent social networks, repeated rejection and consequent restriction of hope and expectation, are both the cause of such problems and a consequence of them (Repper and Perkins 2003). Nonetheless, a poignant definition of social inclusion is that of a service user at the MIND inquiry into social inclusion and mental health problems:

Social inclusion must come down to somewhere to live, something to do, someone to love. It's as simple – and as complicated – as that. There are all kinds of barriers to people with mental health problems having those three things. Dunn (1999), p. 23

Social inclusion cannot, therefore, be seen as a treatment or a therapeutic intervention – it is about rights, choice and opportunities (Bates 2002). Moreover, social workers, with their focus on empowerment and knowledge of community-based services, are often able to provide creative solutions to these difficult social problems.

Social work in a multidisciplinary team

It is widely recognised that all aspects of human life are associated with biological, psychological, social (including cultural and religious) or environmental domains and patients are likely to be experiencing problems in relation to most, if not all, of them. However, professionals working within the major disciplines consider mental health issues in terms of the domains on which their profession is grounded. Figure 19.1 depicts the professions of psychiatry, nursing and social work and demonstrates that all

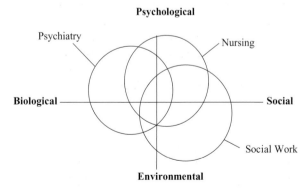

Figure 19.1. Disciplines and domains

Phases of Recovery		Areas of Social Work
Admission and Assessment	**M** **D** **T** **W** **O** **R** **K**	Liaise with community services and other agencies Assess language, cultural and religious needs Explore childcare issues Assist with housing and financial issues Assess and begin to develop family and social relationships Compile a comprehensive social history Consider discharge needs
Continuing Care, Treatment and Therapy	**I** **N** **G** **&** **R** **I** **S** **K** **A** **S**	Encourage patient and carer involvement in service provision Promote anti-discriminatory practice Professional Advocacy and promotion of access to independent advocacy schemes and effective legal representation Prepare Social Circumstances Reports for MHRT Participate in CPA/s117 Discharge Planning Meetings Encourage and facilitate community-based activities Facilitate family and social visits to develop support networks Provide emotional support Provide for cultural, religious and linguistic needs
Pre-discharge	**S** **E** **S** **S** **M**	Devise a care package and obtain funding Arrange best possible accommodation Maximise welfare benefits and assist with financial matters Further assess childcare issues in relation to placement
Community Support	**E** **N** **T**	Continue to develop/evaluate family and social support Provide care/support to deal with problems of daily living Act as Social Supervisor for MHA s37/41 restricted patients Evaluate progress and hand over to community-based team
ENHANCED SOCIAL INCLUSION		

Figure 19.2. The social work model

three are required in order to provide a holistic approach to patient care. Psychiatry, clearly, sits mainly within the biological/psychological domain. Nursing encompasses more of the social domain but, necessarily, extends far into the biological domain because it is concerned with the administration of medical therapies. Controversially, nursing may move further into the biological domain as it increasingly takes on the role of prescribing medical therapy.

Social work focuses on the social, psychological and environmental domains. Indeed, Howe (1998) claims that social work *is* psychosocial work if, by psychosocial work, we mean that area of human experience created by the interplay between the patient's psychological condition and the social environment. Moreover, social work extends further into the social and environmental domains than other disciplines and, consequently, a multidisciplinary team that includes a social worker has greater potential to provide a more holistic package of care (Buckle 2005).

The social work model

The social work model outlined in Figure 19.2 identifies the main areas of work to be undertaken during each phase of recovery from admission to community support (Buckle 2005). Clearly, these phases are neither discrete nor time limited and in the case of short-stay PICUs, depending on the patient's care pathway, may continue after the patient has moved to an acute ward prior to discharge. In the case of longer stay patients in LSUs their social needs are likely to be greater but more time is available in which to meet them.

In addition to the fundamental principles and values of social work, the social work process proposed in this chapter is grounded in the theories of social inclusion, as discussed earlier, and recovery (Repper and Perkins 2003). Recovery refers to the real-life experience of people as they accept and overcome the challenge of being socially disabled by their mental ill health and recover a new sense of self (Deegan 1988). Whether this experience is time-limited or ongoing, the person faces the task of living with, and growing beyond, what has happened to them.

The overall aim is to help people develop their strengths and engage in some form of socially meaningful activity that provides a sense of belonging and allows them to feel that their autonomy is respected in order to rebuild meaningful and satisfying lives. The role of the social worker is, essentially, to promote the social care agenda with a commitment to bringing about positive social change. This means challenging discriminatory practices appropriately and effectively whilst balancing the rights of the individual with the protection of the public.

It is important to emphasise that the ethos of *multidisciplinary working* and *risk assessment* is paramount and permeates the whole social work process. Nonetheless, the success of risk assessment within multidisciplinary teams depends, largely, on good communication to inform others of what is happening (Prins 1999). Social worker participation in risk assessments and risk management plans may be beneficial because professionals in an inpatient setting often tend to overemphasise risk to others as a consequence of regularly dealing with untoward aggressive incidents. Therefore, the involvement of a social worker, as a professional advocate for the patient, has the potential to create a more balanced

argument with regard to patient rights versus public protection (Buckle 2005). Indeed, Cowen (1999) claims that the general denial of rights to people with mental ill health is highly disproportionate to the frequency of criminal acts committed. The remainder of this chapter is devoted to the practice issues associated with anti-discriminatory practice, advocacy, child welfare, the role of 'appropriate adult' and social work prior to admission, before consideration is given to the four areas of phases of recovery outlined in Figure 19.2.

Anti-discriminatory practice

Injustices and inequalities exist throughout societies that are characterised by differentiation and whose people are categorised according to the social divisions of class, age, gender, ethnicity and disability (Thompson 2001). To address these inequalities, anti-discriminatory practice has been a pronounced feature in social work education – more so than that of any other helping profession (Ramon 2001). Consequently, social workers are able to take a leading role in the promotion of anti-discriminatory practice in each multidisciplinary team. This vast topic could occupy a chapter in its own right: indeed, readers may not feel powerful and be wondering how they can make a difference to the inequalities they work with on a daily basis.

In practice, all members of staff have a great deal of power in relation to the patients. The most profound source of power that staff hold over patients is the power to define the situation. If there is more than one view of a situation, such as the patient's suitability for a home visit, the view that will usually hold sway is that of the staff member. This power imbalance enables all team members to do something positive by identifying strongly with the underdog and becoming the champion of the disadvantaged. Indeed, a preparedness to be an advocate, for example by questioning the reasons behind negative responses to patient requests at multidisciplinary team meetings, is part of tackling the discrimination and inequalities (Vaughan and Badger 1995).

Advocacy

The rights of people detained in hospital are severely curtailed. However, advocacy is a process to address the imbalance of power and is necessary where individuals cannot speak up for themselves or make their voices heard by those people in power – namely, the multidisciplinary team (Henderson and Pochin 2001). Two forms of advocacy exist, both commonly used by social workers. Firstly, advocacy in which there is a clear procedural structure for solving the dispute; for example, appealing against the refusal of a welfare benefit which requires a robust, litigious approach. Secondly, advocacy in interpersonal conflicts where there is no apparent solution, such as family disputes, that require constructive negotiation to reach a resolution (Bateman 2000).

Advocacy is long established as a core component of social work and has a direct relationship to anti-discriminatory practice. Nonetheless, social workers cannot be truly independent because of responsibilities to their employer. For this reason, the social worker should ensure an independent advocate or legal representative is available in situations where there may be a conflict of interest. Indeed, the Mental Health National Service Framework (Department of Health 1999) requires people to have access to advocacy services. Nonetheless, in a hospital setting, the social worker with knowledge of policies, procedures and legislation is probably best placed to represent the patient's views at regular meetings where decisions are made that affect their rights and freedom.

Child protection and child welfare

Mental ill health affects whole families and can have very serious consequences for children. The area of child protection is extremely complex and creates tension between the rights of the child and the needs of the parent(s). Moreover, balancing the different perspectives of the professionals and agencies in contact with the family may be difficult. Some professionals may consider their primary responsibility to be for the child, whilst others may focus their attention on the needs of the ill parent (Weir and Douglas 1999).

As with many other inquiries into the death of children, the inquiry into the death of Victoria Climbié focused on the need for all agencies working with children to work together effectively so that positive outcomes for children are maximised (Brayne and Carr 2003). The Children Act 1989 is a complex piece of legislation and the welfare duties are made explicit within it but the concept can be succinctly described thus:

The Children Act 1989 requires everybody to safeguard and promote the welfare of children as far as is possible, because that is the primary and universal duty. [Brayne and Carr (2003) p. 237]

The issue of children visiting patients in psychiatric hospitals is complex. Consequently, such visits should be discussed amongst the multidisciplinary team but, importantly, the decision as to whether the visit should proceed must be in the best interests of the child.

The 'appropriate adult' role

Occasionally, patients need to be interviewed by the police regarding alleged offences. However, it is recognised that although people who are mentally disordered are often capable of providing reliable evidence, they may, under certain circumstances, be prone to providing information that is misleading or self-incriminating (Vaughan and Badger 1995). If there is any doubt about the person's mental state or mental capacity, an 'appropriate adult' should be involved. It is, therefore, difficult to conceive of a situation where an inpatient would be interviewed by the police without an 'appropriate adult' present.

The definition of an 'appropriate adult', in this context, is someone who has experience of dealing with mentally disordered people, such as a specialist social worker or psychiatric nurse and not a police officer (Brayne and Carr 2003). Nonetheless, it is crucial for 'appropriate adults' to be clear about the extent and limitations of their role. They are not expected to simply act as an observer. Above all, it is of crucial importance that the patient understands their right to free legal advice. If, however, the 'appropriate adult' feels the patient is not making an informed choice and legal advice would be advisable, a solicitor should be requested even if the patient does not want one. A useful source of information for anyone undertaking the role is the National Appropriate Adult Network website at www.appropriateadult.com.

Social work prior to admission

The majority of patients will have been subjected to a Mental Health Act 1983 assessment involving an Approved Social Worker (ASW) and, consequently, their social circumstances will have been investigated as part of the process of considering whether admission to hospital is required. The ASW's report should provide information about the individual's accommodation, social networks, daily activities, finances, etc. and contain the views of the nearest relative with whom close links should be maintained. The following case history is indicative of the ASW's role in relation to social care.

Case history A

A mother and two young children were left alone after the father was killed in a car crash. The mother was also caring for an elderly, frail uncle. She became mentally ill and required admission to hospital. The ASW had a duty to make arrangements for the children to be cared for and arranged for their education to continue. Domiciliary care was arranged for the uncle to enable him to continue living in his own home. The family pets were put into kennels and the house made secure. Taking care of these social problems reduced the mother's anxiety and stress thereby enabling her to focus on recovery.

Admission and assessment phase

As soon as possible after admission, the social worker should interview the patient to reinforce their rights

under the Mental Health Act 1983 although they will have previously been explained by medical or nursing staff (Backhouse 2001). It is important to reiterate these rights because the patient may have difficulty comprehending them as a consequence of their disturbed mental state. This is also a good time to explain the social work role especially with regard to professional advocacy and the availability of independent advocacy services.

After admission, patients are often concerned about personal or social matters, such as how they can access their money or who is caring for their home and pets. The practical assistance social workers are able to provide offers an opportunity to engage with patients and build trusting relationships because people are usually willing to engage with professionals if they foresee some tangible benefit. Moreover, working through practical problems inevitably proves to be therapeutic because as each problem is resolved there is usually an incremental improvement in the person's presentation.

Case history B

A young woman was admitted from prison with a history of childhood abuse, frequent self-harm, misuse of alcohol and street drugs and she had been living in a shared house where others exploited her. Her behaviour was problematic with assaults on staff and persistent refusal of medication and care. Nonetheless, discharge planning commenced at an early stage and a representative from an agency providing supported accommodation for vulnerable women visited her to discuss available choices. A change in her presentation soon followed as she realised that an opportunity for change existed.

In cases where, for whatever reason, there has not been a social work assessment, the individual's social circumstances including racial, cultural, spiritual and social needs should be assessed as soon as possible after admission and care plans devised to meet their needs, if possible. A proactive approach is required because patients may not feel confident enough to express their needs and may conform to white cultural norms with regard to dress code, diet, choice of newspaper, etc. For patients in longer stay low secure environments it is useful, at this stage, to compile a social history by gathering information from as many sources as possible including family and other agencies.

Continuing care, treatment and therapy phase

In all probability, the most significant event in relation to an individual's liberty, and consequently one of the more stressful events whilst in hospital, is the Mental Health Review Tribunal (MHRT). The outcome can have a significant effect on the future for both the patient and their family, not only in terms of whether the section is discharged but the recommendations made in respect of future care and treatment (Backhouse 2001). Each MHRT requires an up-to-date social circumstances report and, whilst the authorship is not specified, it is so generally assumed that social workers will provide this information that the Department of Health (2002b) issued a guide to report writing entitled 'Social Circumstances Report by Social Workers for Mental Health Review Tribunals'. The guidance suggests that the following is reported:

- The patient's home and family circumstances, including the attitude of the patient's nearest relative or the person so acting
- The opportunities for employment or occupation and the housing facilities which would be available to the patient if discharged
- The financial circumstances of the patient

Reporting on these areas presents a broad view of an individual's social circumstances but in order for the tribunal to reach a decision on whether it is necessary to detain the patient there are other criteria to be considered. The risks patients pose to themselves and others if discharged are clearly important and, therefore, need to be considered from a social work perspective in addition to medical and nursing perspectives. The report should also consider the patient's needs and whether they could be met

in the community with an acceptable level of risk. Importantly, it should be compiled with due consideration given to the principles of human rights and anti-discriminatory practice, paying attention to race, ethnicity, religion and culture.

Case history C

A young man was admitted after assaulting a neighbour. He lived in a large block of flats close to his parents but they had disengaged because of his threatening behaviour. The neighbours had collectively campaigned for his eviction. As the patient's advocate, using knowledge of housing legislation, the social worker entered into negotiations with the local authority and the resident's association to successfully negotiate continuation of the tenancy agreement. However, the patient remained ambivalent about returning to the flat.

After a series of visits to the family home to provide them with a better understanding of his mental illness they re-engaged with the patient, attended meetings to discuss his care, and his father attended the local carers' group which he found supportive, in the knowledge that he was not alone in this situation.

The above case history demonstrates the problems people experience and the difficult decisions they have to make in order to progress. Practical problems and decisions such as whether to return to existing accommodation are often resolved by adopting a problem-solving approach and working in partnership with the individual. Moreover, the following problem-solving principles can also be applied on a much broader basis, incorporating emotional, psychological, inter-personal and social problems (Thompson 1998):

- Identify aspects of life or current circumstances that are problematic
- Generate a range of possible solutions
- Evaluate the options
- Choose and implement the most appropriate solution

It is widely acknowledged that meeting social, cultural, religious and racial needs is an essential part of care provision. Moreover, the importance of work with families and carers, whilst recognising that some may also be victims, cannot be overstated because family and friends are able to provide support and care that professionals simply cannot. The significance of family, friends and community cannot be overemphasised because the reality for many patients is that they have no friends or community apart from professionals and other service users (Bates 2002; Buckle 2004).

In summary, social workers have an important role in helping patients maintain and develop social ties to the wider community by encouraging appropriate visits and activities. To adequately meet these social needs each PICU should have a social worker as part of the multidisciplinary team and in the case of LSUs the social worker should be dedicated to that team (Department of Health 2002a).

Case history D

A visit to the home of a patient's mother to form links and assist in the compilation of a social history revealed that she had not been coping well for many months due to physical ill health but was reluctant to seek help. A carer's assessment identified her inability to continue as the main caregiver and plans were made for the patient to move into supported lodgings to meet his care needs. An assessment under the NHS and Community Care Act 1990 led to his mother being provided with a domiciliary care service. This situation was understandably difficult for both of them to accept.

Recognition of carers' needs is crucial in order that they are able to cope with demands placed on them when the patient returns to the community. Social workers are often best placed to carry out this type of work with carers because they have more frequent involvement with community-based resources and knowledge of legislation appertaining to provision of statutory services. A useful theoretical model for helping people in situations that require the acceptance of major change, such as giving up the role of main carer or not returning to live at home, is

Egan's three-stage approach which, firstly, *explores* the problem; secondly, helps the person *understand* the situation; and, thirdly, sets the goals before accessing resources to carry out the *action* (Coulshed and Orme 1998).

Predischarge phase

During this phase there is increased involvement with community-based services in order to formulate an agreeable discharge plan. A care plan can then be developed based on the needs/problems of the patient and services or informal care identified to meet the need.

Case history A (continued)

With reference to the first case history, the discharge plan identified the need for continued provision of domiciliary care for the patient's uncle, albeit at a reduced level. The patient's welfare benefits were maximised to alleviate the financial problems and debt counselling was arranged. A multi-agency risk assessment and management meeting was held to consider the risks to the children. Close liaison with the childcare social workers continued in order to implement a successful discharge and gradual safe return to family life in the community. Contacts were also made with a charitable organisation that supports road accident victims.

As referred to earlier, most patients are poor and poverty is associated with social exclusion and high rates of mental ill health (Pierson 2002; Rogers and Pilgrim 2003). Therefore, any practitioner who wants to tackle social exclusion has to focus on maximising the patient's welfare benefit entitlement.

Social workers traditionally take the leading role in providing, monitoring and evaluating packages of continuing care. The process of constructing a 'package' of care services designed to maintain the person in the community is termed care management in the UK (Thompson 1998). In this context, it focuses on utilising individual's strengths and mobilising practical resources from family, neighbours and service providers with the aim of enabling people to live successfully in the community.

Community support

After-care is essential in order that patients cope with life outside hospital and function successfully in the community. The social work focus is on mobilising the identified human and practical resources, and evaluating the care package before handing over this responsibility to a community mental health team. Consequently, during this phase the focus is on continuity of care between inpatient- and community-based services to minimise the stress of moving back into the community because although people want to progress, there are, inevitably, issues of loss, uncertainty and ambivalence.

Conclusion

Social policy in the United Kingdom is placing a greater emphasis on the concept of social inclusion, and supporting people to reintegrate into the community has become an integral part of the work of effective mental health services. From a social work perspective, people with mental ill health want help with ordinary living and support with personal growth and development. They also want well coordinated packages of treatment and care and a plan that takes account of their aspirations for the future (Department of Health 2004). Indeed, social work focuses on the social causes of mental ill health and the need for a social response to the problems people often experience.

Finally, it can be argued that, if people in PICUs and LSUs are to have similar opportunities to others, each multidisciplinary team should include a social worker in order to promote the social care agenda, introduce positive social change wherever possible and, thereby, provide a more holistic service in what is traditionally a health care setting. Without such a service the social needs of these people with mental ill health are likely to remain largely unmet and, consequently, increase the likelihood of further episodes of mental ill health.

REFERENCES

Backhouse R. 2001 Social work. In: Dale C, Thompson T, Woods P (eds) (2001) Forensic Mental Health. Edinburgh: Baillière

Bateman N. 2000 Advocacy Skills for Health and Social Care Professionals. London: Jessica Kingsley

Bates P. (ed) 2002 Working for Inclusion. London: The Sainsbury Centre for Mental Health

Brayne H, Carr H. 2003 Law for Social Workers. Oxford: Oxford University Press

Buckle D. 2004 Social outcomes of employment: the experience of people with mental ill health. *A Life in the Day*, 8(2)

Buckle D. 2005 Social work in a secure environment: towards social inclusion. J Psychiatr Intensive Care 1(1)

Coulshed V, Orme J. 1998 Social Work Practice. Basingstoke: Macmillan Press

Cowen H. 1999 Community Care, Ideology and Social Policy. Hemel Hempstead: Prentice Hall Europe

Deegan P. 1988 Recovery: the lived experience of rehabilitation. Psychosoc Rehabil J, 11: 11–19

Department of Health. 1999 National Service Framework for Mental Health. London: The Stationery Office

Department of Health. 2002a National Minimum Standards for General Adult Services in Psychiatric Care Units (PICU) and Low Secure Environments. London: Department of Health Publications

Department of Health. 2002b Social Circumstances Report by Social Workers for Mental Health Review Tribunals. London: Department of Health Publications. Available online at http://www.dh.gov.uk

Department of Health. 2004 Treated as People: An Overview of Mental Health Services from a Social Care Perspective 2002–2004. London: Department of Health Publications. Available online at http://www.dh.gov.uk

Dunn S. 1999 Creating Accepting Communities. London: MIND Publications

Henderson R, Pochin M. 2001 A Right Result? Advocacy, Justice and Empowerment. Bristol: The Policy Press

Horner N. 2003 What is Social Work? Exeter: Learning Matters

Howe D. 1998 Psychosocial work. In: Adams R, Dominelli L, Payne M (eds) Social Work. Basingstoke: Macmillan Press

Oliver M. 1993 Disabling People and Disabling Environments. London: Jessica Kingsley

Pierson J. 2002 Tackling Social Exclusion. London: Routledge

Prins H. 1999 Will They Do It Again? London: Routledge

Ramon S. 2001 Options and Dilemmas Facing British Mental Health Social Work. Paper presented at Critical Psychiatric Network Conference 2001. Available online at http://www.critpsynet.freeuk.com/Ramon.htm

Repper J, Perkins R. 2003 Social Inclusion and Recovery. Edinburgh: Baillière Tindall

Rogers A, Pilgrim D. 2003 Mental Health and Inequality. Basingstoke: Palgrave Macmillan

Sayce L. 2000 From Psychiatric Patient to Citizen. Basingstoke: Macmillan Press

Social Exclusion Unit. 2004 Mental Health and Social Exclusion. London: The Office of the Deputy Prime Minister

Thompson N. 1998 Social work with adults. In: Adams R, Dominelli L, Payne M (eds) Social Work. Basingstoke: Macmillan Press

Thompson N. 2001 Anti-Discriminatory Practice. Basingstoke: Palgrave Macmillan

Vaughan P, Badger D. 1995 Working with the Mentally Disordered Offender in the Community. London: Chapman & Hall

Weir A, Douglas A. (eds) 1999 Child Protection and Adult Mental Health. Oxford: Butterworth Heinemann

20

User and carer involvement

Kate Woollaston and Stephen M. Pereira

Introduction

This chapter is about the potential for change in inpatient Psychiatric Intensive Care Units (PICU) towards a culture in which users and carers are partners with healthcare professionals to produce the best possible service. Historically, the medical model has presumed that professionals know what is best for the patient. Subsequently there have been difficulties in staff teams' understanding and endorsing of user and carer involvement. However, the inclusion of users and carers in the planning, delivery and evaluation of services is now believed to be crucial and therefore this is an area that needs to be incorporated into practice.

This chapter aims to facilitate this process and first describes current policy on this issue and the evidence on which it is based. Next it addresses staff resistance and ways of supporting staff to reduce this. It then concentrates on patients' involvement in their own care. It then considers the role of user representatives and advocates to assists patients and their involvement services. Finally it discusses the inclusion and support of a patient's carers, which for the purposes of this chapter are defined as a patient's family, friends and loved ones. Throughout this chapter the terms 'patient' and 'user' will be used interchangeably to reflect current practice.

Policies

Numerous policy documents issued by the Department of Health (DoH) stress the need for a patient-centred National Health Service (NHS), including: Partnership in Action (DoH 1998), The National Service Framework for Mental Health (DoH 1999a), The NHS Plan (DoH 2000) and The NHS Improvement Plan (DoH 2004). These papers state that patients should be involved in the planning, delivery and evaluation of healthcare services. In conjunction with this they advocate the importance of patients' being empowered and encouraged to make choices regarding their own health care.

These policies are based on the results of numerous research studies demonstrating that patient satisfaction increases when they are involved in their own care. Specifically user involvement results in a decrease in anxiety and an increase in confidence and understanding. Better relationships with professionals are also reported (Farrell 2004).

Supporting staff

Despite the evidence for user involvement, many research projects describe a discrepancy between policy and practice (Anthony and Crawford 2000;

Psychiatric Intensive Care, 2nd edn., eds. M. Dominic Beer, Stephen M. Pereira and Carol Paton.
Published by Cambridge University Press. © Cambridge University Press 2008

Rose 2003). A survey of user groups and mental health trusts reported that although a variety of methods were employed to involve users, none of these met national standards for user involvement (Crawford *et al.* 2003). This is of great concern and highlights the need to effectively facilitate user involvement.

The mental health trusts and the user groups involved in Crawford *et al.*'s (2003) research identified a wide range of obstacles to this process, these included:

- Concerns that users were not representative
- Staff resistance
- Lack of training
- Lack of coherent strategy
- Limited financial resources

These obstacles should be taken into consideration when planning and implementing methods of user and carer involvement. It is also important to reflect on factors that have been demonstrated to assist this process. The NHS Service Delivery and Organisation Research and Development (SDO R&D) Programme (2004) has documented some of these:

- Training for staff to help them understand the importance of user involvement
- Training for users to enhance their engagement in activities (e.g. meetings)
- An autonomous user group
- Commitment from staff
- A culture that promotes user and carer involvement
- Recognised and understood power differentials
- Adequate resources (time and money)

These findings highlight that user and carer involvement cannot exist in a vacuum. It needs to be in the context of a culture in which professionals feel valued, empowered and supported. To achieve this professionals require general training and support. This is particularly important for staff working with complex, challenging patients. To enhance training for such staff the National Institute for Mental Health in England (NIMHE) (2004) advocate that trained service users and carers are involved in the planning, delivery and evaluation of training concerning the safe and therapeutic management of aggression and

---

Box 20.1. Model of staff support

- Weekly individual supervision
- Weekly reflective practice sessions
- Bi-yearly 'away days' with focused agendas
- Regular training (with trained service users involved)
- Monthly academic sessions, including lectures and the discussion of case studies and journal articles
- Yearly staff surveys concerning job satisfaction, burnout, training needs and management of the unit

---

violence. This is to 'provide staff with a level of understanding/insight and accountability that is related directly to real human experience' (NIMHE 2004, p. 11).

In addition to general training staff need specific training and resources to understand and effectively facilitate user and carer involvement (Walker and Dewar 2001). A model of staff support that could create this culture is shown in Box 20.1. This chapter will now consider the active involvement of PICU patients in their own care and the delivery of services within the unit.

Patient involvement

In addition to the difficulties mentioned above, user involvement on PICUs is impeded by the involuntary status of patients as well as their current mental state. Traditionally it has been assumed that these patients have limited ability to make decisions about their treatment and therefore professionals must act in their best interests. However, Thomas and Bracken (1999) point out that it is very unusual for someone to be irrational in all aspects of their thoughts. Therefore, they caution against paternalism, in which decisions are based solely upon medical reasons without considering personal preferences.

From a patient's perspective their involuntary status may lead to feelings of coercion and disempowerment, with links to resistance (see Chapter 6 for a more detailed discussion). The aim is therefore for patients to feel they are being heard and to enhance a feeling of choice. Christine Bullivant (personal communication, 22 June 2006), user representative and co-founder/manager of Redbridge User Network and User Pressure group (RUN-UP), believes:

It is particularly important that patients detained under the Mental Health Act feel they have a real chance to influence their own care packages and treatment plans.

The National Minimum Standards for General Adult Services in Psychiatric Intensive Care Units (PICU) and Low Secure Environments (Pereira and Clinton 2002) concur with this view and advocate a patient-centred service with a 'non-judgemental, non-patronising, collaborative approach to care' (p. 17). These guidelines suggest:

- Establishing processes in which users can feed back to the service
- User representation in managerial meetings and committees
- User-focused monitoring of the service

A good practice example of the implementation of the National Minimum Standards is the 'Pathways User Empowerment Model' (Pereira 2002). A brief outline of this model can be seen in Box 20.2. This model is based on the principle that users should be able to influence their own care and can be involved in every aspect of the organisation and delivery of clinical services. This principle is demonstrated to be effective in practice by the many positive developments that arose from the patient partnership forum, including the introduction of complimentary therapies and health education programmes. Standards of nursing care were also set through this forum, for example the nurses are now required to have three key working sessions a week with their allocated patients.

The implementation of this model and the subsequent practice developments in Pathways PICU, Chapters House resulted in increased patient satisfaction in all aspects of care and a steady decline in formal patient complaints from six in 1999 to zero in 2002. It also led to the ward team winning various awards, including the DoH, National Awards, Commended Prize for 'Improving the Patient Experience' in 2002 and the 'Best Practice' Commended Award from Primary Care Reports in 2003.

Box 20.2. Pathways User Empowerment Model (Pereira 2007)

- **Patient information pack** – given to all patients on admission. The pack contains general information about the unit, including types of treatment and management strategies that are employed.
- **Patients' concerns log book** – always available on the ward and taken to community meetings.
- **Community meetings** – on Tuesdays and Thursdays with the multidisciplinary team. General issues are discussed; for example, house keeping, the Mental Health Act, staff and social issues. On Tuesdays patients elect a representative to attend the Patient Partnership Forum. On Thursdays the representative gives feedback.
- **Patient partnership forum** – on Wednesdays. Provides a chance to discuss a variety of issues relevant to staff and patients. Enables the dissemination of information between staff and patients. Advocate present to support the patient.
- **Patient satisfaction survey** – an ongoing survey that is given to all patients when they are discharged from the unit. It covers a wide range of areas of concern to patients, including: their treatment, staff interpersonal skills, adverse events, privacy and food.
- **Supportive ward rounds** – key worker meets with the patient beforehand and records their concerns. Advocates are made available to accompany patients and offer support. This is an opportunity for patients to talk in detail about their experiences and for their issues to be taken into careful consideration.
- **Away days** – patients, users' representatives and advocates actively participate.

It is worth noting the presence of outside user representatives and advocates to support patients in the Pathways Empowerment Model. Given the vulnerability of PICU patients it is crucial to involve independent sources of support and these will now be discussed.

The role of user representatives/consultants

Although many authors have noted the benefits of user representatives (Hossack and Wall 2005), there has been some discrepancy regarding the correct terminology and definition of these roles. This chapter will briefly consider these debates before discussing the function of user representatives on PICUs.

User representatives must have experience of using services as either a patient or carer. They are often not paid although many user groups and professionals encourage their training and payment; for guidelines on this see South London and Maudsley NHS Trust (2003). Some user groups employ the term 'User Consultant' to increase the representatives' status and promote payment (C. Bullivant, Personal Communication, 22 June 2006).

In conjunction with this debate there have also been concerns regarding the representativeness of service users who participate in user involvement activities. Bryant (2001) advises distinguishing between representative users and user representatives. He highlights that user representatives are rarely active users themselves and are often dissimilar, in terms of social demographics, to the user group they represent. However, Crawford and Rutter (2004) found that the opinions and concerns of user representatives were similar to those of a sample of current patients. Whilst all of this terminology and debate can be confusing, good practice should include current users and user representatives/consultants in the planning, delivery and evaluation of services on a PICU.

User representatives are more likely to make meaningful contributions to the ward if they feel comfortable on the unit and valued by the ward team; this is also true for advocates. As with user involvement, staff are more likely to create an atmosphere in which these individuals feel welcomed if they are appropriately trained and feel supported (see Box 20.1). Different PICUs may utilise these individuals' knowledge and skills in different ways. A generic model should include user representatives/consultants (ideally ex-PICU patients) on managerial committees, forums and away days. Some guidelines on how to facilitate meaningful user consultant involvement in meetings are shown in Box 20.3.

> **Box 20.3.** Guidelines for working with a user consultant in a meeting (Bullivant 2006)
>
> • It is advisable to have two user consultants present
> • Relevant papers should be available at least one week before the meeting to enable the user consultant to prepare properly
> • Introductions should be made at the start of the meeting
> • Goals of the meeting should be clearly explained
> • Refreshments should be provided
> • Long meetings should include breaks
> • Language should be accessible
> • Other members should be patient and tolerant towards the user consultants, giving them extra time when needed
> • Meetings should not be held in the morning, because some medication impairs functioning early in the day
> • User consultants should be allocated a professional 'buddy' and have pre and post meeting contact with them

The role of advocates

Advocates differ from user representatives/consultants, as it is not essential that they have had personal contact with services, although some of them have. The most common form of advocate is a 'professional' paid advocate, but they can also be volunteers. Nevertheless, all advocates should be trained and independent from mental health services (Action for Advocacy 2004).

The Advocacy Charter (Action for Advocacy 2002) states that their role is to 'help people say what they want, secure their rights, represent their interests and obtain the services they need'. Gentilini (2005) who has been an advocate on a PICU has written in more detail about this role. He states that the primary role of advocacy is to empower patients. This is mainly achieved through listening to patients in a non-judgemental manner and representing them in potentially intimidating situations, for example in ward rounds.

Gentilini (2005, p. 12) puts high priority on advocates being independent and conceptualises this as:

not having any statutory responsibility as regards patient care . . . [they] do not have to make any judgements about what might be best for any individual, only to listen to that individual's own assessment of their needs

He goes on to gives examples of the benefits of this, including giving value-free information regarding treatments, services and the Mental Health Act.

Furthermore, advocates can make users aware of other independent organisations, such as the National Association for Mental Health (**www.mind. org.uk**), Rethink (**www.rethink.org**) and Sane (**www. sane.org.uk**), which all provide information, support and opportunities for action. There are also non-independent resources that users can access; for example, the Patient Advice and Liaison Service (PALS). Every Mental Health NHS Trust now has its own PALS and they can provide information and advice regarding services in the trust to patients and carers.

The relatives of patients with mental health problems have traditionally been neglected and taken for granted in mental health services. This has led to dissatisfaction, which can be detrimental for both user and carer (Walker and Dewar 2001; Cleary *et al.* 2005). Thus, this chapter will now discuss the involvement of carers on PICUs.

Carer involvement on PICUs

Many studies have reported the high levels of distress and caregiver burden experienced by relatives of people with mental health problems (Fadden *et al.* 1987; Östman and Hansson 2004). The enduring nature of this distress has been demonstrated by a longitudinal study, which reported that carers were still experiencing significant psychological distress at the 15-year follow-up (Brown and Birtwistle 1998). In association with this increased levels of mental health problems have been found among carers themselves, most commonly depression (Coope *et al.* 1995).

Given this evidence, recent government policy, including the National Service Frameworks for

Mental Health (DoH 1999a) and the National Strategy for Carers (DoH 1999b), states that services must now consider carers as well as direct users. Carers now have the right to information, support and most importantly their own health needs being met.

In conjunction with these policies the National Minimum Standards for General Adult Services in PICU and Low Secure Environments (Pereira and Clinton 2002, p. 19) state:

Carers should be involved in every appropriate aspect of the patient's care and treatment in order to maximise positive experiences and reduce stigma.

A summary of these standards can be seen in Box 20.4. As clinicians developed these guidelines, they are user friendly and practical to implement.

Broadly, carers' involvement on PICUs can be divided into two areas: their interest and involvement in their loved one's care and their own needs for

---

Box 20.4. Summary of the standards for carer involvement within a PICU/Low Secure Unit (Pereira and Clinton 2002)

- All carers should be involved at the beginning of care through the Care Programme Approach (CPA)
- Written information should be given about all aspects of the PICU
- All identified carers or relatives should be informed within 24 h of admitting or discharging a patient
- Basic demographic information should be checked with carers
- With the consent of the patient, carers can attend weekly ward rounds and express their views
- Carers should be able to request face-to-face meetings with a member of staff
- Crisis plans should include carers
- Risk management plans should include carers
- A carer support network and/or group should exist
- All carers providing substantial care should have their needs assessed and a care plan completed
- All PICUs should have processes and an environment that provide safety, privacy and dignity during visits
- A list of voluntary organisations that provide information and support to carers should be available

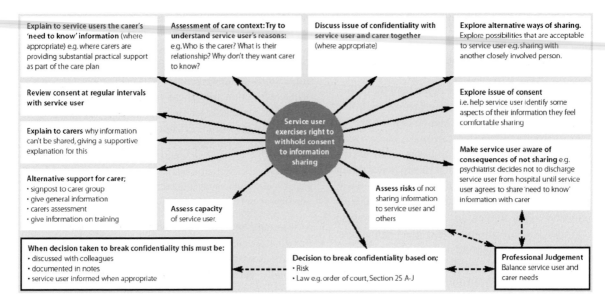

Figure 20.1. Possible strategies for professionals when service users exercise their right to withhold consent to share 'need to know' information with carers (Pinfold *et al.* 2004)

clinical interventions. Mechanisms to enable carers to be involved in their relative's or significant other's care and treatment on a PICU are covered in Box 20.4. There are many ways to support carers and meet their needs; as with patients, much of the effectiveness of these interventions depends on the relationship they have with staff.

Walker and Dewar (2001) interviewed carers and nursing staff; they reported that in their study the two did not have a good relationship. In particular nurses described carers taking out their anger and frustrations on them. This led to staff avoiding carers (which nurses and carers reported). Again this points to the need for staff support and training. Walker and Dewar (2001) also advise having an agreed set of principles and procedures and openly discussing and negotiating involvement with carers.

Recently, the NHS has advocated staff and carers having a reciprocal relationship, in which they both share their knowledge about the user and use their expertise to enhance the care of the patient (NHS SDO R&D Programme 2006). However, users need to feel that staff are being mindful of the boundary

between the confidentiality of their personal information and the support and inclusion of their loved ones (M. Kingsley, personal communication, 26 June 2006).

To help strike this balance professionals can refer to advice issued by the NHS SDO R&D Programme (2006) on sharing mental health information with carers. This paper suggests that information-sharing strategies should be individually tailored, with patients being regularly consulted. It also advises that professionals need to make careful judgements considering the risk of not sharing information and the needs and rights of patients and carers. A diagram featured in these guidelines, which presents strategies for when users withhold consent to share information, is shown in Figure 20.1.

From a psychological point of view, PICU staff should be mindful of the emotional distress that is being experienced by carers (see Chapter 6 for further discussion). For example, Östman and Kjellin (2002) reported that a high proportion of relatives felt isolated and stigmatised. A subset described having suicidal thoughts, which is indicative of the great distress they are suffering. Carers also reported believing the relative would be better off dead and, depending on their relationship with them, wishing they had never been born (parents) or that they had never met them (spouses). It is likely that feelings of guilt would accompany such thoughts and cause distress.

It is therefore essential that PICUs offer carers a space in which they feel heard and supported. This can take the form of individual therapy and/ or a carer's group in which carers can express their thoughts and feelings without feeling judged. Ideally this should be in conjunction with psycho-educational interventions, such as carers' support sessions that can provide information on the nature of mental health problems, triggers, relapse prevention techniques and coping strategies (M. Kingsley, personal communication, 26 June 2006).

Psycho-educational interventions are important, as research has shown links between lack of knowledge about the relative's illness (Barrowclough *et al.* 1987), low self-esteem (Kuipers *et al.* 2006), high carer burden, avoidant coping (Raune *et al.* 2004) and high expressed emotion. High expressed emotion has been found to negatively affect a user's compliance with medication (Sellwood *et al.* 2003), relapse rates (Butzlaff and Hooley 1998) and admissions to hospitals (Honig *et al.* 1995). Therefore, by educating carers and enhancing their coping skills, psycho-educational interventions are beneficial and cost-effective to both carer and user.

Carers should also be made aware of outside organisations that can offer support. Many of these organisations are a useful resource for carers, offering among other services: free counselling, training and 'pampering' experiences. Carers UK (**www. carers.org**) can provide contact details of the carer centre. Carers with more pronounced difficulties and perhaps their own mental health problems might need long-term interventions and therapy. These carers have the right to receive the appropriate assessments, such as Burden Interviews and referrals. Protocols for these should be agreed with the local community mental health teams (Pereira and Clinton 2002).

Conclusion

There is currently a discrepancy between policy and practice regarding user and carer involvement. However, this chapter has highlighted ways in which this discrepancy can be diminished and result in positive practice. Future research should aim to gather outcome measures for involvement strategies to enable the implementation of evidence-based practice.

Acknowledgements

We would like to thank Marc Kingsley and Christine Bullivant for their advice and assistance with this chapter. We are also grateful to Vanessa Pinfold for permission to reproduce the diagram in Figure 20.2.

REFERENCES

Action for Advocacy. 2002 The Advocacy Charter. Retrieved 19.06.06 from: http://www.actionforadvocacy.org.uk (accessed 4 August 2007)

Action for Advocacy. 2004 Advocacy Models. Retrieved 19.06.06 from: http://www.actionforadvocacy.org.uk (accessed 4 August 2007)

Anthony P, Crawford P. 2000 Service user involvement in care planning mental health nurse's perspective. J Psychiatr Ment Health Nurs 7: 425–434

Barrowclough C, Terrier N, Watts S, Vaughn C. 1987 Assessing the functional value of relatives' knowledge about schizophrenia: a preliminary report. Br J Psychiatry 151: 1–8

Brown S, Birtwistle J. 1998 People with schizophrenia and their families. Fifteen-year outcome. Br J Psychiatry 173 (8): 139–144

Bryant M. 2001 Introduction to User Involvement. The Sainsbury Centre of Mental Health. Retrieved 13.06.06 from: http://www.scmh.org.uk/80256FBD004F3555/ vWeb/flKHAL6H9G4N/ $file/introduction+to+user+ involvement.pdf (accessed 4 August 2007)

Butzlaff RL, Hooley JM. 1998 Expressed emotion and psychiatric relapse: a meta-analysis. Arch Gen Psychiatry 55: 184–195

Cleary M, Freeman A, Hunt GE, Walter G. 2005 What patients and carers want to know: an exploration of information and resource needs in adult mental health services. Austr N Z J Psychiatry 39 (6): 507–513

Coope B, Ballard C, Saad K, Patel A. 1995 The prevalence of depression in the carers of dementia sufferers. Int J Geriatr Psychiatry 10 (3): 237–242

Crawford MJ, Rutter D. 2004 Are the views of members of mental health user groups representative of those of 'ordinary' patients? A cross-sectional survey of service users and providers. J Ment Health 13 (6): 561–568

Crawford MJ, Aldridge T, Bhui K et al. 2003 User involvement in the planning and delivery of mental health services: a cross-sectional survey of service users and providers. Acta Psychiatr Scand 107: 410–414

Department of Health (DoH). 1998 Partnership in Action. London: DoH Publications

Department of Health (DoH). 1999a National Service Frameworks for Mental Health. London: DoH Publications

Department of Health (DoH). 1999b National Strategy for Carers. London: DoH Publications

Department of Health (DoH). 2000 The NHS Plan: A Plan for Investment, A Plan for Reform. London: DoH Publications

Department of Health (DoH). 2004 The NHS Improvement Plan: Putting People at the Heart of Public Services. London: DoH Publications

Fadden G, Bebbington P, Kuipers L. 1987 The burden of care: the impact of functional psychiatric illness on the patient's family. Br J Psychiatry 150: 285–292

Farrell C. 2004 Patient and Public Involvement: The Evidence for Policy Implementation. London: DoH Publications

Gentilini L. 2005 The importance of advocacy. Nat Assoc Psychiatr Intensive Care Units Bull 4 (1): 12

Honig A, Hofman A, Hilwig M, Moorthoorn E. 1995 Psychoeducation and expressed emotion in bipolar disorder: preliminary findings. Psychiatry Res 56 (3): 299–301

Hossack A, Wall G. 2005 Service users: undervalued and underused? Psychologist 18 (30): 134–136

Kuipers E, Bebbington P, Dunn G et al. 2006 Influence of carer expressed emotion and affect on relapse in non-affective psychosis. Br J Psychiatry 188: 173–179

National Institute for Mental Health in England (NIMHE). 2004 Developing Positive Practice to Support the Safe and Therapeutic Management of Aggression and Violence in Mental Health In-patient Settings. Leeds: NIMHE

NHS Service Delivery and Organisation Research and Development (SDO R&D) Programme. 2004 Briefing Paper: How Managers can Help Users to Bring About Change in the NHS. London: NHS SDO R&D Programme

NHS Service Delivery and Organisation Research and Development (SDO R&D) Programme. 2006 Briefing Paper: Sharing Mental Health Information with Carers: Pointers to Good Practice for Service Providers. London: NHS SDO R&D Programme

Östman M, Hansson L. 2004 Appraisal of caregiving, burden and psychological distress in relatives of psychiatric inpatients. Eur Psychiatry 19 (7): 402–407

Östman M, Kjellin L. 2002 Stigma by association: psychological factors in relatives of people with mental illness. Br J Psychiatry 181: 149–498

Pereira S. 2002 Focus on Psychiatry. In: Sund B (ed) Hospital Doctor. Surrey: Reed Business Information UK

Pereira S. 2007 Psychiatric Inpatient Practice Development Manual. Cambridge: Cambridge University Press, in press

Pereira S, Clinton C (eds). 2002 Mental Health Policy Implementation Guide: National Minimum Standards for General Adult Services in Psychiatric Intensive Care Units (PICU) and Low Secure Environments. London: DoH Publications

Pinfold V, Farmer P, Papaport J et al. 2004 Positive and inclusive? Effective ways for professionals to involve carers in information sharing. London: National Co-ordinating Centre for NHS Service Delivery and Organisation Research and Development (NCCSDO)

Raune D, Kuipers E, Bebbington P. 2004 Expressed emotion at first-episode psychosis: investigating a carer appraisal model. Br J Psychiatry 184: 321–326

Rose D. 2003 Partnership, co-ordination of care and the place of user involvement. J Ment Health 12 (1): 59–70

Sellwood W, Terrier N, Quinn J. Barrowclough C. 2003 The family and compliance in schizophrenia: the influence of clinical variables, relatives' knowledge and expressed emotion. Psychol Med 33 (10): 91–96

South London and Maudsley NHS Trust. 2003 Patient and Public Involvement Policy: Guiding Principles and Resource Pack. Retrieved on 19.06.06 from: http://www.slam.nhs.uk/about/docs/PPI.doc (accessed 4 August 2007)

Thomas PF, Bracken P. 1999 The value of advocacy: putting ethics into practice. Psychiatr Bull 23: 327–329

Walker E, Dewar BJ. 2001 How do we facilitate carers' involvement in decision making? J Adv Nurs 34 (3): 329–337

PART III

Management of the Psychiatric Intensive Care Unit/Low Secure Unit

Setting up a new PICU: principles and practice

Andrew W. Procter and David Ridgers

Introduction

Throughout the history of mental health care, the methods of managing patients with disturbed and aggressive behaviour have always been important and contentious. This has been particularly the case over recent decades, which have seen major changes in effective therapies and the style of delivery of psychiatric care. Since the 1950s the majority of mental hospital wards have been unlocked and there has been a shift in the philosophy (if not practice) of care towards the community. However, with the increasing development of effective and evidence-based models of community care, it has become apparent that there remain a group of patients whose symptoms and behaviour require special care in a dedicated inpatient unit, usually referred to as a Psychiatric Intensive Care Unit (PICU).

During the 1970s there were a number of descriptions in the literature of PICUs mainly from North America and Australia. The Royal College of Psychiatrists (1980), in its document 'Secure Facilities for Psychiatric Patients: A Comprehensive Policy', recommended a range of secure facilities that were necessary to support local mental health services, including local intensive care units.

In 1991, Dr John Reed led a complex review of services for mentally disordered offenders. By this stage, Government policy had been clearly articulated in the Home Office Circular 66/90. Offenders suffering from mental disorder should receive care and treatment from the health and personal social services rather than in custodial care. This policy of diversion of such offenders from the criminal justice system to health and social services put increasing pressure on the medium secure units, whose inpatient population changed from a heterogeneous group of primarily offenders with some non-offenders, to an almost homogeneous high-risk offender population. This 'squeezed out' any admissions from local mental health units of non-offenders, and also made it more difficult for special hospital patients to be rehabilitated through a Medium Secure Unit.

The Reed Committee (1992) set out five guiding principles for the care of such patients, who should be managed:

- With regard to the quality of care and proper attention to the needs of individuals
- As far as possible, in the community, rather than in institutional settings
- Under conditions of no greater security than is justified by the degree of danger they present to themselves or others
- In such a way as to maximise rehabilitation and their chances of sustaining an independent life
- As near as possible to their own homes or families, if they have them

These five guiding principles should govern the provision of mental health services and are also embodied in the National Service Framework for Mental

Psychiatric Intensive Care, 2nd edn., eds. M. Dominic Beer, Stephen M. Pereira and Carol Paton.
Published by Cambridge University Press. © Cambridge University Press 2008

Health (Standard 5) which proposes that each service user should have, 'timely access to an appropriate hospital bed . . . which is in the least restrictive environment consistent with the need to protect them and the public, and as close to home as possible'.

In the UK there has been increasing recognition of the need for a range of secure services. This has been identified in a number of national and regional documents and initiatives. Even so the National Service Framework for Mental Health recognises that, 'there are gaps in . . . local intensive care provision' and, 'there is a need for more intensive care beds in some inner city areas' (Department of Health 1999).

The closure of large psychiatric hospitals has led to a degree of decentralisation of inpatient facilities to smaller units, often in district general hospitals, each of which requires access to intensive care. As a result of these types of forces, in the UK, many new PICUs are being designed, commissioned and opened. This chapter will address some of the issues which need to be considered by all those who may be involved in the development and opening of a new PICU.

Definition of psychiatric intensive care

For the effective function of any unit, but particularly in intensive care, it is essential that there is clarity about the purpose of that unit and clarity about the treatment plans of the clients.

Psychiatric intensive care is for patients compulsorily detained usually in secure conditions, who are in an acutely disturbed phase of a serious mental disorder. There is an associated loss of capacity for self control, with a corresponding increase in risk, which does not enable their safe, therapeutic management and treatment in a general open acute ward. Care and treament offered must be patient centred, multidisciplinary, intensive, comprehensve, collaborative and have an immediacy of response to critical situations. Length of stay must be appropriate to clinical need and assessment of risk but would ordinarily not exceed 8 weeks in duration. Psychiatric intensive care is delivered by qualified staff according to an agreed philosophy of unit operation underpinned by principles of risk assessment and management (Pereira and Clinton 2002).

Low Secure Units (LSUs) deliver intensive, comprehensive, multidisciplinary treatment and care by qualified staff for patients who demonstrate disturbed behaviour in the context of a serious mental disorder and who require the provision of security. This is according to a philosophy of unit operation underpinned by the principles of rehabilitation and risk management. Such units aim to provide a homely secure environment, which has occupational and recreational opportunities and links with community facilities. Patients will be detained under the Mental Health Act and may be restricted on legal grounds needing rehabilitation for up to 2 years (Pereira and Clinton 2002).

One of the major functions of any treatment is the management of risk associated with the mental illness. That includes risk to the patient's own health or safety, and that of any risk the patient may present to others.

Although there are a number of ways of assessing risk, one way of describing the risk presented by an individual is to consider three distinct aspects of this. These are:

- The *seriousness* of the act which the individual is at risk of committing (i.e. a postulated dimension from minor public order offences, through physical assaults to murder)
- The *immediacy* of the risk (i.e. a dimension of probability of that action occurring within a given time period)
- The *duration* of the risk (i.e. how long the individual will remain at that level of risk)

These aspects of risk translate into the characteristics of the environment and treatment for the individual. Seriousness roughly relates to the level of perimeter security required. Immediacy relates to the intensity and quality of supervision the patient requires and the skills of the clinical team. Duration relates to the prognosis of the mental condition and the anticipated duration of the treatment regime. These three dimensions can be varied independently and serve to describe a range of the components of a comprehensive psychiatric service (Figure 21.1).

In this way the purpose and characteristics of a PICU can be defined according to the needs of individual patients.

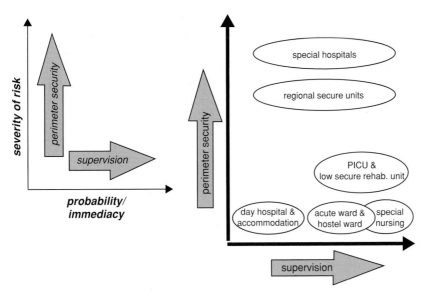

Figure 21.1. Relationship between components of risk and characteristics of secure units. The three dimensions of risk – seriousness, immediacy and duration – roughly translate into the perimeter security, supervision and duration of treatment. At each level of security and supervision there are various types of service for different lengths of treatment, i.e. acute day hospitals and supervised accommodation, acute wards and hospital hostel wards

Needs assessment

The PICU is part of a comprehensive mental health service and even with clear definition need will in part be determined by the range and completeness of the rest of the service.

The first step in the commissioning and opening of a new PICU is the recognition that such a service is required. This frequently involves some form of local population needs assessment. While there are formulaic predictors of population need these are often not as useful as more local ad hoc methods. This is because the requirement for a PICU in a certain area is dependent upon the capacity of other parts of that service to deal with the disturbed mentally ill. Thus measures such as the number of patients in PICUs distant from the local acute inpatient unit or those patients requiring special nursing on general wards probably serve as the best local indicator of the need for a PICU. However, future trends and envisaged changes in service configurations need also to be considered in order to address future demands.

Proposed service description

The population-based needs assessment serves to define the target patient group and from this it is possible to derive all other features of the proposed service. This applies in particular to the characteristics considered above (perimeter security, intensity and quality of supervision, duration of treatment). With this information a detailed service description can be derived. Such a service description must include detailed information regarding admission and discharge criteria and the processes involved in this, as well as the relationship of the PICU to other parts of the general psychiatry service (acute wards and alternatives to hospital admission), rehabilitation services and specialist accommodation for those with severe and enduring mental illness. Particular attention must be paid to the relationship with services for mentally disordered offenders, including the local forensic psychiatry service.

The description of the service also must address the types and duration of treatment and care plans that are likely to be required by the target patient group. This in turn will inform the planning of the staffing of the unit.

The proposal: a planning partnership

Once the need for a PICU has been recognised, a partnership between the commissioners of health services and those who provide them is needed to ensure the effective implementation of a plan. While commissioners have responsibility to ensure that comprehensive services are provided, it is the responsibility of providers to ensure optimum use of resources. At one extreme, a wholly new service may be commissioned, while at the other a provider may reconfigure existing services to create a PICU service within existing budgets. In reality the situation is likely to be somewhere in between these two options. However, it is essential at this stage that the development should take place with a sound financial plan.

This plan will include the consideration of the various options for the PICU. Equally effective PICUs may have very different physical environments and configurations determined according to local need. Thus the first determinant is likely to be the size of the required unit. This can range from an isolatable area within a ward, to a ward or complex accommodating up to fifteen patients. The physical size of the unit will determine the possible sites for the unit. The proximity to referring services will affect the operation of the unit especially with regard to admission and discharge procedures. The possibility of a unit's serving more than one acute admission unit can be considered here and a service which is shared may have advantages in some circumstances over a small, independent unit when demand is low and infrequent. However, this economy of scale and potential for development of specialism among staff must be balanced against the Reed (1992) principle that patients receive care, 'as near as possible to their own homes or families', as well as the potential difficulties of transporting acutely disturbed individuals to a separate and possibly distant unit.

The development of the various options to be considered will involve discussion with architects and/or estates departments. The earlier the dialogue can be started between the planners and clinicians the more satisfactory the outcome is likely to be.

The project manager or management team

One way of establishing a dialogue between the clinicians and architects or designers is to establish a project management team to do this and implement other necessary tasks. While the project management team may have a wide representation of key stake-holders drawn from commissioners, providers (both clinicians and managers), users and others, this group is likely to be too large and unwieldy to successfully oversee the day-to-day management of the project. A solution to this is the appointment of a single project manager. This may be either a senior member of the staff who will work in the unit, or someone seconded from other duties for the duration of the project. Each has its advantages and disadvantages. A member of clinical staff may not have previous experience of this type of work or the skills necessary, but will have the understanding of the purpose and function of the planned unit. Conversely, someone who will not work in that particular unit in the future may have previous experience of opening similar units or of project managing the other services. The important consideration is that the project manager has the necessary skills to complete the work or has access to appropriate support systems to develop these skills throughout the duration of the project.

The project manager must define timescales for each task in discussion with the relevant groups such as architects and builders. The tasks to be achieved include the building design and other estate issues, staffing of the unit, recruitment and training, and the development of policies for the operation of the unit. This latter issue needs to be considered in conjunction with other agencies with which the unit will have operational links as well as addressing meaningful user involvement.

Estates issues

The importance of a dialogue between architects/contractors and clinical staff from an early stage and throughout the entire process cannot be overemphasised. The design of the unit therefore presents a series of compromises. The fittings (door handles, lights, sinks, etc.) are chosen balancing robustness against aesthetic qualities. The internal layout of the ward provides potentially a balance between ease of observation and supervision and the patients' needs for privacy. Building specifications change over time; for more detailed information on the fabric of the building see Pereira and Clinton (2002). An environmental assessment inventory has been developed by Dix *et al.* (2005).

The treatment plans and ward-based activities will determine the rooms and spaces required on the ward. The number of separate and isolated spaces determines the staffing levels required to satisfactorily supervise these activities. Elsewhere in this volume (see Chapter 22) more details of the physical environment of a unit are described, however at the planning stage there is real opportunity to determine these. It is these features and the nature and number of the patient group which determine the staffing requirements of the unit.

New or converted buildings frequently require contractors to return to correct faults which have only come to light once the unit is in use. This is usually anticipated at the time the contract for the work is agreed, and this contract will describe what access the builders will have to the unit after completion to correct such faults ('snagging'). Once the PICU is in operation, it can be very difficult for builders to have safe access to the unit. The presence of the builders and associated noise can exacerbate patients' arousal levels. Tools and other equipment provide a source of potential weapons for either self-harm or harm of others. While it is not impossible for building work to be carried out in an operating PICU, the difficulties of this must be made known to the contractors from the outset, and the extent of access after completion specified in the contract. This is often referred to as a 'no snagging' clause.

There are a number of stages in the planning design and construction of a new building. At each stage the involvement of clinical staff is important. At each stage the involvement of clinical staff is possible and will contribute to the successful outcome of the project. How clinical staff can contribute at different stages in the process is indicated in Table 21.1.

Staffing issues

From the preceding sections it can be seen that the assessment, care planning and treatments required by the target patients will determine the staff required in the unit. It is necessary to consider the professions which need to be represented, and, related to this, the skills required. The size and activities of the unit will determine the absolute numbers of staff of each discipline.

Multidisciplinary team approaches are widely accepted in other sub-specialties of psychiatry as providing effective care delivery for patients with complex needs. The multidisciplinary team is equally effective in the PICU setting. The disciplines of importance include nursing, medical, occupational therapy and other activity-based therapists, psychology, as well as social work. For those patients with severe and enduring mental health problems the involvement of community-based staff in the ward activities is likely to promote long-term engagement after discharge. This may be achieved by, for example, involvement of the community staff as patients start having short periods of leave from the PICU prior to transfer.

How each of the disciplines is provided in the PICU may be a matter for a local solution. However, an identifiable team of the same nurses, doctors and therapists to work with all patients in the PICU will help promote a consistency of approach which may be beneficial in the PICU.

Prior to the opening of the unit the staff identified to work there will require appropriate training in certain areas. This will include general induction into the local service, and training in procedures common to all parts of the service. These topics are likely to include fire procedures, training in the Mental

Table 21.1. Desirable clinical involvement at different stages of a building programme

Stage	Activity	Clinical involvement
Proposal to develop PICU	Size of unit confirmed	Recognition of clinical need
Hospital estates department involved	Initial options considered: • new build versus conversion • site • size possible	Feasibility of patient transfers, access to unit, etc. Outline operational policies to address these points
Architects involved	Confirm space required and layout including perimeter ***and gardens***	Confirm spaces match activities of unit and that layout ensures safe ***observation***
	Detailed room plans developed	Fittings secure and safe
Initial costings produced	Budget renegotiated	Revised plans still appropriate for activities and safety
Plans agreed and tenders sought		Proposed contract includes clauses regarding site access which allow clinical activity in adjacent areas
Contractors appointed		
Preliminary meetings	Confirm contract agreement	Confirm on site arrangements
Building work commences		
Regular progress meetings between contractors and other parties	Monitor progress	Amend plans in line with unforeseen changes and clinical need
Building work finished		
Pre-handover check	Confirm satisfactory completion of contract	Confirm building meets clinical needs
Handover of building to clinical service	Formal acceptance that work has been completed satisfactorily	Involve local estates in preparing building for occupancy
Post-completion correction of problems		Ensure any works do not interfere with safe and effective running of unit

Health Act, and the Care Programme Approach (UK Government Policy) that certain patients have a care plan which is maintained in hospital, in the community and when they cross geographical boundaries. As well as these general topics there are specific skills which are of particular importance in a PICU, such as dealing with violence and techniques of physical restraint.

Having identified a set of core skills required for all staff before the PICU opens, there must also be some process for subsequent appraisal and further training to engender staff development. This will contribute to enhancing staff morale, as well as recruitment and retention of staff. Other factors should be identified at this stage which may improve

recruitment and retention and be incorporated into a policy, possibly in line with other units in the organisation, to provide a variety of clinical experience.

The operational policy

When this includes a mission statement and a statement of the strategic objective of the unit, this is a crucial document to provide all staff with a clear understanding of their role in the care of an individual patient who may present unattractive or antisocial behaviours. As such the operational policy is therefore a key document in promoting staff morale, provided all are aware of its content. The document should include not only the procedural details regarding admission, treatment and discharge, but importantly a description of the philosophy of the unit.

In this planning stage the following topics need to be considered and addressed:

- Philosophy of care
- Description of service users
- Admission policies
- Referral process
- Assessment methods (considering standardised tools)
- Care planning
- Treatment protocols
- Review including liaison with likely discharge placement
- Discharge procedures

User and carer involvement

It is widely recognised that meaningful user involvement is important for the successful running of effective mental health services. Similarly, carers' needs also need to be addressed by these services. The possibility of having user representation on the project management team has been mentioned above; however, this should not stop once the unit is opened, and a process for user involvement in the management of the established unit must be considered.

For an individual patient in the unit advocacy is also important, and some formal advocacy arrangement must be organised. Similarly, the involvement of carers in care plans and the needs of the carers (who may also have been victims) must be addressed by the ward team.

Post-commissioning policy

A well-defined operational policy will ensure that a unit is flexible and adaptable, and continues to develop according to evidence-based practice, and to the changing needs of patient and society, rather than become institutionalised and stagnant. Thus, it must have in place a continuous evaluation and audit of service and all aspects of practice, in line with the

demands of clinical governance (a UK Government requirement to ensure a system for improving, monitoring and standardising quality of care across the country).

The unit may also have an educational role to enhance practice in other settings and thereby possibly prevent the need for transfer of patients to a PICU.

Any ongoing evaluation of the service should include measures not only of the core clinical functions, but also of staff morale and turnover, as a successful unit needs to be sustainable in the long term.

Conclusions

From the preceding discussions it is apparent that while there are a large number of small areas which need to be considered when planning and opening a new PICU, the success of this is dependent on the clarity of the identified purpose of the unit based on an assessment of the local need. If this strategic vision for the unit is then applied consistently in all the subsequent activities the unit is more likely to be successful in the long term. However, the system needs to be flexible and adaptable to respond to changes in local need and developments in practice, and this adaptability must be built into the oragnaisation from the outset.

Acknowledgements

I am grateful to my colleagues Marie LeMaire and Ernie Croft for helpful discussions about the issues raised in this chapter.

APPENDIX 21.1
Example of PICU operational policy

AW Procter and E Croft, **** Ward, Manchester Royal Infirmary

It is important that a PICU meets local needs. Further information that may be useful when formulating a local policy can be found in the National Minimum Standards (Pereira and Clinton 2002).

**** Ward is a ten-bedded Psychiatric Intensive Care Unit serving the **** Healthcare Trust. The ward represents a (low-level) secure environment with a locked door to care for severely disturbed patients on an acute short-term basis. Its concern is to effect as rapid a transfer of patients to open general psychiatric wards as possible: the single most important facilitator of this is the efficacy of its admission procedure.

Admission policy

The aim of the patient's admission must be clearly established from the outset, in order to determine the therapeutic benefit of such a decision and the outcomes expected before the transfer back to the referring ward.

**** Ward will typically only accept patients on a referral basis and after the referring ward has exhausted all methods of managing that patient. As a rule newly admitted patients will not be considered as candidates unless they are well known as having established patterns of creating problems. The decision to refer a patient has also to take into account how that person's overall needs could be best met.

There must be clear therapeutic outcomes sought by the admission rather than solely being one of containment. Where referrals are not regarded as suitable for a PICU, an appropriate plan of care must be formulated with the referring ward, which may include the possible re-referral of that patient at a later date.

Patient characteristics

- Patients suffering from a mental illness and aged between sixteen and sixty-five
- Those patients whose behaviour is so disturbed that it jeopardises the progress and well-being of themselves or others by remaining on a general acute ward

- Those who are severely ill and repeatedly attempting to abscond from the hospital, thereby placing their own or other's safety at risk
- Those who require a degree of privacy and dignity not possible on a general ward

Patients regarded as unsuitable for a PICU environment

- Those with a history of serious violence (e.g. malicious wounding, homicide and other serious offenses such as rape)
- Admissions solely as a result of alcohol or illicit substance intoxication
- Those with organic brain damage

Philosophy of care

The ward's therapeutic milieu places an emphasis upon personally appropriate solutions to patients' problems, focusing in particular upon the relationship between the individual's strengths, problems and beliefs, health or illness status, and his or her world. Intrinsic to this is the view that each person is a unique individual who possesses the potential for maturation, learning and growth in an environment that preserves dignity and fosters mutual respect and acceptance.

Quality care is of paramount importance for severely disturbed patients at the core of which is a multidisciplinary research-based approach, in line with a strict adherence to the mandatory requirements of the Mental Health Act 1983 and the Care Programme Approach.

**** Ward's staffing levels, training and shift patterns necessarily need to enable appropriate, structured responses to acts of violence, self-injury and social disruptiveness. Patients are regarded with compassion and interactions met by calmness, respect and gentleness. Rules are kept to a minimum since we believe discussion and negotiation to be a more beneficial and appropriate medium to encourage the acceptance of responsibility. Similarly, informality among patients and staff is regarded as an important tool in maintaining tensions fostered by the admission at tolerable levels.

Consultant responsibility

When a patient is transferred to **** Ward there is a corresponding transfer of medical consultant responsibility for that persons care. **** Ward benefits from having one dedicated consultant and supporting medical team that works in collaboration with the nursing team and occupational therapist to provide an overall ethos of care.

Nursing perspective

The management of **** Ward fully accepts the finding of the scoping study by the UKCC on 'Nursing in Secure Environments' (United Kingdom Central Council for Nursing, Midwifery and Health Visiting 1999) and will endeavour to incorporate its recommendations into professional practice. In particular:

- Practice standards and procedures – there will be an ongoing concern to develop standards that are supported by research evidence and incorporated into overall performance indicators
- Pre-registration preparation for nursing in secure environments – **** Ward is available for clinical placements of learners to facilitate knowledge and understanding
- With regard to post-registration nursing staff – individuals will be supported in their continuing professional development through clinical supervision, the use of staff appraisal in a facilitative manner, and robust operational policies and procedures which are regularly monitored and updated.

Discharge criteria

Once **** Ward have accepted a patient, the referring ward must designate a liaison nurse to visit the client and monitor his or her progress. When the precipitating problem(s) that necessitated the transfer are resolved to such a degree that the patient would benefit more from an open environment, then he or she has to be returned to the original ward to facilitate progress towards discharge. At this stage that patient's key nurse on **** Ward will effect the transfer of care to the ongoing liaison nurse and, if appropriate, may continue to provide some input to care planning to consolidate the patient's progress.

Discharge criteria

Other policies

There are additional written policies concerning:
- Referrals
- Patient-centred activities
- Commencing leave
- Low stimulus environment
- One-to-ten nursing observations
- Absence without leave
- Searching of patients
- Restraint of patients
- Rapid tranquillisation
- Debriefing following critical incidents
- Preceptorship

REFERENCES

Department of Health. 1999 National Service Framework for Mental Health. London: Department of Health

Dix R, Pereira SM, Chaudhry K et al. 2005 PICU/LSU environment assessment inventory. J Psychiatr Intensive Care 1: 65–69

Pereira SM, Clinton C. 2002 Mental health policy implementation guide; national minimum standards for general adult sevices in psychiatric intensive care units (PICU) and low secure environments. London: Department of Health

Reed Committee. 1992 Review of Health and Social Services for Mentally Disordered Offenders and Others Requiring Similar Services. London: DoH/Home Office

Royal College of Psychiatrists. 1980 Secure Facilities for Psychiatric Patients: A Comprehensive Policy. Council Report. London: Royal College of Psychiatrists

United Kingdom Central Council for Nursing, Midwifery and Health Visiting. 1999 Nursing in Secure Environments: Summary and Action Plan from a Scoping Study. London: UKCC

22

Physical environment

Roland Dix and Mathew J. Page

General philosophy of Psychiatric Intensive Care Low Secure Unit design

The introduction of the National Minimum Standards for General Adult Services in Psychiatric Intensive Care Units and Low Secure Environments (Department of Health 2002) has significantly improved the understanding of the nature of these two types of facilities. The standards were derived directly from the previous edition of this chapter (Dix 2001) and provide a checklist of specifications for physical design characteristics. Further advice may be found in the NICE Guidelines for the Short-Term Management of Disturbed (Violent) Behaviour in Psychiatric In-patient Settings (National Institute for Clinical Excellence 2005). While it is acknowledged that patient characteristics may vary between the two facilities, clinical experience suggests that the design features of both are concordant. Smith (1999) cites four competing needs as being involved in the design of a building: the needs of the commissioning trust, the needs of those managing the building, the needs of those caring for the patients and the needs of the patients themselves. This chapter aims to address those needs, in particular those of the patients and staff.

Much of the design, materials and specifications for the construction of psychiatric hospitals will be well known to NHS trusts' estates departments. Documents such as the design guide for medium secure units (NHS Estates 1993) and accommodation for people with mental illness (NHS Estates 1996) contain detailed guidance for hospital design, much of which is relevant to the PICU and Low Secure Unit (LSU). The Royal College Psychiatrists (1998) report Not Just Bricks and Mortar may also be of use. This chapter aims to provide the clinical context within which PICU/LSU design should be considered. The location, size, operational policy and patient population will vary amongst units. An effective PICU/LSU physical environment needs to be based on broad principles that reflect the type of service one is proposing. For these reasons it is inappropriate to lay down rigid design specifications. This chapter provides experienced-based principles for an effective PICU design, around which individual units may be tailored to meet their specific needs.

For the purposes of this chapter the following statements will constitute the terms of reference for PICU/LSU design.

- The environment will be effective in providing increased safety against aggressive, impulsive and unpredictable behaviour
- The design of the PICU/LSU will make it difficult to abscond and the methods necessary for absconding will be predictable
- The PICU/LSU environment will allow a range of therapeutic activities to take place
- It will provide adequate space and facilities for a homely environment in which a patient can spend the majority of their day; this can be up to 2 years in a LSU

Psychiatric Intensive Care, 2nd edn., eds. M. Dominic Beer, Stephen M. Pereira and Carol Paton.
Published by Cambridge University Press. © Cambridge University Press 2008

These broad statements should be relevant to any PICU/LSU, including those based in local services, and PICUs in Medium Secure Units (MSUs) and special hospitals.

PICU/LSU position and layout

The PICU should preferably be on the ground floor. This will assist in the admission of acutely disturbed patients, and facilitate access to fresh air. One possible benefit often argued for locating the PICU on the first floor is that it may discourage absconding through windows. However, the benefits of locating the unit at ground level are significant and window specifications can prevent absconding. For PICUs/LSUs that are part of hospitals, an entrance to the unit that does not necessitate travelling through the rest of the hospital should be provided. Multiple corridors should be avoided in order to promote unobtrusive observation. Creating shallow-curved alcoves in corridors does not inhibit observation, but does create a less harsh institutional-looking environment. The amount of space to which patients have access is an important factor. Palmstierna *et al.* (1991) investigated the relationship between overcrowding and aggressive behaviour in a PICU. They concluded that aggressive behaviour was more likely in areas of higher patient density. Further evidence that PICUs/LSUs need ample space is provided by Citrome *et al.* (1994), who conclude that length of stay in the PICU is not as brief as may be expected. The NHS Estates Department (1993) design guidance for MSUs suggested that a six-bedded medium-secure PICU should offer 30 M^2 of free access space per patient. When assessing the available space for patients in a PICU, the mistake of including staff areas in square metres should be avoided, six to twelve beds is a good number. There should also be access to an enclosed garden (Dix and Williams 1996; NHS Estates 1996).

Effective designs share a number of general characteristics, e.g. pipes, wires and heating are hidden. Other important characteristics are listed below and illustrated in Figure 22.1.

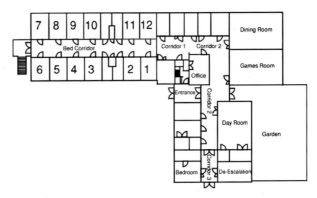

Figure 22.1. Suggested lay out of a PICU

- Wherever possible there should be clear lines of sight. This should also be possible around corners, by means of aligned windows or convex (parabolic) mirrors.
- Corridors are 3 m wide allowing four a breast comfortably.
- Ceiling height is 3 m in some areas, giving the feeling of space.
- The ceiling is fitted with sky lights that allow increased daylight into the main corridors; these should be fitted with suitable glass/film to prevent excessive solar thermal gain.

Security levels

The level of interior and perimeter security is influenced by whether the unit is serving the general adult population or the forensic population. PICUs within or serving a MSU will have security characteristics consistent with the NHS Estates design guide (1993) for MSUs. The same applies for units located within a special hospital. For units serving the general adult population things become a little less clear. It is easy to either over- or under-estimate levels of security for the general adult PICU/LSU. Care should be taken to ensure there is a difference between medium security and the general adult PICU/LSU. Otherwise a unit where expertise and clinical focus are geared towards the general adult population may be placed under pressure to fulfil an inappropriate role, e.g. admit forensic patients with higher security needs. When considering the likely methods that may be used by a patient to abscond, it is a useful exercise to spend at least 2 hs in the unit environment, and ask oneself, 'if I was intending to abscond, how would I go about it?' Following this exercise many of the likely methods will become apparent and preventative steps may be employed. Security issues are described throughout this chapter in the specific areas addressed. All security measures, for example window restrictors, should be as discreet as possible.

Secure garden

The level to which the garden is secure will largely be a matter for the PICU/LSU planning group. Standard operational procedure will generally require a staff presence when the garden is in use. A sensible balance should be drawn between the construction/height of the fence and the oppressive image created by fencing (NHS Estates 1996). Consideration should be given to the proposed patient group and what the garden may be used for. Having the garden of sufficient size to accommodate a sports area, as well as seating and more horticultural areas is advisable.

Main entrance

An air lock design is recommended for the main entrance. This means that the entrance comprises two doors set opposite each other. Once a person has entered through the first door, the second will not open until the first has closed. This may be achieved by means of magnetic lock systems or by synchronised mechanical locks. The main entrance should be located away from the main clinical area. This will help prevent absconding when the entrance is in use. It also helps to remove attention from the main entrance, which is often the focus of drama with regard to absconding attempts.

An airlock system utilising magnetic locks which may be operated via keycards at each door and via

switches in the office is preferable. In many units magnetic plate locks have proved superior to sheer locks, and using two on each door will give the 1200 lb closure pressure necessary to prevent the determined absconder. Doors which open inwards will help prevent people ramming their way out (use of the heavy metal dinner trolley as an aide has been known), provided that the frame and surrounding wall are of adequate strength. Doors should be of a solid core, with a steel skin; if they are locked along the top width, then they will need to be sufficiently solid to prevent flexion at the bottom.

The airlock control system should allow for the following methods of operation:
- Touch / proximity card key
- Push button operation for both doors located within a staff-only station
- An emergency override allowing both doors to be opened at the same time, providing for large numbers of staff to move through the entrance in cases of emergency

Units which include the provision of administration areas should aim where possible to have this independently accessed from the outside, so that clinical staff are not expected to see visitors attending meetings in and out of the airlock entrance.

Fire exits

Fire safety and security are frequently in conflict. The local fire officer must be involved at an early stage of planning (NHS Estates 1993). It is possible for fire exits to be secured on magnetic locks that become inactive when the fire alarm is activated (Dix and Williams 1996). There can be a number of problems with this arrangement. Firstly the system will need to be disconnected from the fire alarm test procedure. Secondly, patients may soon become familiar with this system and simply activate the fire alarm in order to abscond. The most reliable method may be to secure the fire exits on a lock and key. This will require a clear procedure for evacuation in the event of fire.

Fire policies will vary from unit to unit, however a tiered approach is likely to be the most pragmatic;

for instance, in the event of fire, moving all patients and personnel behind one fire door is likely to provide adequate protection in most emergencies. In the event of a prolonged emergency withdrawal to the unit's secure garden may be the next step before evacuating altogether. A contingency, which makes the nearest (preferably lockable) ward available for evacuation, is advisable. In the event of fire exits being used it may be beneficial if they open into a secure area or garden, as the level of confusion caused by an emergency creates an ideal opportunity to abscond.

Windows

Dolan and Snowden (1994) concluded that the majority of escapes from a MSU occurred through windows. While windows offer an obvious target for absconding, they also help the unit to feel less claustrophobic. Any unit design should aim for as much natural daylight as possible into the main clinical areas. The design suggested in Figure 22.1 includes ample outside windows in all rooms, and where appropriate interior windows across rooms. Because of the need for clear lines of sight, outside windows directly into the main corridor are difficult to achieve (see Figure 22.1). To overcome this ceiling sky lights may be used, providing the unit is without a second floor. While windows are an obvious weak point in ward security, Bowers *et al.* (2000b) found that the ability of staff to observe patients and levels of security within wards are not clear correlates for absconding, it is hypothesised that the quality of nursing interventions is more significant.

Polycarbonate, toughened glass and float glasses are recommended. Glass and plastics manufacturers are constantly improving products. Sophisticated glazing panels are available in plastic and glass combinations. The resulting window can be specified as 'bandit proof', shot gun proof, sledgehammer proof and so on (NHS Estates 1996). It is also important for the frame to withstand determined attempts at dismantling. Ventilation is also very important (Mueller 1983) and windows should have a restricted opening of no more than 125 mm. In addition to the window's

standard restrictors the inclusion of a camouflaged durable steel bar, fixed to the outside wall, is also useful. However, provision of a zoned air conditioning system, which can be easily controlled, provides a more secure alternative. In some sitting areas some windows can be placed 700–800 mm above the floor to allow seated outside views. In the extra care area (see below), and possibly other areas of the unit, curtain poles should be avoided. Integral window blinds may be used instead. An assessment of the necessity of any fitting that could be used for suicide by hanging should be undertaken. In areas with inherent difficulties with windows, such as seclusion rooms, they may be located out of reach or consideration may be given to sun pipes, which allow natural light to be transferred through roof spaces, around bends, etc.

Doors

All doors should be of solid core construction of at least 45 mm thickness. Such doors will be durable against abuse and also offer good sound proofing. Lillywhite *et al.* (1995) pointed out the benefits of interview room doors opening outwards. These benefits include prevention of patients barricading themselves in and promoting easy exit. For the interior of the unit it is most beneficial for as many doors as possible to open both ways.

Aggression and access through doors

Areas of high patient concentration are often the location of aggressive incidents (Palmstierna *et al.* 1991). Double doors should provide access to areas from which a patient may require relocation with control and restraint (C&R). This will provide enough width to allow access for a 3 person C&R team. Several authors have identified the dining area and meal times as a focus point for aggressive incidents (Fottrell 1980; Kennedy *et al.* 1995; Hunter and Love 1996). Kennedy *et al.* (1995) found that of eighty incidents of aggression that took place away from the main residential unit, seventy-four took place in the dining room. As a general principle double doors should be installed in rooms such as the day room, dining room, activities room and other areas in which more than two patients gather. For bedrooms a half-leaf arrangement is useful for allowing access to a C&R team. The measurements are shown in Figure 22.1.

Locks

A variety of locks are now available for the modern psychiatric hospital. These include electronic numbered key pads, proximity card locks and the traditional key arrangement. Electronic magnetic locks have the advantage of removing the need for bunches of keys, which often have negative connotations in terms of the authoritarian institution. However, they have several practical problems. Locks operated by the combination key pad have a major disadvantage in that patients soon become familiar with the combination (Dix and Williams 1996). They require the operator to stand directly in front of the key pad to conceal the combination. Also, they often have a time delay between the combination being entered and the lock becoming active. This is also the case for the proximity card lock. The problem here is that once a lock has been activated it is necessary to wait by the door for it to re-engage to prevent a patient following. Also this becomes a problem when struggles occur in doorways. In the case of traditional keys, the female part of the lock should be concave in order for the key to be entered quickly in emergencies. The number of different keys should be kept to a minimum reducing the number that need to be carried.

Technology in this area is progressing apace. The current preference would seem to be key card proximity detectors. These have significant advantages over most systems, the most important being that as each member of staff is issued with a card, should any card be lost, accessibility privileges with that card may be deleted from the computerised access system.

In the near future, face recognition and other biometric security systems will be available at ever decreasing costs. It is important for building designers to remain open minded and creative in assessing the value of new technology, and to communicate their experiences to the wider clinical community.

Where should locks be fitted?

It is desirable to be able to lock off as many of the rooms as possible. Rooms such as the day room and dining area will, for most of the time, remain open for free access by patients. There may be times, however, when it will be necessary for these rooms to be temporarily restricted. The kitchen area presents particular problems and should always be considered a potentially dangerous place. A clear operational policy should describe the use of the kitchen, including the circumstances in which access may be restricted. Obviously, the bathrooms and toilet will need to be lockable from the inside. Staff must be able to override these locks from the outside, with keys held by staff only. Bedrooms may also be locked from the inside with the same precautions as above. It may be useful in promoting responsibility to provide patients with keys to their own rooms, but again this should be with the provision of an override key held by staff. In any room that can be locked from the inside, care should be taken to ensure that the override system will work, even if the interior side of the lock is held.

Observation

Close observation is a frequently quoted reason for admission to the PICU. One-to-one close observation or 'specialing' is a familiar, and often unpopular, practice amongst many nurses. Green and Grindel (1996) found one-to-one close observation to be common practice in eighty psychiatric hospitals in the United States. In their analysis the authors identified several disadvantages including secondary gain and behavioural escalation by the patient. Other authors have also identified one-to-one observation as a problematic procedure lacking clear empirical evaluation of its effectiveness (Duffy 1995; Macpherson *et al.* 1996; Ashaye *et al.* 1997). In their retrospective study, Shugar and Rehaluk (1990) concluded that one-to-one observation in excess of 72 h was particularly problematic and should be avoided. Bowers *et al.* (2000a) found that while close observation was common practice in UK hospitals, policies were often unhelpful and inconsistent. From the available evidence, and in keeping with the experience of many nurses who have performed this procedure, an effective unit design should minimise the need for one-to-one close observation.

Page *et al.* (2004) describe in detail how the provision of infrared closed circuit television (CCTV) may enable less disruptive night-time observation. While this practice is innovative and its use has proved controversial it has been found to have merit within the clinical context. A research project into its efficacy has been published (Warr *et al.* 2005). The system uses infrared cameras in each bedroom which are viewed from a monitor in the office. Patients are allowed to elect whether they are observed via the CCTV or traditional methods, the advantages being increased privacy and less disruption than traditional methods. Many of the preliminary issues are tackled by Dix (2002) and Dix and Meiklejohn (2003).

Closed circuit television may also be used in other areas. Its advantages in the extra care area are discussed below. It can also be used to monitor activity in the unit garden, at entrances to the unit and a high level camera will enable unobtrusive observation of patients on unescorted leave in the grounds. By having a system which records, there will be a photographic record of all visitors and any miscreant activity, such as dropping illicit substances into the unit's garden. A digital recording system is preferable to the more common video systems, as it does not rely on staff's remembering to change tapes on a regular basis. Images are also clearer and can be accessed far more easily.

Figure 22.1 offers a suggestion for a unit design that allows for high levels of unobtrusive observation.

- As many clear lines of sight as possible should be available, avoiding numerous corners and corridors (see Figure 22.1). Interior windows should be aligned where possible (as shown in Figure 22.1) to allow observation across a number of rooms.
- All doors (with the exception of the bathrooms and toilets) should be fitted with a polycarbonate observation panel. This will enhance safety when moving around the unit by ensuring that the staff and patients can see the other side of doors.
- Bedrooms and bathrooms should be fitted with a louver-type window controlled from the outside by a key mechanism. There have been reports of louver windows being broken and the laminate creating a catapult effect, causing glass to be thrown from the frame with force. An additional piece of polycarbonate on the outside should prevent this phenomenon.
- Bedroom lights should be controlled by switches with a dimmer, one located inside and the other outside the room. This will allow for night time observation.
- In areas where corridors meet or there are not clear lines of sight, convex mirrors can be fitted at ceiling level to allow views around corners.

Facilities for managing the most acutely disturbed patient

Patients who demonstrate extremely unpredictable and assaultative behaviour present particular management problems. Throughout the history of mental health care seclusion was often the solution for this type of behaviour (Renvoize 1991). In recent years the use of seclusion has been questioned for its clinical, ethical and practical value (Hamil 1987; Angold 1989; Tooke and Brown 1992). Kinsella and Brosman (1993) suggested the use of an extra care area (ECA) as an alternative to seclusion. This is defined as a closely supervised living space, away from the main clinical area, in which a single patient may be nursed away from the rest of the patients (Dix 1995). Curran *et al.* (2005) also provide detailed guidance on the composition and design of an ECA. The NHS Estates building note number 35 (1996) advises the project group for a new PICU to decide on the need for a seclusion room. If the extra care option is chosen it should be used for the shortest possible time, as extended use is prone to producing the same negative effects as one-to-one observation (Kinsella and Brosman 1993). National Institute for Health and Clinical Excellence (2005) guidance for the management of violence requires all inpatient units to have access to seclusion facilities.

Recent debate has focused on the use of seclusion as an alternative to prolonged restraint following deaths due to postural asphyxiation (Patterson and Leadbetter 2004).

Figure 22.1 shows an ECA, which could also include a seclusion room, or, if preferred, a de-escalation room in which staff remain with the patient, rather than locking the patient in.

Extra care area composition

Unless staffing levels will allow staff to be dedicated to the ECA, it should be possible for the ECA to be part of the unit, and not physically separated. In terms of the number of staff needed, there is a danger of creating a ward within a ward. Figure 22.1 shows an ECA separated by double doors, which could be fixed open to allow the ECA to become part of the unit. In the ECA a higher level of safety is needed than anywhere else in the unit. Care is necessary to ensure that items which could be used as a weapon are avoided.

The ECA should be able to provide for the daily living needs of a single patient. This will require the following, all in close proximity to each other:
- A seclusion/de-escalation room (see below)
- A toilet and shower facility
- A sitting room with simple furnishings
- An entrance to the ECA directly from outside the unit, for the admission of acutely disturbed patients
- Access to the garden
- An intercom system to the main office

Design of seclusion/de-escalation rooms

- This room should be located in the ECA of the unit
- It should have a single, moulded vinyl safety bed

- The size should allow for at least 7 m^2 and a ceiling clearance that cannot be reached by jumping or standing on the safety bed
- The room must be able to withstand determined attack and damage
- The walls and floors should be lined with a welded seam vinyl surface
- The door should be of solid core design of a least 55 mm thickness, with an observation panel, double glassed with high-grade 5 mm polycarbonate
- It should be possible to see into the whole room from the observation panel, without any hidden corners
- Ventilation/heating should be provided through air vents placed at ceiling level out of reach; noise levels generated by this equipment must also be minimised
- The placement of infrared CCTV cameras in this area enables staff in the ward office to monitor the situation
- A recording system may also be useful for reflection/debrief and as protection for both staff and patients from false allegations of abuse

Recreation and occupational therapy

The value of planned therapeutic activity amongst patients in the institutional setting has long been accepted (Aumack 1968). There is strong evidence that psychiatric institutions are poor performers in ensuring that therapeutic activity is high on the agenda (Drinkwater and Gudjonsson 1989; Standing Nursing and Midwifery Advisory Committee 1999). Correlation between aggression and inactivity has also been established (Lloyd 1995). With the inevitable preoccupation with safety and containment, a PICU/LSU may be amongst the most guilty of psychiatric settings in failing to provide adequate resources for therapeutic activity (Zigmond 1995). Best (1996) dramatically demonstrated the value of activity for bringing about positive changes to disturbed behaviour in the PICU setting. An effective PICU/LSU design will have given the provision of therapeutic activity an equal status to safety and security. Page (2005) describes the profile of a new low secure service and adequate numbers of staff to patients.

Recreation/activity facilities

Figure 22.1 includes:
- A games room in which a pool table, table tennis table and, exercise bike may be placed
- A games room in which board games, art equipment and stereo equipment is placed
- A day room and sitting room equipped with television and video
- Access to an enclosed garden area

For the most part activities will be undertaken with the direct support of staff. Individual assessments will indicate the amount of staff intervention required (Best 1996). When not in use or as clinically indicated, these areas may be locked off. Use of activity equipment and facilities should be supported by standard operational procedures (SOP) (see below). Activity programmes must include collaboration between nursing staff, and occupational and sports therapists. Electrical sockets and TV aerial points in bedrooms are useful for patients wanting to listen to music alone. There should be the provision for the power to be disconnected by staff if additional safety is required.

Furniture and fittings

The unit environment should be made as homely as possible. Wall mounted pictures, pot plants and non-moulded furniture promote a relaxed environment without presenting a major risk to safety. Poster-type pictures may be fixed to the wall on a back board covered with polycarbonate. Some units may wish to surround the television and video with a polycarbonate-fronted protective case. In the experience of the authors protection of this type may encourage attacks towards the television, rather than deterring them. The unit should be fitted with a pay telephone to which the patients have free access (Department of Health 2002). This could be on a portable trolley, allowing for it to be removed in the event of consistent inappropriate use.

The unit should be decorated in pleasant homely colours, paint must be vinyl and should be tolerant of scrubbing in case of dirty marks and stains. Carpets should also be used where possible to prevent an 'institutional look'; however, these must be of a very high quality and should be both burn and stain resistant.

Staff and patient safety

Personal alarm systems carried by staff that, when activated, alert others to an emergency are useful. The basic principle of these systems is a signal sent from a hand unit to a wall- or ceiling-mounted sensor which has an audio visual output. These units operate by ultrasonic, infrared or radio signals. The technology in this area is rapidly developing and new products are constantly entering the market. When considering which product will be most effective, a demonstration by the manufacturer is a necessary step. The following common problems should be avoided:
- Systems that are too directionally sensitive resulting in the need to point the hand set directly at the receiver
- Systems where the hand set is over powered, resulting in the activation of several receivers confusing the exact location of the emergency
- Systems that are under sensitive, resulting in the need to press the hand unit several times before the alarm is sounded

Wall-mounted emergency buttons with audio visual output are also a necessary fitting. These should be installed in addition to the hand-held systems as they also offer protection for the patients. A button should be placed in all rooms and at regular intervals in corridors. There should be the provision for the system to be de-activated centrally in the event of persistent inappropriate use by patients.

Systems are now available which rely on all signals being processed by a personal computer (PC). This has significant advantages in that all events are recorded and can be audited later (a questionnaire can be set up on the PC, and circulated after every incident). Using an integrated system which allows control/isolation of water and electricity is also advantageous. It is also possible to have a portable alarm which, when activated, causes the PC to make a pre-recorded telephone call on the hospital's emergency system announcing a psychiatric emergency.

Communication systems

Two-way radios are recommended, as they are useful for communication around the hospital and on escorted leave. They are also of particular value in other situations, for example searching for a patient who has absconded. Again a variety of products are available with new equipment entering the market. For extended range it is necessary for a booster transmitter to be installed on top of the building. Standard industrial units are relatively inexpensive and offer good performance and reliability. With booster units these radios are capable of working over a 10-mile radius. Regular servicing is imperative as batteries will need replacing every 12–18 months. For longer distance escorted leave, a mobile phone is recommended, pre-programmed with the numbers of the ward, the hospital reception and the police.

Transport

Access to a dedicated vehicle is highly recommended. It should be of a suitable size without having an institutional look; so-called multi purpose vehicles (MPVs) or people carriers are ideal and more comfortable than minibuses.

The vehicle should be suitable for a variety of purposes such as taking patients on escorted leave, the unit holiday and searching for and retrieving the absconded patient.

Robustness is a consideration, as inevitably the vehicle will receive a harder working life than when in domestic use.

Safety must be a consideration; a vehicle with a higher European safety rating should be preferred.

Standard operational procedure

The value of equipment and managing the physical environment may be optimised by developing standard operational procedures (SOPs), which are widely used by organisations faced with complex management situations. They describe a standard response to situations that commonly occur, and for which contingency plans are needed. They are designed to promote confidence in the staff for dealing with difficult situations, maximising the therapeutic options that may be considered. The following is an example of a SOP in the event that a patient becomes disturbed, or attempts to abscond while on escorted leave.

1. During every episode of escorted leave, the escort will carry a radio and/or mobile telephone. The mobile phone must also be carried if the destination is over 1.5 miles away.
2. Before leaving the unit the escort will ensure a second radio is held by a member of staff and that both are switched on and working. The escort will state the intended destination and approximate duration of leave.
3. If there is a deviation from the stated plan or expected duration of leave, the escort will inform the unit.
4. If the patient becomes disturbed or attempts to leave the escort, take the following actions:
   - Attempt verbal negotiation
   - Failing this, contact the unit and assess the appropriateness of physical intervention; only attempt physical intervention if safe to do so
   - If physical intervention is inappropriate, follow the patient at a safe distance, contacting the other staff by radio with situation reports at 5-min intervals

Standard operational procedures are used to support staff in the use of equipment and maintaining a safe environment. They should be kept as simple as possible and taught to all the unit staff (including medical and paramedical team members). In terms of the physical environment, other areas where the development of SOPs should be considered are:

1. Preparing the ward environment for an acutely disturbed admission
2. Interviewing or negotiating with a potentially aggressive patient
3. Use of the ECA

Future innovations

Most scientific advancements relevant to PICU and LSU design are in the area of security. In the coming years more products will come available and they will all probably become more affordable.

Such innovations might include:

- Use of face/iris-recognition access systems, as this has huge advantages over keys and cards, namely they cannot be lost
- Use of thermal imaging CCTV to assess someone's temperature and vital signs without disturbing them
- Use of Global Positioning Systems for locating staff, patients and vehicles when away from the unit.

While much of the above will not sit comfortably with many mental health practitioners because of their institutional connotations, they should not be ignored. It is essential that front-line clinical staff remain open minded and pragmatic about the environment they work in and possibilities for improvement.

Conclusion

In a chapter of this size it is not possible to describe every detail of the ideal PICU/LSU physical environment. The design guidance offered is not overly prescriptive but is intended to provide the principles on which PICU/LSU design can be based.

During her study of nurses' perceptions of a new PICU, Gentle (1996) identified dissatisfaction with the physical environment as a major issue. Taj and Sheehan (1994) also found high levels of dissatisfaction in the architectural design of a new acute unit. After only 6 months they recommended major design changes. In a statistical comparison of a ward atmosphere and staff attitude between a PICU, a regional secure unit and an acute ward, Squier (1994) commented that in the PICU:

Organisational structure and programme clarity were diminished, which indicates the difficulty staff have maintaining order and organization.

It is essential that the planning of a new PICU/LSU involves a detailed and careful analysis of the physical environment. For those planning a new PICU development, it is highly recommended that several visits are made to established units to consider the environment's strengths and weaknesses. Joint working between clinicians and architects is also essential. A design will only be a success if both parties work collaboratively. Once a new unit is operational, it should be considered as an inherent part of planning that the physical environment will be modified and developed.

REFERENCES

Angold A. 1989 Seclusion. Br J Psychiatry 154: 437–444

Ashaye O, Ikkos G, Rigby E. 1997 Study of the effects of constant observation of psychiatric in-patients. Psychiatr Bull 21: 145–147

Aumack L. 1968 The patient activity checklist: an instrument and an approach for measuring behaviour. J Clin Psychol 25: 134–137

Best D. 1996 The developing role of occupational therapy in psychiatric intensive care. Br J Occup Ther 59: 161–164

Bowers L, Gournay K, Duffy D. 2000a Suicide and self harm on inpatient psychiatric units: a national survey of observation policies. J Adv Nurs 32: 437–444

Bowers L, Jarret M, Clark N, Kiyimba F, McFarlane L. 2000b Determinants of absconding by patients on acute psychiatric wards. J Adv Nurs 32 (3): 644–649

Citrome L, Green L, Frost R. 1994 Length of stay and recidivism on a psychiatric intensive care unit. Hosp Community Psychiatry 45 (1): 74–76

Curran C, Adnett C, Zigmond A. 2005 Factors to consider when designing and using a seclusion suite in a mental hospital. Hospital development. Sidcup: Wilmington Media Limited

Department of Health. 2002 Mental Health Policy Implementation Guide: National Minimum Standards for General Adult Services in Psychiatric Intensive Care Units and Low Secure Environments. London: Department of Health

Dix R. 1995 A nurse led psychiatric intensive care unit. Psychiatr Bull May: 285–287

Dix R. 2001 The physical environment. In: Beer MD, Pereira SM, Paton C (eds) Psychiatric Intensive Care. London. Greenwhich Medical Publications

Dix R. 2002 Observation and technology: logical progression or ethical nightmare. Nat Assoc Psychiatr Intensive Care Units Bull 2 (4): 22–29

Dix R, Meiklejohn C. 2003 Observation and technology: questions and answers. Nat Assoc Psychiatr Intensive Care Units Bull 3: 39–49

Dix R, Williams K. 1996 Psychiatric Intensive Care Units: a design for living. Psychiatr Bull 20: 527–529

Dolan M, Snowden P. 1994 Escapes from a medium secure unit. J Forensic Psychiatry 5 (2): 275–286

Drinkwater J, Gudjonsson G. 1989 The nature of violence in psychiatric hospitals. In: Howells K, Hollin C (eds) Clinical Approaches To Violence. Chichester: Wiley, pp. 287–305

Duffy D. 1995 Out of the shadows: a study of the special observation of suicidal psychiatric in-patients. J Adv Nurs 21(5): 944–950

Fottrell E. 1980 A study of violent behaviour amongst patients in psychiatric hospitals. Br J Psychiatry 136: 216–221

Gentle J. 1996 Mental health intensive care units: the nurses experience and perceptions of a new unit. J Adv Nurs 24: 1194–1200

Goldney R, Bowes J, Spence N, Czechowicz A, Hurley R. 1985 The Psychiatric Intensive Care Unit. Br J Psychiatry 146: 50–54

Green J, Grindel C. 1996 Supervision of suicidal patients in adult inpatient psychiatric units in general hospitals. Psychiatr Serv 47 (8): 859–863

Hamil K. 1987 Seclusion: inside looking out. Nurs Times 83 (5): 174–179

Hunter M, Love C. 1996 Total quality management and the reduction of inpatient violence and costs in a forensic psychiatric hospital. Psychiatr Serv 47 (7): 751–754

Kennedy J, Harrison J, Hillis T, Bluglass R. 1995 Analysis of violent incidents in a regional secure unit. Med Sci Law 35 (3): 255–260

Kinsella C, Brosman C. 1993 An alternative to seclusion? Nurs Times 89 (18): 62–64

Lillywhite A, Morgan N, Walter E. 1995 Reducing the risk of violence to junior psychiatrists. Psychiatr Bull 19: 24–27

Lloyd C. 1995 Forensic psychiatry for health professionals. Therapy in practice. London: Chapman and Hall

Macpherson R, Anstee B, Dix R. 1996 Guidelines for the management of acutely disturbed patients. Adv Psychiatr Treat 2: 194–201

Mueller C. 1983 Environmental stressors and aggressive behaviour. In: Green R. Donnerstein R (eds) Aggression; theoretical and empirical reviews, volume 2. Issues in Research. New York: Academic Press

Musisi S, Wasylenki D, Rapp M. 1989 A Psychiatric Intensive Care Unit in a psychiatric hospital. Can J Psychiatry 34 (3): 200–204

National Institute for Clinical Excellence. 2005 Short Term Management of Disturbed (Violent) Behaviour in Psychiatric In-patient Settings. NICE Guidelines. London: NICE

NHS Estates. 1993 Design Guide: Medium Secure Psychiatric Units, NHS Estates. Leeds: Executive Agency of the Department of Health

NHS Estates. 1996 Accommodation for people with mental illness. Health Building Note 35: Part 1 – the acute unit. Leeds: Executive Agency of the Department of Health

Page M. (2005) Low secure care: a description of a new service. J Psychiatr Intensive Care 1(2) 89–96

Page M, Meiklejohn C, Warr J. 2004 CCTV and night-time observations. Ment Health Pract 7 (10): 28–31

Palmstierna T, Huitfeldt B, Wistedt B. 1991 The relationship between crowding and aggressive behaviour in the psychiatric intensive care unit. Hosp Community Psychiatry 42 (12): 1237–1240

Patterson B, Leadbetter D. 2004 Learning the right lessons. Mental Health Practice. 7 (7): 12–15

Reed Committee. 1992 Review of Health and Social Services for Mentally Disordered Offenders and Others Requiring Similar Services. London: Department of Health/Social Services Office

Renvoize E. 1991 The association of medical officers of asylums and hospitals for the insane, the medico-psychological Association, and their presidents. In: Berrios G, Freeman H (eds) 150 Years of British Psychiatry 1841–1991. London: Gaskell, pp. 29–75

Royal College of Psychiatrists. 1998 Not Just Bricks and Mortar. London: Royal College of Psychiatrists

Shugar G, Rehaluk R. 1990 Continuous observation for psychiatric in-patients. Comp Psychiatry 30 (1): 48–55

Smith M. 1999 Designed for living. Ment Health Care 2 (11): 367–369

Squier R. 1994 The relationship between ward atmosphere and staff attitude to treatment in psychiatric in-patient units. Br J Med Psychology 67: 319–331

Standing Nursing and Midwifery Advisory Committee. 1999 Mental Health Nursing: 'Addressing Acute Concerns'. London: SNMAC

Taj R, Sheehan J. 1994 Architectural design and acute psychiatric care. Psychiatr Bull 18: 279–281

Tooke K, Brown J. 1992 Perceptions of seclusion: comparing patient and staff reactions. J Psychosoc Nurs 30 (8): 23–26

Warr J, Page M, Crossen-White H. 2005 The appropriate use of closed circuit television (CCTV). Observation in a secure unit. Bournemouth: Bournemouth University (ISBN 1-85899-184-6)

Zigmond A. 1995 Special care wards: are they special? Psychiatr Bull 19: 310–312

23

Managing the Psychiatric Intensive Care Unit

Phil Garnham

Introduction

The Psychiatric Intensive Care Unit (PICU) is a place of rapid and constant change, with high levels of arousal experienced by staff and patients alike. Although the pace of change may be less rapid on a Low Secure Unit (LSU), other problems are very similar.

Effective management can ensure that key principles are not lost or compromised by a pressurised environment and that all actions and care are carried out within the context of safe practice.

One measure of effective management is the consistency with which the unit retains its place on the continuum between therapy and containment. The roles of the ward manager and multi-professional team are crucial in this process.

The increasing role of PICUs and LSUs in today's modern mental health provision has resulted in implementation guides developed by the Department of Health. These identify guidelines and evidence-based practice in support of the National Service Framework for Mental Health (Department of Health 1999a). The Mental Health Policy Implementation Guide: National Minimum Standards for General Adult Services in Psychiatric Intensive Care Units (PICU) and Low Secure Environments (Pereira and Clinton 2002) and Adult Acute Inpatient Care Provision (Department of Health 2002a) will be referred to within this text.

Key principles

- A clear sense of purpose for the unit is known and owned by the staff, and communicated clearly to patients
- The purpose of the unit is to manage acute mental ill health episodes and then return the patient to a more appropriate care setting
- As far as possible and practicable, patients and their relatives are actively involved in their care and how it is delivered to them
- Staff at all levels are consulted and involved in the decision-making process with regard to the running of the unit
- Staff are given full support for career development and the promotion of excellence in practice
- The functioning of the unit is subject to regular audit and appraisal in order to develop and improve care given to patients
- The principles of clinical governance should be adhered to, namely monitoring the effective quality of clinical care
- The principles of risk assessment and management are adhered to

For any local approach to be achievable and effective, consideration should be given to national approaches. The National Service Frameworks for Mental Health (Department of Health 1999a) sets out standards in five areas to, 'reduce variations in practice and deliver improvements . . .'.

Psychiatric Intensive Care, 2nd edn., eds. M. Dominic Beer, Stephen M. Pereira and Carol Paton.
Published by Cambridge University Press. © Cambridge University Press 2008

Table 23.1. National standards and service models

Standard one	Mental health promotion
Standards two and three	Primary care and access to services
Standards four and five	Effective services for people with severe mental illness
Standard six	Caring about carers
Standard seven	Preventing suicide

The chapter on 'Effective services for people with severe mental illness' (Department of Health 1999a) makes frequent reference to psychiatric intensive care and low secure services, e.g. gaps in provision (p. 49); access to hospital (p. 62); and monitoring of milestones (p. 68).

Where do the PICU and LSU fit within the local management structure?

A fundamental question which must be addressed is where the PICU and LSU should be situated managerially. That is, do they form part of the acute service, the forensic services, community respite, etc.? The only definite answer is that they do not belong in Older Adults services!

Local services will differ in their function and form; therefore, the decision as to where these units should be situated is best left to local opinion. However, the author believes that the acute psychiatric inpatient services are best suited. Here they will share managerial and philosophical input. Indeed, most of the patients of the PICU will be drawn from these clinical areas. For some services, LSUs and PICUs may benefit from being in the same management structure as forensic services. The decision should be firmly based in a recognition of the recovery needs of the patient group.

Guidelines for care

At times, PICUs and LSUs will be frantic and chaotic places. This problem may be compounded in PICUs where staff may have little or no warning of an admission. Invariably, the patient will be experiencing acute psychiatric or drug-induced symptoms, or will be expressing feelings of acute anxiety, distress, threat or fear. The nature and definition of the admission will lead to the patient's feeling uncertain, frightened and experiencing a loss of control. At times like this the staff may often feel unable to take control of their immediate environment, or frozen by the anxiety of the unknown. It is all too easy, when faced with adversity, to 'batten down the hatches' in a need for certainty and the danger is that patients are forgotten in this crisis, leaving them isolated and uncared for. This can lead to an increase in symptoms experienced by the patient and a subsequent rise in the level of disturbance. Staff will need to feel confident and in control of the admission process, which will then enable a consistent, confident and caring approach.

It is essential then that the ward area can provide a structured, responsive and understanding environment. Patients will respond better to a setting where they feel that their emotions and experiences are contained or held safely. The staff group need to understand clearly what the expectations of their role are and be confident in exercising their ability to care for the individual's needs. An accurate assessment of the patients' needs, often under difficult conditions, is essential to the success of the admission process. The patient may be experiencing a lack of understanding, resentment and occasionally hostility. It is the nurses' role to reassure the patient as soon as possible that they are in a safe, caring and understanding place. Unit policies and guidelines should reflect this approach. Identifying areas where guidance is required, such as search procedures, levels of observation and day-to-day duties, will help the staff to work safely and consistently. These policies and guidelines will also need to provide a degree of delegation to the staff, so that they feel permitted to exercise individual or team decisions within certain previously defined parameters, such as the ability to reduce or increase leave status or adjust individual guidelines.

A comprehensive list of policies that should be available on PICUs and LSUs can be found in the National Minimum Standards for General Adult Services in Psychiatric Intensive Care Units and Low

Secure Environments (Pereira and Clinton 2002).
Some of the more significant ones are detailed
below.

Operational policy

Every unit needs one. It should reflect the local
approach to PICU whilst encompassing any larger
service frameworks, e.g. Mental Health Nursing:
'Addressing Acute Concerns' (SNMAC 1999a) and
Practice Guidance: Safe and Supportive Observation of Patients at Risk (SNMAC 1999b) and Mental
Health Policy Implementation Guide: Developing
Positive Practice to Support the Safe and Therapeutic Management of Aggression and Violence in
Mental Health In-patient Settings (NIMHE 2004). It
should be practical, accessible and realistic. A sample
operational policy can be found in the Appendix to
Chapter 21.

Working practice manual

This document should exist as a frame of reference
for all staff working in the PICUs and LSUs and should
remain accessible to healthcare assistant and consultant alike. It should be relevant and up to date
and serve as the main practice area document for
induction and ongoing practice and development.
The working practice manual should be evaluated,
reviewed and updated on a yearly basis. Everyone
should be made aware of it, and the practice laid out
within it adhered to.

The following is a list of relevant areas to which
the working practice manual needs to pay particular
attention. The author has tried to cover the diverse
and constantly changing needs of this challenging
patient group.

Admission policy

This will reflect the needs of the admitting population as well as any services and agencies that may
be involved. It should give clear guidance for staff

Table 23.2. Restricted items

Strictly forbidden	May be allowed but usually held by staff
Illegal drugs	Money
Weapons, e.g. knives (injury/self-harm)	Lighters
Scissors/pen knives	Razors
Alcohol	Jewellery
Solvents	Electrical goods
Glass bottles	Any medication
Matches	
Lighter fuel	

and be capable of implementation (see Appendix to
Chapter 21 for sample policy).

Visiting policy

This needs to be sensitive to patients' and relatives' needs, whilst offering the clinical team a sense
of control over access to the unit. Specific attention should be given to the child protection policy
and child visitors. Any restrictions placed on visitors
must be consistent with the Human Rights Act 1998
(UK Parliament 1998).

Restricted items

Patients or relatives may try to bring items onto
the unit which, without staff being aware, may
cause problems or complicate an already problematic situation. These need to be clearly identified to
staff, patients and relatives alike and clear demarcation made between strictly forbidden items and
items which may be helpful to a patient's care,
but that staff need to know about or have control
over.

It is important to note that the list in Table 23.2
shows possible options and is not exhaustive. What
is a safety issue for patient A, may not be for patient B.
There is no substitute for a comprehensive individual
assessment based on a thorough understanding of
the patient's behaviour and need.

Keys

Whether electronic or good old-fashioned keys, staff need to be aware of how they work, who can have one and what to do if one is missing, or not working. A common sense but strict policy will enable staff to maintain safety, whilst avoiding a key-dominated environment. All new staff should have an agreed, signed induction, before they are allocated a key or left to operate any system.

Kitchen/servery

The policy should cover access to these areas, spelling out the criteria, with clear guidelines on how the assessment should be made. Particular attention should be paid to the patient's current and ongoing mental state, behaviour, understanding of responsibility and ability to use the environment safely. If sharp knives are to be used, then a full risk assessment should be undertaken and documented using the aforementioned criteria and including a skill-based activities of daily living assessment.

Staff/patient call alarms

The team needs to know how and when to summon assistance and what each individual's responsibility is at any given time. Regular testing should occur and a record of this kept; and as a matter of course all staff should be inducted into the effective use of the alarm system immediately.

Privacy and dignity

The unit will require a privacy and dignity policy in line with recommendations laid out in Women's Mental Health: Into the Mainstream (Department of Health 2002b).

Searching patients

As this is a contentious area regarding individual privacy and dignity and the responsibility of profession-

Table 23.3. Leave granting

Type of leave	Authorisation
Clinic garden leave	The team is expected to identify any issues of risk and plan for or implement strategies to minimise risks. This can be given at the discretion of the nursing team
Hospital grounds	The decision to grant leave should occur as part of the management decisions made through the ward round
Leave outside of the hospital grounds	The decision to grant leave will always be made by the multidisciplinary team within the context of a ward round. The only exceptions to this will be in the case of emergency medical treatment

als, staff will need to be clear on what is permissible and what is not, and to know particularly what other course of action is available to them if a search cannot be undertaken.

Clinic checks

Staff need clear direction on what area needs checking and how often. A record should be kept.

Escorts

This policy will need to indicate the balance of responsibility staff have to safeguard themselves whilst providing a safe experience for the patient. Breaking down in table form and clearly identifying who is responsible for what is often helpful, as shown in Table 23.3.

Absence without leave (AWOL)

Clear guidelines, processes and protocols on the reporting and searching of AWOL patients is needed.

Police liaison may be of benefit when the unit suddenly needs to call upon them, or vice versa. Useful guides for Police Liaison Protocol can be found from the London Development Centre for Mental Health, Pan-London Flowcharts for Protocols: Service User Missing from Hospital or other Heathcare Setting.

Restraint (see Chapter 9)

The unit's policy should reflect the Mental Health Policy Implementation Guide: Developing Positive Practice to Support the Safe and Therapeutic Management of Aggression and Violence in Mental Health In-patient Settings (NIMHE 2004).

The UKCC Nursing in Secure Environments: Summary and Action Plan (1999) and The Royal College of Psychiatrists' (1998) Management of Imminent Violence Occasional Paper OP41 will be also be of use, as they provide the precursors to the above.

The Positive Practice Guidelines will provide a clear framework and way forward. The resources required to deliver this framework will need to be made available within the unit or organisation, leaving staff with a clear sense of their role and responsibility. Training in breakaway techniques is essential and an accepted approach to the therapeutic management of violence and aggression identified.

Regular training and refreshers should be provided every 12 months for breakaways and restraint training and these need to be built into a staff induction package, which is linked to the ongoing professional development of the staff team.

Seclusion (see Chapter 8)

Not all units will opt to use seclusion. Where they have, a clear policy and monitoring statement need to be made. The Royal College of Psychiatrist's guidelines (1998) on the Management of Imminent Violence and the Mental Health Act Code of Practice 1983 (Department of Health 1999c) can offer a good framework. Where units opt out of the use of seclusion, it must be made clear to staff what alternatives are to be used, along with any resource and training implications. Again the Royal College guidelines can help in the therapeutic management of potential violence and aggression.

Observation/monitored supervision

The PICU will be mindful of its approach to close observation. Managing the delicate balance between maintaining a patient's personal safety (at a time when they are usually not able to manage it for themselves), whilst avoiding a custodial or punitive approach to care is a skill that is developed through supervision, support, education and experience. Poorly implemented observation can produce anger, resentment and frustration, often leading to an exacerbation of the behaviour the observation is trying to prevent.

The lack of any evidence towards the effectiveness of observation has led Baxter and Cutcliffe (1999) to propose a move away from 'defensive practices, such as observation' towards the 'human needs of the individual'. However, current practice in many settings is to establish clear criteria for observations in an attempt to minimise inconsistency and maximise safe practice. Any policy must reflect the needs of the patient and give clear/sound guidelines to the practitioner.

As referred to previously in this chapter, Practice Guidance: Safe and Supportive Observations of Patients at Risk (SNMAC 1999b) is 'intended to be a template for local services to use in developing protocols and practice'.

Risk assessment (see Chapter 12)

This will need to follow in line with any trust hospital policy and, whilst providing a framework within the clinical area, should inform staff of the issues around risk assessment. Some way of formally recording any risk assessment should be produced and rigorous evaluation, monitoring and communication of results need to be encouraged.

It is helpful for any approach to set clear guidelines as to standard risk assessment points which should be addressed in any decision-making process. These areas will include:

- Past behaviour
- Current mental state
- Alcohol and drug use
- History of violence
- History of suicide/self-harm
- History of absconding
- Relapse indicators
- Protective factors

Other factors may be appropriate given a particular individual's circumstances and these should be included and documented in any risk assessment process.

Drug and alcohol use

This area is a sensitive and complicated one. The team should be addressing issues such as, 'Why do patients abuse or misuse? How has this developed? Can it be understood? Can it be prevented? If it cannot be prevented, can it be minimised? Can patients be helped to use alcohol more appropriately, or do they need to be stopped?'. All these issues have differing answers depending on the person who asks the question and the person to whom the question is directed.

Given such a complicated set of issues, a policy will need to balance the need to prevent a crime being committed against the long-term well being of the patient. A policy should offer clear guidance to staff on what to do in the case of the taking and supplying of non-prescribed drugs or substances, but it may also encourage a positive and inquisitive approach to the nature of behaviours. The application of the law and boundaries of confidentiality will have to be considered within any policy framework.

Any policy statement will have to balance the therapeutic use of alcohol, e.g. for social or recreation purposes, against its potential for misuse.

If alcohol and drug consumption are to be monitored and the results used as a therapeutic aid, then a rigorous but sensitive process of taking specimens will need to be adopted. Patient's privacy and dignity will need to be maintained, whilst at the same time ensuring that the specimen produced is not tampered with. Anyone with experience of drug and alcohol care in institutions will know some of the lengths patients will go to in order, to produce a negative urine specimen.

The ward environment

In order to ensure that the environment provides high-quality therapeutic interventions balanced against a safe environment, the provision of a structured environment is essential.

Of course it could be argued that any combination of effective interventions can, together, make up a safe and structured environment. However, it is often not the case that this occurs by chance. It is not the author's intention to provide an exhaustive list of possible elements for an effective structure, but to provide a back bone upon which a safe, united, responsive and flexible environment can be created. It is all too easy to settle on a particular approach, which has proven safe, but this cannot always continue to be ensured and can often lead to a custodial and negative approach to patient care. It is essential that the staff team remain alert to all changes that can occur within the environment. They will then remain responsive to the needs of the immediate situation and to those of individual patients.

There will be many other factors that can contribute, but a basic structure is essential. Below are a number of elements essential to the development of an environment that, by its nature, is structured and safe, yet responsive to individual needs.

Buildings should be purpose-built and should allow good observation. The Nursing Office should preferably be at the centre of the unit where all day areas, bedroom corridors, recreation and assessment areas can easily be observed. The unit should be well lit with plenty of natural daylight, providing individual living space, with sturdy, well-maintained and decorated rooms.

Management of the ward should be structured, with a clear hierarchy as to who makes decisions, whilst allowing involvement from all staff, with each grade and discipline being clear about their role and function.

The shift system should be clearly defined and the structure adhered to. For example all nursing staff should attend handovers to maintain a consistent care approach with good communication. To assist in this process it would be helpful for the multidisciplinary team to meet before the oncoming shift, to discuss and share observations, check out quality and accuracy of reports and plan for information to be handed over. This will aid team cohesion.

The shift will also benefit from having a coordinator, whose duty it is to plan and organise the shift, receive and manage information and be aware of all staff and patient changes.

Crucial to this structure is the consistent and effective use of a Communication Book, Diary and Shift Meeting Minutes and a commitment from all staff to update themselves at the start of each shift.

An individualised handover, where the nursing report is read out to the patient, is a good time for staff to meet and discuss progress with the patient. It will also bring the oncoming staff immediately up to date with the patient's progress.

Regular staff meetings should be facilitated by the ward manager with the intention of including the nursing team in policy- and decision-making processes, fostering ownership of the environment and disseminating any local or national developments. These meetings will need to identify a purpose and direction to avoid them becoming over critical.

It is desirable to recruit staff with an appropriate attitude and personality and attributes such as the following:

- Non-judgmental
- Patient-focused
- Self-aware
- Reflective
- Able to treat patients with dignity and self-respect
- Committed to self-development
- Demonstrate an understanding of patients' situations

Lowe (1992) identifies the following categories as ways to make therapeutic interventions more effective:

- Personal control
- Staff honesty

- Providing face-saving alternatives
- Setting limits
- Use of structure
- Facilitating expression
- Monitoring
- Timing
- Calming
- Confirming messages
- Use of non-verbal skills

The integration of the above skills into a secure setting where the nursing team manage potentially difficult behaviour is discussed further in Conlan *et al.* (1997).

Staff mix

Wherever possible, the staff group needs to reflect the age, gender and cultural mix of the patient group. However, in reality, this is often difficult to achieve with any consistency and hence concentrating on the above recruitment aspects may compensate for any shortfall.

Internal rotation

Rotas should be organised to maintain consistency and yet mix staff together, e.g. a rota system that enables small teams to work together for the majority of time, but that overlaps with other small teams. This will enable teamwork and a sense of belonging within the staff group, whilst avoiding the development of fixed attitudes and inconsistent approaches.

Therapeutic programme

This will need to reflect the needs of the patient group and be flexible enough to accommodate local changes within the patient group. Any programme will benefit from a focus-based plan which enables the ward community to interact together, encouraging socialisation and awareness of the needs of others. Providing occupation can enhance self-esteem, reduce boredom and decrease irritability, minimising the potential for violence and aggression.

Multidisciplinary input

The multidisciplinary team (MDT) will need to adopt a cohesive, consistent and influential position. All disciplines will be represented, provide structured and informative feedback and, where appropriate, be prepared to endorse team decisions.

Case-management review system

The unit requires a space or place whereby the team can reflect on patient care and progress. Particularly in the PICU, where rapid turnover of the patient group may occur, it can often be difficult to spend lengthy amounts of time discussing each individual. The team will have to balance the need to review acute symptom management, whilst maintaining a focus on future options. It is easy to become reactive rather than pro-active. This indicates the need for an efficient review system which allows for team discussion and patient involvement. A system which allows for monthly reviews of patient care (if longer term care is occurring) whilst enabling weekly management can help. The reviews concentrate on history, progress, risk management and discharge planning, whilst the weekly management meeting concentrates on day-to-day risk, care plan and leave issues.

Empowerment of nursing via assessment and decision-making schemes

There should be weekly summaries of patient progress, and wherever possible pre-admission nursing assessments, thus primary nurse responsibility is supported and respected by effective delegation, with MDT responsiveness.

Effective multi- and interdisciplinary working

The care team needs to be able to agree on risk assessment factors and communicate this to the patient, relatives and professionals such as social workers, probation officers, GPs, the community psychiatric nurse, and other members of community teams.

Regular attendance from any or all of the above at case reviews and discharge meetings will greatly enhance the consistency and effectiveness of follow-up treatment.

Evidence-based practice and research

The care team must ensure that their practice is based upon contemporary research and is subject to clinical audit. The audit process has to be viewed in the wider context of Clinical Governance set out in The New NHS (Department of Health 1997) and A First Class Service: Quality in the New NHS (Department of Health 1998), whilst taking into account the needs of the local service. This is very important in order to ensure that high-quality care is delivered, and the unit strives toward being a 'centre of excellence' whilst meeting the needs of its patients and staff.

To focus on incident monitoring, use of seclusion, restraint and staff sickness will give a picture of the current atmosphere within the environment, but will only be of use if this is looked at within the wider context of staff recruitment and retention, induction, professional development and job satisfaction, whilst evaluating ward milieu, patient resources and patient satisfaction.

The nature of the patients cared for by PICUs and LSUs suggests that key areas of research could be the use of seclusion, control and restraint, rapid tranquillisation and the variables of race, gender and time of day of incidents. All incidents, or reports of 'near miss' incidents, that occur in the unit should be routinely analysed on a quarterly basis. This will start to build up a picture of where flash point areas occur and will enable ward managers to prioritise resources and target educational areas.

Education and training plan

It is important that education and training focus upon the needs of the patient group which, by definition, will also meet staff needs. When planning training sessions, thought must be given to the symptoms experienced by patients, both as a result of their illness and their treatment (side-effects). Evidence-based interventions and sociological issues such as lifestyle and coping responses should be included. The training approach needs to be responsive to issues not often experienced or particular diagnoses that staff do not work with regularly. In this way the unit can provide training that enables the staff to do their job better, feel that they are supported by their organisation in what they do and demonstrate the same sensitive and responsive approach to its staff training needs as it hopes to do with its patient group. The use of a Personal Development Review will assist in identifying the training needs of the staff group as well as of individuals.

Wherever possible training should be interdisciplinary in order to share and amalgamate different experiences and skills. In fostering reflective practice, significant carers can be encouraged to present case reviews with the team, to encourage appraisal of care and promote good practice.

As educational needs are manifold, it is useful to attempt to systematise the service's response to its need. It is important that the unit manager is clear and supportive about its approach to education.

Risk assessment

This will need to reflect the type and nature of admissions, be realistic as to what can be achieved and encourage the development of a format in which information can be managed effectively.

Risk management

Linking risk assessment material into the latest care planning and Care Programme Approach (CPA) (Department of Health 1999b) documentation will enable the MDT to look at the patient in a dynamic and objective way thus enabling a care management approach which can be pro-active and responsive to individual needs.

Staff inter-personal skills

Training opportunities which offer the team the opportunity to role-play symptom experience, and

understand and use effective and appropriate communication skills, whilst enabling the sharing of experiences, feelings and responses, can enable a team to develop into a more coherent unit, which will have a positive impact on the quality of care delivery. Courses such as the Association of Psychological Therapies (APT) workshops on the 'Reinforcing Appropriate, Ignoring Difficult Behaviour (RAID)' system for working with Challenging Behaviour or: 'How Not to Get Hit – Preventing Face to Face Violence' can be of great use to team confidence and their sense of cohesion.

Management of violence and aggression

The ability to deal with face-to-face issues and de-escalation techniques is just as important as an understanding of the theoretical origins of violence and aggression. Also, the ability to appreciate the use of a therapeutic milieu and the impact of the structure and environment upon the ward's atmosphere will greatly enhance the team's attitude to the workplace and influence the unit positively (Royal College of Psychiatrists 1998). The Mental Health Policy Implementation Guide: Developing Positive Practice to Support the Safe and Therapeutic Management of Aggression and Violence in Mental Health In-patient Settings (NIMHE 2004) provides an excellent framework for creating a positive culture and policy approach to the therapeutic management of violence and aggression.

Breakaway techniques/control and restraint/care and responsibility

The approach to physical restraint and containment is a difficult area which generates more discussion than there is room for here. The PICU/LSU will need to establish an approach that is mindful of its patients' needs and rights, whilst offering the staff group some autonomy and control over their environment. A training strategy that empowers its staff group to approach potentially dangerous situations in a positive and confident manner is less likely to rely upon the use of seclusion and restraint. Enabling the staff to utilise breakaway techniques and control and restraint techniques will remain viable only whilst adequate refresher training and staff resources are present. However, a cohesive and robust attitude to this area will inevitably produce a team that is comfortable in its abilities whilst prepared to reflect upon its actions. This can lead to a positive approach to the treatment of a potentially difficult patient group.

Furthermore the unit needs to have strategies in place to ensure that its staff are 'culturally' competent through reflecting the equality and diversity issues highlighted by the Independent Inquiry into the Death of David Bennett (Norfolk, Suffolk and Cambridgeshire SHA 2003).

Team building

Although often not cheap, team building and empowerment training can contribute to a team's sense of identity, purpose and cohesiveness. Team empowerment training or away days can offer value for money if set in the context of a wider strategy.

Individual, group and family work

Concentrating on providing a broad but basic level of understanding in the above areas, linked to a treatment philosophy encompassing the same, can provide and maintain effective staff interventions. The team will often be balancing the roles of care-giver and custodian. Having confidence to provide information with a preparedness to listen to concerns and issues from patients and their relatives, linked to a clear treatment goal, can enable the staff group to convey warmth and understanding, whilst feeling in control.

Advocacy and empowerment

Advocacy and empowerment are areas recognised as essential to the feeling of involvement (Sang 1999) and a sense of being listened to, that will assist greatly in the patient's recovery. Empowerment can allow the patient access to information about their rights and treatment and can facilitate the patient to have a degree of control over treatment received.

Advocacy can enable users of services to influence practice and give the patients a voice that can be heard, to support them through difficult times. The issue of advocacy and nursing is stated in the UKCC guidelines (1999) as follows:

5. Work in an open and co-operative manner with patients, clients and their families, foster their independence and recognise and respect their involvement in the planning and delivery of care.

This is not often as straightforward when applied to PICU/LSU nursing. Given the increasing likelihood that some patients detained under the Mental Health Act (Department of Health and the Welsh Office 1983) will have used illegal substances, often in an attempt at self-medication prior to admission, issues of confidentiality may make nurses experience an apparent conflict between policies and guidelines on the one hand and the patient's best interests on the other, making it difficult for them to remain objective or independent at times.

Exploration, training and reflection will be essential if the nurses are able to pick up on the nuances and subtleties of advocating for this patient.

Formal advocacy may well be served better when provided by outside agencies who are seen as separate from the local service structure, such as MIND groups or the National Schizophrenia Fellowship. The PICU would do well to encourage and invite such groups into its organisation to agree local protocols and assist in improving access and feedback.

The development of Patient Advocacy Liaison Services (PALS) within mental health and learning disabilities services has created a direct link with patient experience and organisational response, creating a closer and more responsive relationship between the provider and user of services.

Mental Health Act

With the increased use of both the civil and the criminal parts of the Mental Health Act, the PICU/LSU will require a comprehensive package of Mental Health Act and Code of Practice (Department of Health 1999c) training to enable its staff to be confident

Table 23.4. Summarising a training approach

Safety and security	Therapeutic intervention	Patient empowerment	Legislation and statutory requirement
Team empowerment	Individual work	Advocacy	Mental Health Act
Risk assessment	Group work	Empowerment	Health and safety
Care and responsibility training	KGV symptom scale assessment	Daily living skills	Fire evacuation training
Use of environment and structure	Inter-personal skills	Motivational interviewing	Control of Substances Hazardous to Health (COSHH)
Induction	Family work	Compliance therapy	Cardiopulmonary resuscitation (CPR)
Management of violence and aggression	High-dose neuroleptic usage	Relapse prevention	First aid
Risk management	Atypical anti-psychotics	Substance misuse	Care Programme Approach (CPA)
Breakaway	Early warning signs Cognitive symptom intervention		Mental health law
Relevant further and higher education			

and competent in these areas. In increasing the staff's confidence the service will enable the team to spend more time concentrating their efforts on assessing and nursing the needs of their patients.

NB The Mental Health Bill (UK Parliament 2007) is proposing changes to the existing Act making recommendations to utilise the advantages of the community treatment aspects of restriction orders across a wider spectrum and these proposals will need to be kept under review. A more detailed discussion of the implications for nursing practice can be found in Ashmore and Carver (2000).

High-dose neuroleptics, emergency medication management and atypical antipsychotics

Input from pharmacy staff on the increasing developments and changes relating to psychopharmacological treatments will enable the team to offer the most effective and appropriate treatment regimes, enhancing the quality of patient care and creating positive experiences for staff and patients.

Evidence-based interventions

Access to medication management training, early warning signs, cognitive interventions for schizophrenia (Wykes *et al.* 1998), relapse prevention (Marlatt and Gordon 1985), motivational interviewing (Miller and Rollnick 1991), compliance therapy (Kemp *et al.* 1997), KGV symptom scale assessment (Krawiecka *et al.* 1977) and the social functioning scale (Birchwood *et al.* 1990), amongst others, will enable the staff to gain a better understanding of symptomatology, to choose more effective interventions and disseminate them throughout the team.

Since the first edition of this book the National Institute for Health and Clinical Excellence (NICE; www.nice.org.uk) has produced a number of clinical guidelines which should become part of any treatment approach. They include guidance on acutely disturbed behaviour, eating disorders, schizophrenia and self-harm.

Formal training

The organisation will need to maintain strong links with its healthcare training provider or local nurse training university, to ensure that the education provided remains appropriate to the context of the healthcare area and provides practitioners who are best equipped to deal with the demands of the day. The unit service should endeavour to offer its experience and involve itself in the provision of training.

The Thorn courses for psychosocial interventions, cognitive-behavioural therapy and medication management are courses of particular relevance.

It is important for the service to remain aware of the skill and experience mix of its staff group and, whenever possible, utilise them as a training resource to develop any areas of team inexperience. This will enable the core staff group to influence and facilitate improvements in the quality of care given.

Of course the staff group will not be able to cover all areas and resource management will be an ongoing issue in the prioritisation of training needs, but the use of a focused approach can aid management. It is important that the service remains aware of the skill and experience mix of its staff group and utilises them as a training resource to develop areas of inexperience, whilst empowering its core staff group to influence the quality of care given.

To aid recruitment and retention of staff the service should ensure that the staffing budget has taken into account sufficient provision to enable staff to undertake further education and training at a local or higher level from education providers to enhance skills, confidence and understanding.

Staff support

In an environment that is turbulent, constantly changing and very stressful, there is a clear need for structures that offer staff support and the opportunity for staff to explore their practice (Minghella

and Benson 1994). These structures can take various forms: they can be informal or formal, but there must be a forum that all staff recognise as being consistent and safe in which they can express their views. The role of the manager is to ensure that these meetings take place and to encourage as many staff as possible to attend. There will be occasions when the manager and members of the multi-professional management team should attend and be part of the team, but there will also be times when the rest of the team needs space away from 'management'.

One of the most useful and difficult to achieve skills of a manager is knowing when to attend and when to allow space. This facilitates the balance between a supportive manager and an overcontrolling one. The unit itself and how it is allied to the needs and dynamics within the staff group will affect whether the manager should be present or not. There are no hard and fast rules. Perhaps one of the best ways of getting it right as often as possible is to make a habit of asking the staff group what their expectations of you, as the manager, are. If these expectations are unreal, this should be gently highlighted to the staff group and then the whole team can explore and identify more realistic expectations. These should be achievable and will not then lead to the staff team feeling let down by the manager, or to the manager feeling frustrated or having let down the team.

Some mechanisms for staff support are detailed below.

Induction and mentoring

This is vital for all new staff. PICUs and LSUs can be alarming places on first contact; it has already been stated that there is a need for consistency. The process of induction and mentoring will enhance this, as well as providing support for new staff in the environment. It is useful to have a formal record of the induction process, to which the individual can refer to and which can be tailored according to the individual's need based on their experience, grade, skills and competencies.

The role of mentor or preceptor for newly qualified staff is a very meaningful one and it is vitally important that the person assuming the role is equipped to do so, and elects to assume such a role, rather than having it thrust upon them. Support and ancillary staff also need support, structure and induction.

Reflective practice

All staff should be encouraged to maintain their professional portfolio to enable them to reflect upon their practice (Palmer *et al.* 1994).

Shift meetings

The author believes that every nursing shift should have a space set aside for a shift meeting. This should be at the same time each day, for each shift. All staff on duty, from all disciplines, should attend, and the patients should be informed that staff are not available for this period. The content of the meeting is informal and should concentrate on the business of the day, but will inevitably allow staff to reflect on recent incidents and the strategies employed to deal with them. It will also allow a space for ventilation of feelings about current patients and their behaviour, which will assist the staff in going back to face the patients again, and engage in therapeutic interactions.

Facilitated staff group

Where possible, the unit should employ an outside facilitator, brought in on a monthly basis, to chair an open session for staff. This is designed to allow staff the opportunity to explore current issues that may be causing division in the care team.

The facilitator may have a psycho-dynamic or psycho-therapeutic background and no clinical experience of the environment. A different strategy would be to employ a clinician with relevant experience who could act as advisor and reflect on the team's practice from an objective perspective.

Both these options have relative merits and disadvantages, but the crucial point is that an outsider comes into the staff group on a regular basis and

assists with some of the criticisms of insularity and isolationist practice that may be levelled against staff.

Team building

For a newly developed unit with a brand new team this is an imperative. However, even well-established teams can benefit from space away from the unit, facilitated by a team-building expert to assist them in examining how they function as a team.

Clinical supervision

The issue of clinical supervision is of great importance to all staff who are involved in the day-to-day care of patients. It is particularly important in areas of high stress where patients may be difficult to treat, such as the PICU/LSU. Various models for clinical supervision have been proposed (Butterworth *et al.* 1998); the chosen model should reflect the views and wishes of the majority of staff. With a relatively small staff, there is merit in debating whether the clinical supervision should be offered by external staff. This allows for free expression thus not allowing staff to feel inhibited by talking to their work colleagues. The suitability of the supervisor is important as this prevents the potential clash with the annual staff appraisal. The operative phrase here is 'suitability' of the supervisor. It should be possible to make a reciprocal arrangement with another local team. Even if they work in another specialised field, e.g. elderly care, they may be able to offer a useful focus to the PICU team members.

Post-incidents debrief and support

The link between untoward incidents and incidence of staff sickness and absence is well documented, allied with the increasing recognition of post-traumatic stress disorder (PTSD) amongst healthcare staff. This indicates that a strategy for dealing with serious incidents in a structured way may be advantageous (Chapter 11 in Wykes 1994).

The strategy for this must include some or all of the following:

- Immediate post-incident debrief for all staff involved, facilitated by a senior clinician who was not directly involved.
- Immediate debrief for patients and opportunity to discuss their concerns.
- Structured post-incident debrief within 3 days for all staff involved. This is from two clinicians who are not from the PICU/LSU, and who have skills in such work.
- Individual sessions, fixed term for staff most closely involved or who request such input. This is again from an outside clinician and is totally confidential.
- Access to a confidential, independent counselling service.

Stress busters

The trust/hospital may wish to consider offering an activity for the staff group that will assist in reducing stress, e.g. discounted local gym membership or a similar approach that has been identified as beneficial by the staff group.

Annual appraisal and review

Every employee should have an appraisal at least annually. This should, if possible, be a self-appraisal and should focus on identifying practice deficits and developing a training package to overcome these. Annual appraisal or personal development will enable the manager and his or her staff to have face-to-face dialogue and identify a training plan.

Audit of strategies

The manager of the unit should ensure that there are in place methods of auditing the quality of care given to patients and the quality of staff support available in the unit. To audit care effectively, it is important to have a clear structure and purpose for the unit, with particular areas of demarcation mapped out. It is then straightforward to audit against them. Any subsequent changes can be measured against initial results, demonstrating whether a change has pro-

duced a positive or negative result. The use of staff and patient satisfaction questionnaires should be used widely and also a system set up whereby cross-audit occurs, e.g. one unit auditing another along agreed criteria, to enable comparison and the sharing of knowledge. Methods for evaluating the quality of staff support should include confidential leaving questionnaires for staff who resign. An analysis of numbers of leavers, as a proportion of the staffing establishment, is a useful measure. Areas such as PICUs and LSUs do have a high staff turnover, and in order to continually develop the unit's needs, new staff will always be required. However, there should be a balance in turnover and stability to ensure consistency. Recruitment to PICU/LSUs can be difficult and a high level of staff vacancies can lead to escalating stress, and increasing sickness. Staff satisfaction questionnaires that are anonymous and administered by an outside agency can be a useful gauge of that nebulous but so important entity staff morale. The canvassing of existing staff on education and training issues, service structures and local decisions can also increase staff well being.

Staff–patient ratios

Although there are no nationally agreed criteria for unit staffing and there are different ways of providing psychiatric intensive/low secure care, certain common sense rules need to be applied. Whether provided within the acute psychiatric unit or in a purpose-built unit, practicalities of staff and patient safety should remain high on the agenda.

The Mental Health Policy Implementation Guide: Adult Acute Inpatient Care Provision (Department of Health 2002c) states:

5.3.2 Quality care is dependent on effective relationships not only with service users but also between staff. There needs to be a stable and consistent inpatient ward team, staffed to accommodate the needs for structured therapeutic service user engagement, staff training, supervision and practice development in addition to the more formal or routine duties of ward staff. Indeed there is evidence from some services that staffing levels incorporating structured engagement and practice development can considerably diminish the use of bank and agency staff, improve morale, recruitment and retention of staff and be more acceptable to users.

5.3.8 We do not make specific recommendations on the nursing establishment required for an inpatient ward. There is no simple formula for calculating the nursing and multidisciplinary staffing requirement. This is influenced by a number of complex factors, such as ward size, the configuration of local services, existing staff skills, the availability of support. Needs are not static and are subject to local variation. The work of Acute Care Forums and collaborative development networks will identify appropriate staffing establishment benchmarks as an early priority in implementing this guidance.

5.3.9 While we are not in a position to recommend any specific staffing establishment requirements it is clear from the evidence and feedback from service users and staff that many of our inpatient wards do not have appropriate staffing levels with the skills required to achieve the necessary standards of care. Commissioners of inpatient services will need to review current establishments, informed by benchmarking exercises, and in many cases will need to direct significant extra investment into inpatient services, staffing and training to overcome current serious service deficits.

It is clear from the above guidance that units are empowered to identify local service requirements and put in place an effective but flexible structure consistent with the changing demands of PICUs and LSUs.

Conclusion

Obviously many of the proposals outlined in this chapter have a cost implication, but they should not be discounted for this reason. In the long run, many of the strategies proposed can be cost saving. For the PICU/LSU to maintain standards of care to some of the patients most in need of this care, a modern, well-trained and supported workforce with positive attitudes and an open-minded approach to their work can do much to work towards the high quality of care that these patients require.

Useful information

The National Institute for Mental Health in England
Blenheim House
West One
Duncombe Street
Leeds LS1 4PL
www.nimhe.org.uk

The National Institute for Health and Clinical Excellence
www.nice.org.uk

The Association for Psychological Therapies
APT
PO Box 3
Thurnby
Leicester LE7 9QN
UK
Tel: 0116 241 9934
www.apt.co.uk

MIND
Tel: 0345 660 123
web: www.mind.org.uk

National Schizophrenia Fellowship
Tel: 0207 330 9100
web: www.nsf.org.uk

Acknowledgements

Thanks to Debbie Coleman for her valuable contributions to the chapter in the first edition of this book.

REFERENCES

Ashmore R, Carver N. 2000 Mental Health Practice (Feb) 3 (6)
Baxter P, Cutliffe J. 1999 Mental Health Practice (May) 2 (8)
Birchwood M, Smith J, Cochrane R, Wetton S, Copestake S. 1990 The social functioning scale. Br J Psychiatry 157: 853–859

Butterworth T, Faugier J, Burnard P. 1998 Clinical supervision and mentorship in nursing, 2nd edn. Cheltenham: Stanley Thornes

Conlan L, Gage A, Hillis T. 1997 Managerial and nursing perspectives on the response to inpatient violence, 7. In: Crichton J (ed) Psychiatric Patient Violence: Risk and Response. London: Duckworth

Department of Health. 1997 The New NHS: Modern, Dependable. London: HMSO

Department of Health. 1998 A First Class Service: Quality in the New NHS. London: HMSO

Department of Health. 1999a National Service Frameworks. Mental Health. Modern Standards and Service models. London: Department of Health

Department of Health. 1999b Effective Care Co-ordination in Mental Health Services: Modernising the Care Programme Approach – A Policy Booklet. London: HMSO

Department of Health. 1999c Mental Health Act 1983: Code of Practice. London: HMSO

Department of Health. 2002a Mental Health Policy Implementation Guide: Adult Acute Inpatient Care Provision. London: Department of Health

Department of Health. 2002b Womens Mental Health: Into the Mainstream. London: HMSO

Department of Health and the Welsh Office. 1983 Mental Health Act 1983. London: HMSO

Kemp P, Hayward P, David A. 1997 Compliance Therapy Manual. London: Institute of Psychiatry

Krawiecka M, Goldberg D, Vaughan M. 1977 A standardised psychiatric assessment scale for rating chronic psychotic patients. Acta Psychol Scand 55: 299–308

Lowe T. 1992 Characteristics of effective nursing interventions in the management of challenging behaviour. J Adv Nurs 17: 1226–1230

Marlatt GA, Gordon RG. 1985 Relapse Prevention. London: Guilford Press

Miller WR, Rollnick S. 1991 Motivational Interviewing: Preparing People to Change Addictive Behaviours. London: Guilford Press

Minghella E, Benson A. 1994 Developing reflective practice in mental health nursing through critical incident analysis. J Adv Nurs 21: 205–213

NIMHE. 2004 Mental Health Policy Implementation Guide: Developing Positive Practice to Support the Safe and Therapeutic Management of Aggression and Violence in Mental Health In-patient Settings. Leeds: NIMHE

Norfolk, Suffolk and Cambridgeshire Strategic Health Authority. 2003 Independent Inquiry into the Death of David Bennett. Cambridge: Norfolk, Suffolk and Cambridgeshire Strategic Health Authority

Palmer A, Burns S, Bulman C. 1994 Reflective practice in nursing. Oxford: Blackwell Science

Pereira SM, Clinton C. 2002 Mental Health Policy Implementation Guide: National Minimum Standards for General Adult Services in Psychiatric Intensive Care Units and Low Secure Environments. London: Department of Health

Royal College of Psychiatrists. 1998 Management of Imminent Violence. Occasional paper OP 41. London: Royal College of Psychiatrists

Sang B. 1999 Service user movement. The customer is sometimes right. Health Serv J 109: 22–23

SNMAC Standing Nursing and Midwifery Advisory Committee. 1999a Addressing acute concerns – report by the Standing Nursing and Midwifery Advisory Committee. London: Standing Nursing and Midwifery Advisory Committee

SNMAC Standing Nursing and Midwifery Advisory Committee. 1999b Safe and supportive observation of patients at risk. London: Standing Nursing and Midwifery Advisory Committee

UK Parliament. 1998 The Human Rights Act 1998. London: The Stationery Office

UK Parliament. 2007 Mental Health Bill. London: The Stationery Office

UKCC. 1999 Nursing in Secure Environments: Summary and Action Plan from a Scoping Study. London: United Kingdom Central Council for Nursing, Midwifery and Health Visiting

Wykes T. 1994 Violence and Health Care Professionals. London: Chapman and Hall

Wykes T, Tarrier N, Lewis S. 1998 Outcome and Innovation in Psychological Treatment of Schizophrenia. New York: Wiley

24

Multidisciplinary teams within PICUs/LSUs

Andy Johnston and Stephen Dye

Introduction

Multiprofessional working is essential within health care environments. Successive legislation in the UK (Department of Health and Social Security 1977; Department of Health 1990, 1999, 2000, 2001) and, more significantly for the purposes of this book, the National Minimum Standards for Psychiatric Intensive Care (Department of Health 2002) have attempted to outline methods of both implementing and positively running these interactions. Despite this, the development of high-quality and well functioning teams remains a continuing goal.

This chapter outlines the developmental history of the multidisciplinary team (MDT) principle within the UK, discusses some potential problems, elaborates on what makes a successful team and why working within a truly MDT is beneficial within a Psychiatric Intensive Care/Low Secure Unit (PICU/LSU). It also describes roles within the team and finally how teams can remain effective.

Definition of a multidisciplinary team

Mohrman *et al.* (1995) define a team as, 'a group of individuals who work together to produce products or deliver services for which they are mutually accountable. Team members share goals and are mutually held accountable for meeting them, they are interdependent in their accomplishment, and they affect the results through their interactions with one another. Because the team is held collectively accountable, the work of integrating with one another is included among the responsibilities of each member'.

There is no one definition of an MDT and formal definitions in the wider literature do not accurately describe those recognised as mental health teams. Ovretveit (1995) argued that, 'a multidisciplinary team without differences is a contradiction in terms' and defined multidisciplinary mental health teams as 'a group of practitioners with different professional training, employed by more than one agency, who meet regularly to coordinate their work providing services to one or more clients in a defined area' (Ovretveit 1993 p. 9), whereas Opie (1997) regards this as merely *interdisciplinary* teamworking. Perhaps it is best to examine Onyett *et al.*'s (1994) statement '. . . actual features of the organisation and operation of mental health teams appear not to lend themselves to meaningful categorisation when you look at what they *actually* do, rather than what they *aim* to do'. He argues (2003 p. 4) that one should use a rather permissive definition of mental health teams but to, 'remain aware that in order to achieve specific outcomes, teams will need to be tightly defined, designed and managed'.

The medical profession has traditionally dominated the care of mentally unwell individuals. This may have been because much of the care was provided within institutional settings run by doctors.

Psychiatric Intensive Care, 2nd edn., eds. M. Dominic Beer, Stephen M. Pereira and Carol Paton.
Published by Cambridge University Press. © Cambridge University Press 2008

Psychiatric hospitals are no longer run by psychiatrists supported by 'attendants' and part-time voluntary 'lay almoners'. However, simple proliferation of different types of staff does not necessarily bring cooperation or team work. Different ways of interdisciplinary working have developed, ranging from those led by consultants in ward rounds (in which the main decisions of patient care are made) to those that make fully developed MDT decisions with regular meetings, have a degree of role blurring and shared responsibility. We will advocate that, in a PICU/LSU environment, a multidisciplinary-led service with shared goals agreed by a team is an option that can be successful.

History

In 1965, when Enoch Powell (the then Minister of State for Health) gave a speech signalling the intention to close the old 'watertower' asylums, he was also signalling the advent of community multidisciplinary teams as we know them today. Indeed, history has shown that, in psychiatry, the principle and practice of multidisciplinary working has tended to emanate from community settings, whereas hospital care has continued to be provided in an interdisciplinary fashion based upon a medical model. As PICU/LSU are relatively recent sub-specialities, they are ideally placed to provide high-quality patient care in a multidisciplinary fashion within an inpatient environment, building upon the experience gained from community MDT working. Thus it is essential that the developmental history of community mental health teams (CMHTs) and lessons learnt about multidisciplinary working are examined.

Ten years after the 'watertowers' speech, the components of a comprehensive, integrated mental health service were specified for the first time in the white paper 'Better Services for the Mentally Ill' (Department of Health 1975). This placed emphasis on provision of a comprehensive range of local services rather than closure of asylums (making reference that these should not shut until appropriate local services had been developed). The policy was

exceptionally hazy about timescales and this was borne out in practice: despite a extensive decrease in the number of 'asylum' inpatients and a change in the nature of services, by 1986 the closure score of asylums was one.

The trend of community-based interventions continued; in 1981 the green paper 'Care in the Community' (Department of Health and Social Security 1981) began by saying, 'Most people who need long term care can and should be looked after in the community. That is what most of them want for themselves and what those responsible for their care believe to be best'. The development of this type of system inevitably meant an increase of staff (and of different professional types) based in community settings. This entailed communication between staff and interdisciplinary working.

In 1988, the Spokes Report into the care and treatment of Sharon Campbell (Department of Health and Social Security 1988) recommended that health and local authorities should have joint responsibility for the aftercare and follow-up of hospital patients and that this included regular multidisciplinary review meetings. The case provoked a media campaign that castigated community care and the inquiry could be considered to be the initiation of the Care Programme Approach (a system of care delivery relevant to the care and support of people with mental health difficulties). One of the confusions surrounding the Care Programme Approach was the uncertainty between social care agencies and health care agencies regarding the difference between it and case management: both shared the same core tasks and were concerned with coordinated assessment of health and social care needs. This uncertainty was addressed in 1995 (Department of Health 1995) with the document 'Building Bridges', which elaborated the need for multidisciplinary and interagency working and remarked, 'For people subject to the CPA, in essence the key worker and care management functions are the same'.

In 1997, the Sainsbury Centre produced a report entitled 'Pulling Together' (Sainsbury Centre for Mental Health 1997). This recognised that staff should be ready to work in multidisciplinary teams but that available training did not reflect the services to be provided. In the foreword, Rabbi Julia Neuberger stated, 'We feel strongly that narrow sectional interests have to be abandoned to make the system work'. At the same time, the report encouraged teams to, 'value the diversity of professions and that developments should take place within existing professional frameworks'. To some, these two statements may seem contradictory and acceptance of the philosophy encompassing both statements has been one of the difficulties in establishing fully functional multidisciplinary team working.

The National Service Framework (Department of Health 1999) emphasised that the quality of assessment of individuals with severe and enduring mental health difficulties is enhanced when undertaken jointly by members from a health and social care background. We would go further by suggesting that it is improved when performed by members from different professional backgrounds per se and that in PICUs/LSUs this should be the norm.

With the advent of assertive outreach *teams*, crisis resolution *teams* as well as early intervention *teams*, multidisciplinary working seems to be here to stay and thus it is imperative that it works well. Both the history of development of CMHTs and the lessons learnt provide an ideal opportunity to study the components of a successful MDT within PICU/LSU. It is our opinion that PICUs/LSUs are in an ideal position to fully develop team-working processes given that they deal with such a specific patient group and have dedicated staff of different disciplines.

Criticism

Some critics have stated that MDTs are by their very nature and historical roots an ineffective and unproductive way to deliver services: 'At the planning stage the "need" for community MDTs is usually assumed rather than argued in a coherent way . . . [it is] driven by ideology rather than evidence of effectiveness' (Galvin and McCarthy 1994). Watson (1994) stated that, 'cooperative working is not something that can be achieved by legislation alone and it has rarely been

totally achieved in practice', but why is that? The relationship between ideology and reality needs to be examined.

The closure of large institutions was not arrived at by means of evaluative studies or by careful examination of community needs, but simply because it seemed reasonable and attractive from several points of view and because it had an obviously humane feel about it. The same lack of evaluation before being put into practice appears to have applied to working in MDTs. Perhaps this was understandable since community working necessitated not only more staff but also an increased variety of more highly trained staff and thus development of interdisciplinary working was an inevitable consequence.

Community mental health teams were conceived because of apparent benefits in achieving community care (Couchmann 1995; Chalk 1999; Gibb *et al.* 2002). These included multidisciplinary assessment and case allocation according to need as well as integrated, multidisciplinary care and access to a wide range of skills. Theoretically there were also benefits of skill sharing, support and good staff morale. However, the majority of research highlights problems within CMHTs including ambiguous roles and responsibilities, and general problems with interagency and multidisciplinary working (Lucas 1996). These result in communication difficulties, leadership conflict as well as poor team management.

Norman and Peck (1999) have proposed four main reasons for poor inter-professional working: loss of faith in the system within which practitioners work, strong adherence to uni-professional cultures, absence of a strong and shared philosophy and mistrust of managerial solutions. They also provided ways to improve MDT working which included clarifying accountability and responsibility, and also ways to draw upon theory to help understand team effectiveness, role clarification and to enhance role relations (Peck and Norman 1999). Roles and responsibilities of mental health staff are integral to the professional persona and are likely to be defended vigorously. Professionals can seek to distinguish their roles which may result in inflexible boundaries and disputes about areas of practice and to mistrust within MDTs.

Can it work?

Looking at the roles of teams in organisations generally, Mohrman *et al.* (1995) found that working in teams enabled organisations to rapidly develop and deliver high-quality products and services cost-effectively, allowed the organisation to learn and retain learning more effectively, promoted innovation through the cross-fertilisation of ideas, achieved better integration of information and saved time by having tasks undertaken concurrently.

In a review of teamworking in healthcare teams, Opie (1997), as well as mentioning similar problems to those already described, remarked on advantages that can result. These included development of quality care for patients through the achievement of coordinated and collaborative inputs from different disciplines; improved, better informed and holistic care planning; higher productivity; the development of joint initiatives; increased staff satisfaction and professional stimulation; and, consequently, more effective use of resources.

As part of a larger scale study of healthcare teams in the UK, Borrill *et al.* (2000) examined 113 CMHTs using a stakeholder-derived formulation of effectiveness (Richards and Rees 1998; the stakeholders included patients, carers, advocates, practitioners, policy makers, managers and researchers). She found the teams that worked well together were more effective, more innovative and that effective inter-team communication was associated with better mental health of team members (see Box 24.1).

Box 24.1. Features associated with effectiveness (Borrill *et al.* 2000)

- Clarity of and commitment to objectives
- High levels of participation
- Commitment to quality
- Practical support for innovation
- Fewer part-time workers
- Clear leadership

Box 24.2. Examples of challenges associated with leadership (Onyett 2003)

- Professional autonomy vs accountability to management
- Integrating different disciplines (some of which may be employed by other agencies)
- Achieving effective carer/user involvement in services
- Working with traditional medical leadership roles
- Diversity of skill mix and background amongst team members

The issue of leadership in mental health teams is complex and has many difficulties (Box 24.2) but there seems to be no doubt that clear leadership is essential and this will be discussed further when considering how to form a high-quality team.

Laidler (1994) highlighted the importance of professional respect for successful multi-professional working. The ability to maintain and own profession-specific skills and to develop flexibility around common skills are necessities for coherent teamwork and development of a shared ethos when working with service users. Gibb *et al.* (2002) suggest there are three key processes at work in developing a team's practice: team building, role negotiation and trans-disciplinary decision-making. In addition, many researchers have emphasised that a crucial principle of successful multidisciplinary working is to focus the efforts of the team on only one particular patient group (e.g. Ovretveit 1993; Miller *et al.* 2001). This is a key aspect of work within PICU/LSU and needs to be clear within the operational policy of such a team. It gives both stakeholders and staff a clear notion of the type of individual who will be best served by this specialised service.

From this, the team can develop distinctiveness and have a starting point for resolution of any conflict between team and professional identities. Onyett (2003, p. 119) states, 'The social psychology of groups . . . suggests that the best outcomes will result when practitioners are able to identify both with the team and their own profession. This is more likely to occur when they are clear about the aims of the team *and* their own personal role as a practitioner'. This sits well with the apparently contradictory statements of the Sainsbury Centre mentioned previously and is vital in the successful functioning of a PICU/LSU team.

One further essential component to a successful multidisciplinary team mentioned in the 'Pulling Together' report and by others (e.g. Test and Marks 1990) is the issue of interdisciplinary training. This encourages role expansions rather than 'turf guarding' and arguments over who is responsible. PICUs/LSUs provide an ideal opportunity to develop truly interdisciplinary training programmes that also act as successful team-building exercises.

Developing a team approach within PICU/LSU

Team effectiveness cannot be assumed, teams need to be designed to be effective. To fully embrace a multidisciplinary approach within these teams requires developing and implementing an ethos of shared vision with the teamwork philosophy at its core. Fundamental to this is an understanding and acceptance of the roles and responsibilities of each team member as well as continuous effective communication in order to facilitate collaborative working practice when delivering patient care. Also essential is an effective approach to ensuring that treatment approaches agreed by members of the 'planning component' of the team are translated and understood by members of the 'delivery component'.

Whyte and Brooker (2001) identified that several authors have attempted to create categories of teamwork that may clarify some of the confusion surrounding multidisciplinary teams. For example, Ovretveit (1996) described five dimensions of teamwork (Box 24.3) and suggested that by using each of these dimensions, a team can measure (and therefore promote understanding of) its functioning.

Some problems encountered by MDT members are related to 'role blurring' or 'role overlap'. This can occur when teams are unclear about the differences in professional roles and there exists an overriding ethos that, 'most of the tasks within the team can be carried out equally well by any member of the team'. A shared interdisciplinary understanding of

> **Box 24.3.** Dimensions of teamwork (Ovretveit 1996)
>
> - Degree of integration among professionals
> - Extent to which a team collectively manages resources (according to patient needs or along professional boundaries)
> - Membership issues
> - Processes defining a patient's interactions with the team and how decisions are made
> - Processes by which a team is managed

each other's cultures, working methods, roles and responsibilities promotes collaboration, team effectiveness and cohesion. However, the idea that staff from different disciplines can easily identify different spheres of competence and allocate work accordingly is, perhaps, a naive one.

In terms of clarifying roles, a useful team exercise is for each discipline to describe what knowledge, skills and responsibilities they have specific to their profession and those which are common to other disciplines. Furthermore, each professional group could describe how they see other disciplines' roles within the team. It needs to be emphasised that this should be performed in a method that stresses positive role expectations, as the negative side may lead to statements such as 'he/she is NOT doing this/that' and split the team. Information gained should be used to inform and support a clearer understanding of professional-specific roles and help prevent blurring or unhelpful role overlapping.

Role clarification fits neatly with the recommendations made by the Sainsbury Centre in Pulling Together: that all individuals within a team should share core competencies but some should have specialist capabilities. This was taken further in their publication The 'Capable Practitioner' (Sainsbury Centre for Mental Health 2001) in which a capability framework was illustrated (that outlined skills, knowledge and attitudes required by practitioners) and extended to examine context-specific application within specific service settings.

Harrison (1990) emphasised successful interaction and communication. He suggested that there are only good and bad psychiatric teams and that the qualifications and academic standing of the psychi-atrist (for example) has little relevance if he or she is unable to work with other team members to provide a comprehensive and effective service. Indeed, in their study about MDT decision-making processes, Ford and Farrington (1999) suggested that the MDT decision-making forum was consultant dominated in terms of the amount said and particularly the decisions made. They go on to suggest that if the principles of MDT working are to have any effect, all healthcare professionals should feel comfortable in expressing uncertainty and doubts about such important clinical decisions. We would argue that, in addition, successful MDT working also relies upon 'reflexivity' within the team: West (1996) defined this as, 'the extent to which team members collectively reflect upon the team's objectives, strategies and pro-cesses, as well as the wider organisation and environ-ment, and adapt them accordingly'. The ability of a range of people to develop the reflection and enquiry skills that allow them to talk openly about issues that give rise to conflict without becoming defensive is crucial to an effective and capable team maintaining a high level of function.

Anecdotal evidence would suggest that within psy-chiatric intensive care, team membership turnover may be as high as 40% every two or three years. The ability to define and clarify professional roles, promote greater understanding of expectations and accountability as well as close, appropriate commu-nication and trust between professionals will help to ensure that the team is fluid, has an ability to embrace change, and grow as a result.

Team members' roles and responsibilities

Common responsibilities

In addition to the importance of individual role clar-ification, Michalon and Richman (1990) identified the importance of PICUs themselves developing a clear identity and role. Therefore it is important to ensure that when we consider the roles and respon-sibilities of team members, we also consider their 'common' responsibilities in the context of an agreed

---

Box 24.4. Examples of common team roles/responsibilities

- Input into decision-making
- Engaging with patients
- Communicating information
- Promoting the unit's philosophy
- Induction of new team members
- Development of others
- Supporting relatives/carers
- Accepting referrals
- Referral assessments[a]
- Communicating outcomes of assessments
- Admission protocols
- Care and treatment planning
- Risk assessment
- Progress reviews
- Emergency management of disturbed behaviour

[a] Participation in referral assessments should be a common responsibility (each discipline will bring its own perspective completing a referral assessment thus enabling a more thorough, rounded and complete assessment).

---

service operational policy (shared vision). Within a PICU MDT, the *shared focus* is caring for patients who are usually experiencing the most acute phase of their illness.

It is fair to suggest that, irrespective of discipline or professional background, we all wish to deliver good-quality, evidenced-based care and treatment to our patients. The complexities of this are vast and incorporate team members using professional-specific skills, knowledge and experience. In identi-fying common roles and responsibilities, we should consider the tasks of the team (for examples see Box 24.4).

Professional-specific responsibilities

When considering 'professional-specific' roles it is important to gain an overview of the wider context. In this, we refer to the way in which legal limita-tions, professional codes of practice and employ-ment contracts can assist or hinder the team or organisation's views and their work. For example, a consultant psychiatrist may have a contractual obligation to oversee and coordinate patient care. However, nowhere is it stated in any legal or national framework that a consultant is accountable for the practice of a qualified individual from another professional discipline (Ovretveit 1993). In much the same way, a unit manager may carry 24-hour responsibility, but he/she is not accountable for others' individual practice.

Certain responsibilities are clearly professional specific and cannot be carried out by qualified individuals from other professions. It is important to identify these when reviewing a team's function. For example, medical staff have professional-specific powers under the Mental Health Act, as do social workers (ASWs) and nurses. In relation to the prescribing of medication, this is generally a medical/doctor-specific responsibility, though nurse prescribing of certain drugs is legislated for and operational in some areas. A doctor is professionally responsible for diagnosing a patient using recognised criteria, however the information required in making a diagnosis may be provided by many other disciplines. A nurse may provide preceptorship or mentorship to a student or junior colleague, though the individual's learning supports professional growth and the team as a whole.

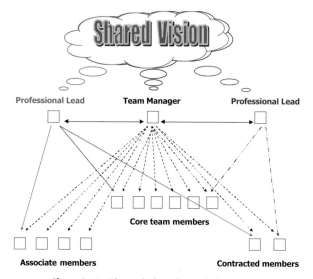

Figure 24.1. The multidisciplinary-led team

Team roles

Team leadership/management

Many problems that teams face are as a result of ineffectual leadership or ill-defined responsibility, accountability and authority of the 'leader'. The importance of clarifying the roles and responsibilities of the team leader should not be underestimated. Within PICU/LSUs, teams tend to be either medically led or nurse led. Few fully embrace multidisciplinary leadership in their approach to treatment, care delivery and service development, or consider how this could work given the limitations of most 'management or professional structures'. We would argue that leadership within the team could and should perhaps be jointly provided by the senior members of the team. To be led in a multidisciplinary fashion with leaders fully signed up to a joint ethos of care potentially provides greater clarity for team members and helps provide a collective sense of ownership within the team. For this to succeed, extremely clear profession specific and operational-specific roles within the team's senior members are needed, e.g. management role versus consultant role versus lead nurse role.

It is not necessary or even appropriate for the leader to formally manage individuals from other disciplines. Whether a service MDT is led by a consultant psychiatrist or a senior nurse is immaterial, the important aspect is clarity of leadership and the qualities it brings. We are a long way off formal multi-professional appraisals, though team and service objective setting is a useful way forward in promoting team development and responsibility. The role of the leader is one of facilitating team cooperation/collaboration and achieving the best outcomes from combined efforts.

Responsibilities allied to this role are ensuring that the team is functioning according to operational/service policy, organising and coordinating team members' contribution to the care and treatment of the patient group and maintaining an overview of clinical service delivery to ensure patient and team needs are met. Figure 24.1 demonstrates how this might be achieved: the core team members (for example nurses, unit dedicated occupational

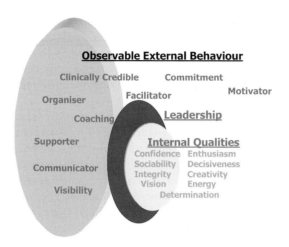

Observable External Behaviour

Clinically Credible   Commitment

Organiser   Facilitator   Motivator

Coaching   **Leadership**

Supporter   **Internal Qualities**

Communicator   Confidence   Enthusiasm
Sociability   Decisiveness
Integrity   Creativity
Visibility   Vision   Energy
Determination

Figure 24.2. Leadership qualities diagram

therapists, healthcare assistants, other therapists, administrators and technical instructors) being directly managed by the team manager although professional leadership is also essential. Associate team members may include junior doctors, psychology assistants and social workers. The time contributed by, and clinical input of, these individuals would be coordinated and supported by the manager; however, issues relating to professional practice and performance, once identified, would then be addressed via professional leads. Whilst each member is accountable to the manager in terms of adhering to team policy and ensuring that agreed time and function are being provided, each retains clinical responsibility for their own work, supervised by their professional heads. The manager therefore coordinates the functions/tasks of the associate members.

Examples of contracted team members are: pharmacists, sessional therapists, project workers or domestic staff. This group are contracted to serve on the team on a part-time basis. Having a team manager does not mean that practitioners lose their autonomy. On the contrary, an effective team manager will encourage individual autonomy within the shared framework and focus of the team.

Leaders and managers require strong leadership skills to influence others and facilitate change (Figure 24.2). The manner in which they conduct this can be observed in external behaviour and is driven by internal qualities. Effective leaders are clear and straightforward in their interactions with others and demonstrate predictable consistency when dealing with the performance of others.

Role of the psychiatrist

A multidisciplinary approach requires that the psychiatrist functions as a team member and shares overall clinical responsibility with the team manager for monitoring patient treatment and staff delivery of clinical services. In real terms he/she is the organiser of the overall medical care of the patients. The psychiatrist must engage with the patients often enough to carry out necessary therapeutic tasks and to establish and maintain a working relationship.

Despite the multidisciplinary nature of care that is required, each discipline will bring its own area of expertise to the team and have a clear role. Whatever the model of leadership within the service (medical, nursing or multidisciplinary) there must exist a close and unified relationship between the senior staff of the unit and the consultant psychiatrist. The role of junior doctors within a unit will inevitably vary, dependent on their grade, but examples are shown in Box 24.5. The consultant psychiatrist will have specific responsibilities, examples are shown in Box 24.6.

Box 24.5. Examples of junior doctor roles

- To be a key member of the multidisciplinary team, providing medical input
- To take part in referral assessments
- To complete medical admission procedures
- To provide day-to-day reviews and management of patients
- To participate in the multidisciplinary team patient review meetings
- To participate in referral meetings
- To write medical reports and present cases in the hearings for Hospital Managers and Mental Health Tribunals under the supervision of the consultant
- To provide necessary support to the unit staff
- To take an active role in service development
- To liaise with others, providing information on psychiatric intensive and low secure care

> **Box 24.6.** Examples of consultant psychiatrist roles
>
> - Providing necessary support to unit staff
> - Taking lead role in the multidisciplinary team for the unit
> - Medically leading referral assessments
> - Supervising/advising other medical staff on the day-to-day management of the patients
> - Leading/taking a key role in the multidisciplinary team patient review rounds
> - Taking a key role in team weekly referral meetings
> - Writing medical reports and presenting cases in hearings for Hospital Managers and Mental Health Tribunals
> - Taking an active role in coordinating, planning and implementing care planning arrangements
> - Providing regular supervision for junior doctors and facilitating their appraisals
> - Taking an active role in developing the service and representing it
> - Ensuring the clinical governance structures are medically robust and working adequately and monitored appropriately through clinical audit
> - Liaising with medical colleagues, providing information on psychiatric intensive and low secure care

Role of the nurse

It is easy to view the role of nursing as simply undertaking certain given tasks. For example within PICUs and LSUs, as in other areas, the nurse would be responsible for all stages of the nursing process: to act as primary/named nurse for a given number of patients or to fulfil the role of care coordinator/keyworker. The role of the nurse, however, also has a major impact on the functioning of the rest of the MDT, particularly in promoting a healthily functioning environment.

The therapeutic role of the nurse encompasses many functions/characteristics and can be described as proactive and reactive. The nurse–patient relationship is the basis of all nursing activity and can act as an instrument to facilitate self-learning and promote a patient's recovery. Through this relationship the nurse can facilitate professional closeness (caring and empathy), advocacy, education (mental health promotion) and identify other areas of need to support the patient on the journey to recovery. These functions promote the development of fundamental trust between care giver and care receiver, which in turn allows the necessary understanding, integrity, honesty, reliability, responsibility and accountability to grow.

Kitson (1985) identified three integral components of the nurse–patient relationship. Firstly, a need for commitment from the nurse to provide the support necessary to sustain the patient's emotional, practical and time dimensions. Secondly, the possession of appropriate knowledge and practical skills that contribute to the performance of 'caring' activities; and thirdly, that the total interaction is given direction through respect for the patient.

Unlike other professions, nurses are continuously present throughout a patient's stay within hospital. The nurse's presence has been defined as a powerful phenomenon, and has been described as an elusive concept: challenging to measure in quantitative terms yet recognised by both nurses and patients (Martin, 1995). Nurses undertake to provide safe, stable and supportive relationships as well as environments to allow the patient to feel safe, 'cared for' and protected to an extent that enables them to engage in treatment. This function underpins the nursing role and is both proactive and reactive in nature. The nurses' constant presence allows them to be sensitive to and react to a patient's mental state and behaviour at any given time in order to aid retrieval of stable mental health, in essence supporting the patient.

Similarly, nurses provide the role of supporting other disciplines within the MDT in their work with patients. Whether this is providing a safe environment for them, providing information about patients, escorting patients to/participating with patients in occupational activity, or administering medication. This functional role is what holds healthcare services together and supports team members from other disciplines in delivering care and treatment.

Nurses' ability to tolerate 'being with' and to understand the patient and his/her behaviour, to whatever degree possible, in a humane, considered manner and to translate that experience into meaningful information is a very sophisticated activity. This activity supports the entire team in its level of functioning and ability to deliver effective treatment for patients in the most acute episodes of illness. Given the focus of PICU/LSU care, it is a role that is empathic, skilled and extremely valuable.

Role of the clinical psychologist

The contribution of clinical psychologists can be extremely beneficial. Historically, clinical psychologists were not very involved in the inpatient environment – this used to be the domain of the 'medical model'. In the days of the large institutions, psychologists would for example perhaps run token-economy programmes with individuals or groups of patients. In recent years this has changed and psychological therapy approaches are deemed appropriate even for psychotic patients. Consequently the role of clinical psychologists has expanded into acute ward environments. In addition, many nurses have acquired a considerable amount of psychological therapy skills, often taught to them by clinical psychologists.

Within the NHS clinical psychologists have always had a rather privileged 'outsider' role, which has often led to their being undervalued and criticised by professionals who spend most of their time on the ward, i.e. nurses and doctors. However, this outsider role can be highly beneficial. The high-intensity, locked atmosphere of the unit not only contains patients' destructive psychoses, but also psychologically traps patients and staff. An experienced, psychotherapeutically orientated clinical psychologist could apply his/her expertise to the ward environment, including supervision, joint therapy with staff, guidance and de-briefing of staff, and fulfil a useful psychological second-opinion function for patients. In addition the senior clinical psychologist could also be available to help ward management with the often delicate balancing act of managing the unit, which may include 'conflict resolution.'

We could also argue for a more team-centred role for a junior clinical psychologist. There is clearly a need for psychometric assessments such as neuro-psychological screening, which can help enormously in the process of treatment and discharge planning. We would also see a team-based clinical psychologist as instrumental in providing an ongoing psychological perspective to the work of occupational therapists and to many nursing activities such as hand-over, key-worker sessions, and involvement of relatives. The ongoing observation and evaluation of interactions between patients, between staff and between staff and patients could also serve as a safeguard against 'trapped' dynamics becoming destructive. And last, but not least, the PICU environment is one of constant change and this flow of change needs to be managed, which includes ongoing learning. Clinical psychologists should be able to contribute to these processes.

Role of the pharmacist

It is essential that pharmacists providing a service to a PICU are actively integrated in the MDT and regularly attend ward rounds, hand-overs or team meetings. In this way, the pharmacist is continually (preferably daily) updated with the change in each patient's condition, particularly with respect to insight and any risk assessments.

The pharmacist should also screen all the prescriptions every day to advise on: potential drug–drug or drug–food interactions; maximum doses, especially where high-dose prescribing or combinations occur, physical monitoring requirements and their frequency, the need to obtain consent for a given medication. Also, wherever possible the pharmacist should be available to discuss any concerns the patient may have with the individual and/or their carers.

The role of the occupational therapist

Occupational therapists (OTs) use meaningful activity to assess, develop and facilitate optimal functioning and promote occupational balance. Often when patients are admitted to a PICU/LSU they are able to participate in a functional lifestyle. This can be due to disturbed behaviour, acute psychotic symptoms and associated high levels of risk.

Box 24.7. Pharmacist roles include

- Recommending appropriate treatment options taking into account the physical and mental state of the individual, in particular any risk factors
- Advising on suitable formulations of prescribed medication especially where concordance is questioned
- Advising on the preparation and reconstitution of specific agents, e.g olanzapine intramuscular injection is a dry powder for reconstitution, unlike any other agent regularly used in psychiatry
- Provision of appropriate written information on medication for the patient when 'informed consent' is being sought, e.g when valproate is used for prophylaxis of mania, an off-label use which is not described in the manufacturer's patient information leaflet
- Providing professional advice on the individual's prescribing plan to Mental Health Act Commission Second Opinion Appointed Doctors where Form 39 consent is sought
- Advising other members of the MDT on the potential implications of side-effects of medication on their work with the individual, e.g. discussion with dietician and sports/activity coordinator the potential for weight gain with atypical antipsychotics

In a PICU/LSU setting OTs work within the MDT and contribute to the holistic assessment of the patient's presentation and their needs. In this setting OT's pay particular attention to how a patient's presentation affects their ability to participate in their chosen roles, routines and meaningful activities.

Occupational therapists use a variety of standardised and non-standardised assessments. Currently a number of OTs use The Model of Human Occupation (Kielhofner, 2001) on which to base their intervention. This model has a number of standardised assessments suitable for use within the PICU/LSU setting, e.g. Assessment of Communication and Interaction Skills (ACIS), Assessment of Motor and Processing Skills (AMPS) and the Volitional Questionnaire (VQ) to name a few. Use of observational assessments has value in this clinical area as patients are often unable to participate in longer interview style assessments due to the acute nature of their illness.

Occupational therapists contribute to risk assessment and management of patients through observation of patients in a variety of situations, e.g. social groups, activity-based groups and domestic activities of daily living such as cooking. These assessments contribute to a holistic assessment of the patient. The OTs contribute to the overall assessment through continuous liaison and feedback to the rest of the MDT.

Often there may be a shortage of OTs, and in turn this often means that OTs are not fully represented in PICUs. It is recognised within the National Minimum Standards that OTs are an important part of the MDT and essential within LSUs. In PICUs there has been some debate regarding the relevance of occupational therapy with this particular patient group due to the patient's acute presentation. Occupational therapists working within the PICU setting generally find it a rewarding area to work and feel valued by the MDT and, more importantly, the patient group.

The role of the social worker

Principles of human rights and social justice are fundamental to social work. This involves identifying, seeking to alleviate and advocating strategies for overcoming structural disadvantage, hardship and suffering. The overall aim of the work is to overcome social and environmental barriers to discharge and, if possible, change any adverse circumstances that contributed to the patient's hospital admission. Consequently, it is essential that the social worker interacts actively with the MDT by attending ward rounds and CPA meetings. Moreover, the social worker is ideally placed to provide information appertaining to the patient's family and social network, which is crucial to risk assessments.

Initial social work contact is often with an Approved Social Worker (ASW) as part of a Mental Health Act assessment. The statutory duties are clearly defined but after the patient is admitted to hospital, the social care is often passed to either another social worker from the relevant community team or the dedicated social worker in longer-stay low secure environments.

Box 24.8. Social worker's roles include

- Undertaking approved social work assessments and arranging admission under the MHA (1983). Arranging for the patient's property to be protected (National Assistance Act 1948).
- Promoting anti-discriminatory practice and providing a social perspective to all aspects of care including assessment of social and cultural needs.
- Engaging with the patient's family or significant others to build support networks and assess risks in relation to discharge planning. Undertaking carer's assessment of need.
- Assisting with accommodation issues and promoting change if beneficial to the patients.
- Taking the lead role in non-statutory childcare work, and liaising with Social Services Departments in the case of statutory child protection issues.
- Assisting with financial problems, including welfare benefits and debts, helping to remove stressful situations upon discharge.
- Providing social circumstances reports for Mental Health Manager's Reviews and Mental Health Review Tribunals. Preparing the patient for the meeting and promoting independent advocacy and legal representation.
- Attending MDT meetings and CPA reviews, maintaining a focus on discharge planning. Representing the patient's and family views and advocating on their behalf to bring about social change. Accessing community care funding for packages of care in the community.

The social work contribution to an MDT in relation to the domains in which the team works with patients is discussed further in Chapter 19 and examples of the role are shown in Box 24.8.

Team morale

Teamwork is not the panacea for all ills; however, a well-developed team can make positive differences to patient care and be both challenging and rewarding to work within. Good teamwork does not just happen. Instructing groups of staff that they are now a team will not promote or sustain effective teamwork.

Box 24.9. Blanchard's characteristics

- **P**urpose & values
- **E**mpowerment
- **R**elationships & communications
- **F**lexibility
- **O**ptimal performance
- **R**ecognition & appreciation
- **M**orale

The question of how to keep a team motivated requires complex and multifaceted responses. Key areas to address would include: interdisciplinary training, team-building events, robust communication strategies and the provision of visible performance data reporting the activity, treatment outcomes and continued developments within the service (there are many more!).

Blanchard (2001, pp. 143–144) captures some of these elements and uses the acronym PERFORM to describe some of the characteristics of a high-performing team (Box 24.9).

Attaining high performance and good morale requires providing a clear purpose with shared values and goals, unleashing and developing skills (*empowerment and flexibility*), creating team power (*relationships and communication*), and keeping the accent or focus on the positive (*recognition and appreciation*).

One of the key aspects of effective multidisciplinary team functioning is communication. Many studies in this area have tended to focus on particular aspects of team communication such as power within relationships (Fried 1989) and conflict arising from the degree of involvement of team members (While and Barriball 1999). How a team facilitates communication and shares information will impact on all aspects of team-working and care provision. Each team should consider how to increase the frequency and quality of communication both within it and between it and other teams (see Box 24.10). This should improve the team's engagement and thus quality of care.

A communication system will only be successful if it is viewed as beneficial to all members. Many teams

---

Box 24.10. Team communication

- Does the team **rely** on a weekly/monthly meeting to convey information and maintain the focus of the team?
- Do senior members of the team actually work in a manner that embraces the shared vision? Actions speak louder than words.
- What are the teams preferred modes of communication (both internally and externally)? Do we know? What are the options?
- Does the team have a system which encourages critical analysis of the work and embraces new ideas?
- As a team, do we act upon ideas for development and support innovation? Without this, ambivalence can develop.

(and organisations for that matter) make efforts to ensure that information is passed downward (from management). However, team members listen more effectively when they themselves believe they are listened to. Upward communication channels tend to be less robust.

Many teams have regular team meetings in which information is shared. The effectiveness of these meetings will differ from team to team, depending on many things, not least how the meetings are structured. Without a defining focus, many team meetings may develop into 'letting off steam' forums, which, in the short term, may offer some limited benefit. However, one manner in which to keep the accent on the positive could be to encourage all team members to attend meetings and provide one idea/suggestion or innovation for improvement for discussion. In terms of promoting a shared vision, this may assist team members in remaining focused on their overall aim whilst actively contributing to developments. It may also improve overall morale providing that developments/improvements are implemented and sustained.

There are many recognised approaches to team-building and some useful tools for measuring how your team is functioning. Whyte and Brooker (2001) studied twenty-one teams from secure environments across the United Kingdom using the Onyett Team Membership Questionnaire (TMQ: Onyett *et al.* 1997) which contains twenty-nine items rated

on a five-point semantic differential scale. They concluded that to work effectively in a multidisciplinary manner within secure environments required a combination of organisational legitimacy, a willingness by professionals to engage with each other, inter-professional skills and motivation, an enhanced knowledge base of contemporary treatment approaches, and leadership and training related to how to be a member of a team. They suggested that one or more of these factors were absent in the teams struggling to be effective.

The Team Membership Questionnaire is a dynamic tool and can provide both quantitative and qualitative data. We have provided a more simplistic tool as a starting exercise to assess where your team is now (see Box 24.11). The information collated can be used as a building block to support team growth and identify areas for improvement. Initially ask every member of your team to score the statements using the ratings provided. It is important to agree the timescale to be considered, e.g. the previous 6 months. Team members should be asked to rate as individuals. Facilitators should decide beforehand whether data are provided anonymously, or whether further information is required, e.g. grade, discipline, etc.

Once the rating exercise has been completed, compare scores and identify areas in which the team is doing well. Discuss why this might be. The development areas will be clearly identified and, as a team, discussion and planning should be focused on what action is required to bring the ratings up in the areas of concern.

Clearly, this exercise is only a start, but it is one way of valuing individuals' input and identifying areas which the team can collectively address to promote team-working and their effectiveness. This type of exercise should also assist in identifying poor systems which, if cured, would be a step towards conquering poor morale.

Disagreements and resolution

There are many possible sources of conflict within a PICU/LSU setting and also in its relationships

Box 24.11. Basic team-working questionnaire

1. **SHARED VISION** – *degree to which there is clear ownership of the mission statement and operational policy*   **Rating**   1 2 3 4 5
2. **OBJECTIVES** – *degree to which clear objectives are in place for the team as a whole*   **Rating**   1 2 3 4 5
3. **INFORMATION** – *degree to which I feel that: Organisational, Management and Clinical information is available to support the team in doing its job*   **Rating**   1 2 3 4 5
4. **COMMUNICATION** – *degree to which I feel inter-colleague (multi-professional within team) communications are effective*   **Rating**   1 2 3 4 5
5. **RELATIONSHIPS WITH OTHER TEAMS** – *degree to which professional working relationships with other teams are constructive and supportive of the team in conducting its activities*   **Rating**   1 2 3 4 5
6. **POLICIES and PROCEDURES** – *degree to which existing systems are helpful in supporting the team in conducting its activities*   **Rating**   1 2 3 4 5
7. **SUPPORT and SUPERVISION** – *degree to which cooperation and supportive relationships are demonstrated within the team*   **Rating**   1 2 3 4 5
8. **RECOGNITION and ACHIEVEMENT** – *degree to which 'good work' is recognised and rewarded*   **Rating**   1 2 3 4 5
9. **INNOVATION** – *degree to which new ways of working are generated and result in positive change*   **Rating**   1 2 3 4 5
10. **EMPOWERMENT** – *degree to which I feel confident to make suggestions or try out new ideas*   **Rating**   1 2 3 4 5
11. **INVOLVEMENT** – *degree to which I feel involved in the decision-making processes that affect the team's functioning*   **Rating**   1 2 3 4 5
12. **DEVELOPMENT** – *degree to which I feel my professional development is geared towards supporting the activities of the team*   **Rating**   1 2 3 4 5

Scale:
1 – Very poor   2 – Poor   3 – Fair   4 – Good   5 – Very good

with professional stakeholders. Being part of a team brings its own challenges when dealing with disagreements. Discussions and decision-making take time, and individuals' personalities can become entwined in this process (which may help or hinder the procedure).

Disagreements can occur between many different people/elements (see Box 24.12). The nature of these conflicts can be emotional, factual, constructive, destructive, argumentative, open or suppressed and the content can encompass a host of issues, e.g. admissions or treatment programmes, diagnosis or discharge arrangements, the team's structure.

As the team grows, so will its members' abilities to build on their personal skills and experiences in handling disputes. A key approach is to minimise the emotive element and to substitute it with a rational pragmatic approach when seeking resolution.

Management by consensus is not always the most effective manner in which to address certain

Box 24.12. Possible foci of disagreements

- The leader and individual team members
- The leader and the whole team
- Individual team members
- The lead nurse and lead doctor
- The whole team and the organisation's management
- The team and its stakeholders

issues. Sometimes individual team members will be required to make decisions or take action not concordant with the team ethos or contradictory to the operation of the unit. The manner in which these types of disagreements are addressed has an impact on inter-personal/professional relationships and requires careful analysis of the underlying issues.

When addressing disagreements, it is important to find common ground and be mindful that the team's purpose is to serve the needs of its patient group. In line with current good practice, each unit should have a 'working practice manual' containing all policies and procedures relating to the unit, its function and the manner in which service is delivered. The manual should have been arrived at through wide consultation and provides a useful starting point in resolving disagreements.

Since many PICUs/LSUs offer a referral-based service, it is not uncommon for disagreements to arise with other service areas or senior management regarding admissions, predominantly out of 'working hours'. As with any service, it is important to keep statistical data relating to the unit's activity and operation. This information can prove invaluable when trying to resolve conflict with external stakeholders. Resolution of disagreements can often lead to improvement in practice or systems that benefit patients. For example, following disputes concerning the issue of 'out of hours' admissions, one unit has implemented training packages for other staff to assess suitability for admission and this, combined with a defined patient pathway, has led to a smoother and more responsive service. Another unit has implemented a defined person on each shift to perform assessments.

Staying effective

Some aspects of how to remain effective as a team have already been discussed in team development. Should a team or individuals within it reach 'burnout' it is important that both team development and its process of trying to remain effective are examined. It is evident that these are continuous processes and, for teams to remain effective, they and their procedural framework need to adapt to internal and external changes. The complexity of team relationships and how individuals within the team (and the team itself) relate to outside influences should not be underestimated. One of the most difficult aspects of teamworking within PICUs/LSUs is the ability to adapt to continually changing circumstances whilst flourishing and holding true to the core vision. This is essentially about the team's capability and capacity to change effectively.

Whilst much has been written about change management and to fully discuss it is outside this chapter's remit, some key principles pertinent to PICUs/LSUs should be outlined. Within any multidisciplinary team there are multiple stakeholders both involved in and contributing to its effectiveness and method of working. Each brings its own diverse actions, incentives, motivations and judgements. This makes it a complex system that could result in chaos. This possibility can be minimised by the development of robust standards, guidelines and approaches to best practice as well as team-based training and educational interventions. Implementation of these within complex systems requires multiple approaches that make use of experience, creativity, innovation and experimentation.

Experience of working within PICUs and LSUs comes not only with time spent in such an environment but, more importantly, the ability to reflect upon this time. Questions such as 'What has benefited patients?', 'What hasn't?', 'How have you reacted to certain situations and why?' as well as numerous others are important. Time spent within team-building exercises allowing individuals to consider these, as well as a robust system of individual supervision are necessities if a team is to remain functioning well. Creativity and innovation within the boundaries that are set for both the team member and the team should be encouraged and, if facilitated well within systems, will lead to strengthening and increased morale. This links with experimentation: if something works well then positive reinforcement will enable teams to improve. If something has not worked well, lessons that are invaluable for team development and improved patient care may result. An example may be a team member engaging with a particular patient who has an interest in gardening to improve a unit's outside space. This could lead to money being sourced to make the outside area more pleasant and a horticulture ward group that is attended by staff and patients.

Also vital to sustaining performance level is continuous quality improvement. Ultimately it is the judgements made on service provision that are critical. Having the correct people making those judgements on the best available information is of paramount importance. Teams should therefore be built around patients, but if they are only involved in monitoring and evaluating poor services then the purpose of patients making those judgements is defeated. Patients need to be involved in the planning of services, training of staff, staff development as well as monitoring, researching and evaluating the service. Patient participation is vital and needs to go beyond mere tokenism. For further information, Hutchison (2000) has suggested ways in which this can occur.

Quality assurance systems require the establishment of standards set within a clear framework. Until recently there have never been such standards for the achievement of high-quality PICU/low secure care. Although there may be a danger that high levels of specification can work against creativity, the development of National Minimum Standards should be welcomed within an area that has traditionally been ill-defined. These standards help provide impetus for improvement of team working and hence service provision, but for these improvements to occur and be sustained, local quality assurance initiatives working in a cyclical fashion need to be introduced (see Box 24.13).

For the team to flourish, individual PICU/low secure MDTs should address these issues in a manner that reflects local arrangements, issues and difficulties. Successful teamworking will prosper with structured use of clinical improvement cycles.

Box 24.13. Quality assurance should: (Onyett 2003, p. 236)

- Demonstrate that the service is doing what it is meant to do
- Consider improvements rather than only correcting deficits
- Aim to achieve high performance from the outset
- Involve front-line staff as key players
- Focus on building the capacity of staff to become more effective (e.g. through personal development plans)
- Involve patients at all levels of the quality assurance process

---

Conclusion

As today's healthcare delivery system evolves, all levels of professionals are learning that a team approach is both efficient and effective for providing quality patient care. Teamwork ensures that the multidisciplinary members deliver intensive, continuous and coordinated care and treatment within an agreed framework of professional accountability. This ensures that results of the team's collective approach are greater than the sum of its individual members' efforts.

Most team members are skilled in their profession-specific work. However, within basic professional training, little emphasis is placed on how to successfully work within teams. This has possibly led to the difficulty of each profession at times perceiving the others with perplexity, bemusement, confusion and occasionally mistrust. If the history of the somewhat patchwork introduction of team working is also considered, it is no surprise that some individuals have had a negative view of multidisciplinary working.

The traditional role of the medical consultant managing and leading teams is changing; some PICUs/LSUs are nurse led, some medically led. We would argue that by having a narrow focus, PICUs/LSUs are in an excellent position to develop teams that are truly multidisciplinary, with defined roles for all team members not only within the care provided by the team but also in its own development and operational management. This can only be achieved through careful planning, robust appraisal and development procedures (for both the team and individual members), effective mechanisms of quality assurance and, most of all, by constantly having the patient and his/her needs at the forefront of the team's objectives.

Acknowledgements

We are extremely grateful to the following for their contributions on the roles of different professions: Dave Buckle, Tracy Holmes, Trudi Hilton, Reinhard Kowalski and Hannah Lukacs.

REFERENCES

Blanchard K. 2001 High Five. New York: Harper Collins

Borrill C, West M, Shapiro D, Rees A. 2000 Team working and effectiveness in health care. Br J Health Care Manage 6(8): 364–371

Chalk A. 1999 Community mental health teams: reviewing the debate. Ment Health Nurs 19: 12–14

Couchmann W. 1995 Joint education for mental health teams. Nurs Stand 10: 32–34

Department of Health. 1975 Better Services for the Mentally Ill. London: HMSO

Department of Health. 1990 NHS and Community Care Act. London: HMSO

Department of Health. 1995. Buiding Bridges: A Guide to Arrangements for Inter-Agency Working for the Care and Protection of Severely Mentally Ill People. London: HMSO

Department of Health. 1999 National Service Framework for Mental Health: Modern Standards and Service Models. London: HMSO

Department of Health. 2000 The NHS Plan – A Plan for Investment. A Plan for Reform. London: HMSO

Department of Health. 2001 Health and Social Care Act. London: The Stationery Office

Department of Health. 2002 National Minimum Standards for General Adult Services in Psychiatric Intensive Care Units (PICU) and Low Secure Environments. London: Department of Health Publications

Department of Health and Social Security (DHSS). 1977 The National Health Service Act. London: HMSO

Department of Health and Social Security. 1981 Care in the Community: a consultative document on moving resources for care in England. London: DHSS

Department of Health and Social Security. 1988 Report of the committee of inquiry into the care and after-care of Miss Sharon Campbell. London: DHSS (Cm 440)

Ford K, Farrington A. 1999 Risk assessment. Assessing dangerousness in regional secure units – decision making in the multidisciplinary team. Ment Health Care 2(6): 201–204

Fried BJ. 1989 Power acquisition in a health care setting – an application of strategic contingency theory. Hum Relat 41: 915–927

Galvin SW, McCarthy S. 1994 Multi-disciplinary community teams: clinging to the wreckage. J Ment Health 3: 157–166

Gibb CE, Morrow M, Clarke CL, Cook G, Gerting P, Ramprogus V. 2002 Transdisciplinary working: evaluating the development of health and social care provision in mental health. J Ment Health 11(3): 339–350

Harrison P. 1990 Multidisciplinary teams and how to survive them. Occasional paper for Community and Rehabilitation Section. London: Royal College of Psychiatrists

Hutchison M. 2000 Issues around empowerment. In: Basset T (ed) Looking to the Future: Key Issues for Contemporary Mental Health Services. Brighton: Pavillion Publishing/Mental Health Foundation

Kielhofner G. 2002 The Model of Human Occupation. Theory and Application. Baltimore: Lippincott, Williams & Wilkins

Kitson A. 1985 Education for quality. Senior Nurse 3(4): 11–16

Laidler P. 1994 Stroke Rehabilitation: Structure and Strategy. London: Chapman and Hall

Lucas J. 1996 Multidisciplinary care in the community for clients with mental health problems: guidelines for the future. In: Watkins M, Hervey N, Carson J, Ritter S (eds) Collaborative Community Mental Health Care. London: Arnold, pp. 351–370

Martin P. 1995 Nurse–patient relationship. In: Martin P (ed) Psychiatric Nursing. Harrow: Scutari, pp. 271–281

Michalon M, Richman A. 1990 Factors affecting length of stay in a psychiatric intensive care unit. Gen Hosp Psychiatry 12(5): 303–308

Miller C, Freeman M, Ross N. 2001 Interprofessional Practice in Health Social Care. London: Arnold

Mohrman SA, Cohen SG, Morhrman AM. 1995 Designing Team-Based Organisations. San Francisco: Josey Bass

Norman IJ, Peck E. 1999 Working together in adult community mental health services: an inter-professional dialogue. J Ment Health 8(3): 217–230

Onyett S. 2003 Teamworking in Mental Health. Basingstoke: Palgrave MacMillan

Onyett SR, Heppleston T, Bushnell D. 1994 A national survey of community mental health teams. J Ment Health 3: 175–194

Onyett S, Pillinger T, Muijen M. 1997 Job satisfaction and burnout among members of community mental health teams. J Ment Health 6: 55–66

Opie A. 1997 Thinking teams thinking clients; issues of discourse and representation in the work of health care teams. Sociol Health Illn 19(3): 259–280

Ovretveit J. 1993 Coordinating Community Care: Multidisciplinary Teams and Care Management. Buckingham: Open University Press

Ovretveit J. 1995 Team decision making. J Interprofess Care 9: 41–51

Ovretveit J. 1996 Five ways to describe a multidisciplinary team. J Interprofess Care 10: 163–171

Peck E, Norman IJ. 1999 Working together in adult community mental health services: exploring inter-professional role relations. J Ment Health 8(3): 231–242

Richards A, Rees A. 1998 Developing criteria to measure the effectiveness of community mental health teams. Ment Health Care 21(1): 14–17

Sainsbury Centre for Mental Health. 1997 Pulling Together. The Future Role and Training of Mental Health Staff. London: SCMH

Sainsbury Centre for Mental Health. 2001 The Capable Practitioner. London: SCMH

Test MA, Marks IM. 1990 Commentary on Chapter 17. In: Marks IM, Scott RA (eds) Mental Health Care Delivery: Innovations, Impediments and Implementation. Cambridge: Cambridge University Press, pp. 254–256

Watson GB. 1994 Multi-disciplinary working and co-operation in community care. Ment Health Nurs 14: 18–21

West MA. 1996 Reflexivity and work group effectiveness: a conceptual integration. In: West MA (ed) Handbook of Work Group Psychology. Chichester: Wiley

While A, Barriball L. 1999 Qualified and unqualified nurses' view of the multidisciplinary team. J Interpersonal Care 13(1): 77–89

Whyte L, Brooker C. 2001 Working with a multidisciplinary team in secure psychiatric environments. J Psychosoc Nurs 39(9): 26–34

25

National Standards and good practice

Stephen Dye, Andy Johnston and Navjyoat Chhina

Introduction

By the very nature of its practice, psychiatry today continues to be influenced not only by mental health professionals but also by the framework within which care and treatment are delivered. In the UK this includes legal [e.g. The Mental Health Act dealing with compulsory detention of patients (Department of Health 1983)], social (e.g. family and carers), user involvement (e.g. user groups) and political interventions (e.g. Department of Health guidelines). Given the rights of patients enshrined within statute and other government guidance, e.g. Care Programme Approach (Department of Health 1999a), in no other subspeciality is the interface with legal, ethical, political and social issues more acute than within locked Psychiatric Intensive Care Units (PICUs). Yet astonishingly, up until relatively recently, it is the one area within which these issues had been most neglected. The publication of the UK National Minimum Standards (NMS) (Department of Health 2002) gave clinicians, managers and commissioners a framework to deliver high-quality services and care to some of the most severely and acutely unwell patients treated by the mental health system. This chapter will outline development of the standards, summarise and review their structure and content, as well as describe evidence of practice in UK PICU and Low Secure Unit (LSU) settings.

National Association and need for Standards

In the UK, the National Association of Psychiatric Intensive Care Units (NAPICU) was established in 1996. Its key aims are to advance psychiatric intensive care and low secure services, improve mechanisms for the delivery of psychiatric intensive care, audit effectiveness and to promote research, education and practice development within the speciality. Formation of NAPICU gave rise to discussion amongst clinicians regarding standards of care, ethical issues, definitions of these units and the patient group served. A survey published in 1997 (Beer et al. 1997) highlighted the disparity between units in the UK (see Box 25.1). This gave rise to further debate and in 2001 the Department of Health commissioned the PICU Policy Research and Development Group, based at North East London Mental Health NHS Trust (NELMHT), to produce national PICU Standards. To achieve this, a PICU and Low Secure Practice Development Network consisting of a multidisciplinary group of professionals and user representatives from around the UK was formed that identified and agreed standards and general good practice guidance for psychiatric intensive care and low secure services. This led to the publication by the Department of Health of the 'National Minimum Standards for General Adult Services in Psychiatric Intensive Care Units (PICU) and Low

Psychiatric Intensive Care, 2nd edn., eds. M. Dominic Beer, Stephen M. Pereira and Carol Paton.
Published by Cambridge University Press. © Cambridge University Press 2008

Box 25.1. UK National Survey Findings
(110 units) (Beer *et al.* 1997)

- Eighty-eight units locked their doors at all times
- Forty-six of those units accepted informal patients
- Forty-eight of the eighty-nine units accepting prison transfers also accepted informal patients
- Seventy-two units accepted a mix of intensive care and chronic or challenging behaviour patients
- Sixty-five units had a male-to-female ratio of 4:1 and a further twenty-five units a ratio of 5:1 or more male patients to every female patient
- Eight units had a ratio of at least ten male patients to every female patient
- Seventy-six units did not have a policy for administration of high-dose neuroleptics either for rapid tranquillisation or longer-term treatment in 'treatment resistant' patients
- Twenty-two units did not have a policy for the practice of control and restraint and fifteen did not have a policy for seclusion
- Thirty-two units had no policy for searching patients or visitors
- Twenty units did not have an admission/exclusion policy
- Fourteen units did not have a junior doctor
- Twenty-nine units did not have a dedicated consultant providing overall clinical responsibility for that unit
- Thirty-two units had no occupational therapist
- Forty-six units had no pharmacist input
- Fifty units had no psychologist input
- Forty-nine units had no social worker
- Ninety-eight units had no other therapy (e.g. art therapy)

Box 25.2. PICU definition

Psychiatric intensive care is for patients compulsorily detained usually in secure conditions, who are in an acutely disturbed phase of a serious mental disorder. There is an associated loss of capacity for self-control, with a corresponding increase in risk, which does not enable their safe, therapeutic management and treatment in a general open acute ward.

Care and treatment offered must be patient-centred, multidisciplinary, intensive, comprehensive, collaborative and have an immediacy of response to critical situations. Length of stay must be appropriate to clinical need and assessment of risk but would ordinarily not exceed 8 weeks in duration.

Psychiatric intensive care is delivered by qualified staff according to an agreed philosophy of unit operation underpinned by principles of risk assessment and management.

Low secure definition

Low Secure Units deliver intensive, comprehensive, multidisciplinary treatment and care by qualified staff for patients who demonstrate disturbed behaviour in the context of a serious mental disorder and who require the provision of security.

This is according to an agreed philosophy of unit operation underpinned by the principles of rehabilitation and risk management. Such units aim to provide a homely secure environment, which has occupational and recreational opportunities and links with community facilities.

Patients will be detained under the Mental Health Act and may be restricted on legal grounds needing rehabilitation usually for up to 2 years.

Secure Environments Mental Health Policy Implementation Guide' in April 2002 (Department of Health 2002).

Format of National Minimum Standards (NMS)

The introduction comprehensively defines PICUs and LSUs (Box 25.2) and describes the background and development of the standards. The NMS are then organised into fifteen sections (Box 25.3). Following this, there is a short section regarding implementation as well as a list of contributors and acknowledgements. There are also seven appendices

(Box 25.4) that provide further details, guidance and recommendations addressing the implementation of particular standards.

The document supplies an all-encompassing framework on which to base services; it provides transparency with regards to expectations as to what should be delivered, and gives guidance on how to provide care in what is a challenging area of psychiatric practice. Each main section is divided into:
- Rationale for developing standards of that nature
- Standards pertaining to that topic
- Good practice guidance relating to the topic

> **Box 25.3.** The Standards
>
> 1. Admission criteria
> 2. Core interventions
> 3. Multidisciplinary team (MDT) working
> 4. Physical environment
> 5. Service structure – personnel
> 6. User involvement
> 7. Carer involvement
> 8. Documentation
> 9. Ethnicity, culture and gender
> 10. Supervision
> 11. Liaison with other agencies
> 12. Policies and procedures
> 13. Clinical audit and monitoring
> 14. Staff training
> 15. PICU/low secure support services

> **Box 25.4.** Appendices
>
> 1. Core interventions
> 2. MDT working
> 3. Physical environment
> 4. User involvement
> 5. Policies and procedures
> 6. Clinical audit
> 7. Staff training

Within each subheading there are simple-to-refer-to numerical references that ensure easy auditing and communication (for example, Standard 10.2.1 states that, 'Clinical supervision should occur at a minimum of once every 2 weeks . . .'). This provides every reader with a simple reference point with which to convey information to others.

The NMS offer clear operational definitions of both psychiatric intensive and low secure care. A mutually agreed definition leads to consistency in service operation and is the most important factor to the efficient running of such services. It is crucial to define roles within the framework of providing psychiatric care in a locally sensitive fashion. Failure to do so is an invitation to confusion within a system and to potential poor practice. The interface between open acute, intensive care, long-term low secure,

intensive rehabilitation and forensic units must be clarified and the definitions provided by the NMS go some way to address this.

The classifications described in the NMS also lead to clarification of practice issues in a number of different areas, which are further addressed within the document. Many of these topics are covered elsewhere in this book (e.g. physical environment, multidisciplinary working, liaison with other agencies). This chapter focuses upon factors affecting practice and how these are addressed by the NMS.

Good practice issues

Admission criteria and legal status of patients

Standard 1.3.2: Patients will be detained under the appropriate completed assessment/treatment section (not admitted on Sec 4, 5/2, 5/4, or 136) of the mental health act/order

As was shown above (Beer *et al.* 1997), a significant proportion of units accept informal patients (patients who are not compulsorily detained). Whilst there may be sound clinical reasons for this, it does raise the issue of the rights of informal patients in locked units and their treatment in the 'least restrictive environment' possible (National Service Framework for Mental Health; Department of Health 1999b) especially with regard to autonomy in terms of leave from the ward, possessions and visits from relatives, to name but a few. Continuing consent to residence and treatment is often assumed but this has been challenged notably by the 'Bournewood' case that was brought before the European Court of Human Rights (*HL* v *UK* 2004) which resulted in a judgement that it is unlawful (without prior authorisation) to provide care or treatment for an informal, incapacitated patient in a way that amounts to deprivation of liberty (for further discussion see Laidlaw and Buckle 2006).

Some units that admit informal patients have established procedures whereby patients who are informal sign a declaration on a daily basis agreeing to stay on the ward. This begs questions as to who decides on the capacity of a patient to give this consent, how often this is assessed and how capacity status is recorded. It has been recognised (Sugarman and Moss 1994) that a large proportion of informal patients admitted to general psychiatric wards did not know they had the right to refuse treatment and anticipated being instructed, pressurised or restrained if they tried to do so or attempted to leave the ward. One might strongly argue that these figures are likely to be higher for informal patients who are treated within locked wards.

The NMS aim to reduce these discrepancies between units in the UK by firstly establishing whether patients admitted to PICUs are suffering from a 'serious mental disorder'. They outline in a clear, succinct manner the criteria for admission as well as additional inclusion and exclusion criteria. The good practice guidance also makes reference to the UK National Service Framework (Department of Health 1999b) when stating that care should be given in the least restrictive environment possible. The Standards also instruct that patients cared for within PICUs or LSUs are detained under an order of the Mental Health Act that formally has admitted them to hospital for a period of time and that enables some form of treatment. There are units that admit patients who have been detained or held under emergency Sections of the Mental Health Act (e.g. Section 4 or Section 5) if they meet the unit's own admission criteria. The rationale for this is that PICUs should be able to respond to emergencies. However, there are also many potential difficulties surrounding this; for example, the lack of power to legally treat patients (except under common law), and that a number of patients who are detained under other sections (e.g. Section 136, Section 5/2) are not subsequently formally detained.

It is impossible to deliver appropriate psychiatric care in a unit that accepts all types of patients who are acutely disturbed or demonstrate challenging behaviours. The NMS therefore aid services by stipulating a number of exclusion criteria; for instance, having a primary diagnosis of substance misuse, dementia, or learning disability.

The NMS only give brief mention to assessment prior to admission and follow-up support following

---

Box 25.5. Examples of tools used by some PICUs in assessment

1. Brief Psychiatric Rating Scale (Overall and Gorham 1962)
2. Overt Aggression Scale (Yudofsky *et al.* 1986)
3. Beck Depression Inventory (Beck *et al.* 1961)
4. Young Mania Scale (Young *et al.* 1978)
5. Pierce Suicidal Intent Scale (Pierce 1981)
6. KGV (Krawiecka *et al.* 1977)
7. HoNOS (Wing *et al.* 1998)

---

non-admission. These are major areas in the smooth functioning of, and good service provided by, high-quality units. For example, some units use additional tools when performing assessments (see Box 25.5). Again, it is important to recognise that PICUs do not operate in isolation but are part of a complex system of provision of psychiatric care within a local organisation, and thus to be overly prescriptive with certain Standards may do more harm than good. For example, Standard 1.2.2 states: 'Patients will only be admitted if they display a *significant* risk of aggression, absconding with associated *serious* risk, suicide or vulnerability . . . in the context of a *serious mental disorder*'. These phrases can be interpreted diversely by different individuals and thus give rise to debate. It is therefore left to each unit, with their expertise and that of colleagues within their stakeholder groups, to develop (in a transparent fashion) individual assessment structures that suit their own needs and those of their organisation.

Long- and short-term admissions

PICU definition: . . . Length of stay . . . would not ordinarily exceed 8 weeks

Low Secure definition: . . . Patients will be detained . . . needing rehabilitation usually for up to 2 years

The distinctive tenets underlying psychiatric intensive and low secure care need to be considered uppermost when admission structures and procedures are developed. It is here that the NMS come into their own and provide clear directions. For each unit, the definition of intensive care/low secure care as given in the introduction to the Standards must form one of the cornerstones for admission criteria as there are obvious distinctions between intensive care and low secure care.

Units that accept a mixture of patient groups, with different clinical needs, treatment and recovery foci, often provide a compromise of care for all groups of patients. The treatment plans and needs of the acute group of patients are reviewed with immediacy and more regularly than those of longer-term patients. This potentially leads to the care of the latter group of patients being neglected. It is clinically well accepted that the longer-term disturbed, or complex needs patient and the acutely disturbed patient require a substantially different philosophy of care. The NMS make a purposeful distinction between the differing types of unit and the care that should be delivered (*Standard 1.5.1: 'Differences in function between PICUs and Low Secure environments need to be taken into consideration when implementing the above standards'*). Within some Standards, however, commonalities that both types of patients share are appreciated: e.g. *Standard 1.2.1: 'Patients admitted to the PICU/Low secure environment will have behavioural difficulties which seriously compromise their physical or psychological well-being, or that of others and which cannot be safely assessed or treated in an open acute inpatient facility'*.

Forensic patients

Due to a more proactive approach within the penal system in identifying psychiatric disturbance (e.g. court diversion schemes), a greater proportion of patients with either past histories of violence or exposure to it are being admitted to PICUs (Atakan 1995). A study outlining admissions to PICUs in London (Pereira *et al.* 2005) revealed that 65% of patients admitted showed physically aggressive behaviour as part of their clinical profile (including reasons for admission or a violent forensic history) and a substantial proportion (17%) were detained under forensic sections of the Mental Health Act (Department of Health 1983), most commonly Section 37 (a hospital admission order made by the court), or Section 37/41 (a hospital order with

Home Office restrictions). PICUs and LSUs need to be aware of the limitations of their service in safely managing such patients and the NMS again aid services by stipulating the following exclusion criteria: *Standard 1.4.1: 'The patient is assessed as presenting too high a degree of risk for a low secure environment: some may require admission to forensic services. Restricted patients should not be accepted unless there is provision to transfer them to an open ward if warranted by their clinical condition'*. This both highlights the level of security to which such units are designed and that restricted patients can stay longer than is clinically required within such units. The fact that, in Pereira *et al.'s* (2005) survey, some patients were admitted under a Restriction Order probably reflects local pressures for PICUs to accept all categories of difficult patients. The NMS do, however, allow for reasoned debate and discussion amongst clinicians and managers to occur regarding such admissions.

Diversity

*Equality (defn): The state of being equal (OED), **i.e. no differences***
*Equity (defn): The quality of being fair and impartial (OED), **i.e. respecting differences***

It is essential that that all service users treated within health services are identified as individuals, and recognised as having differing and distinctive daily needs. Nowhere is this more apparent than within mental health services and nowhere within mental health services is this more necessary than in secure settings (as illustrated by the Bennett inquiry; Norfolk, Suffolk and Cambridgeshire Strategic Health Authority 2003). The combination of acute mental illness and deprivation of liberty in a setting of security makes respecting a user's individual needs more important and significant. The difference between equality and equity is vital; the NMS specifically highlight areas of ethnicity, culture and gender and give guidance on a number of different aspects ranging from environment (e.g. *Standard 9.2.8: Gender specific areas for activities, e.g. bathroom, toilet,*

Table 25.1. Staffing on PICUs

	London Survey PICUs[a] (%) (n = 17)	UK National Survey PICUs[b] (%) (n = 170)	London Survey Low Secure Units[a] (%) (n = 16)	UK National Survey Low Secure Units[b] (%) (n = 137)
Consultant covering PICU/LSU only	88	20	94	27
Occupational therapist	82	48	81	58
Clinical psychology	65	24	63	50
Social worker	24	21	56	46

[a] Pereira *et al.* (2005)
[b] Pereira *et al.* (2006)

bedroom, lounge), to staffing (*e.g. Standard 9.2.4: A commitment to ensuring that the ethnicity of staff members reflects that of their patients*), to practice (e.g. *Standard 9.2.2: Any assessment tools used should be sensitive to the ethnic and gender needs of the patient*) and to availability of information, equipment and services (e.g. access to interpreters, religious/ethnic documents). In conjunction with relevant statutory law [e.g. Race Relations Act (Home Office 2000), Disability Discrimination Act (UK Government 2005)] and other Health Service documentation [e.g. Safety Privacy and Dignity in Mental Health Units, Department of Health 1999c], the NMS offer every service excellent guidance on how to meet individual patient need.

Multidisciplinary working and clinical leadership

In the 1997 national survey (Beer *et al.* 1997), nearly 45% of units included did not have psychologist, pharmacist or social worker input allocated to them; 30% did not have an occupational therapist; and 90% lacked other types of therapy input (such as art therapy). One-third of PICUs did not have a consultant with overall responsibility for the PICU. At that time, this may have partly reflected the lack of clarity of the role of a PICU within general adult services. If specific and clear guidelines are in place for the use of a PICU, then clear clinical leadership would ensure efficient and appropriate use of the facility. Chapter 24 makes

reference to different types of leadership within PICU settings with specific reference to multidisciplinary leadership and professional leads sharing the vision of an appropriate psychiatric intensive care service.

The NMS outline the staff required for best practice (*Standard 5.2.1: All PICU/Low secure units should be staffed by the following core services: medical, nursing, psychology, occupational therapy, social work, pharmacy, dedicated social worker especially for long stay low secure environments*). With regards to leadership, Standard 5.2.2 makes reference to the fact that each unit should have, at a minimum, a dedicated lead clinician (medical or nursing) with authority to make decisions regarding all aspects of unit operation. It goes on to recommend that each unit should have a dedicated consultant who has specific and enough sessions to provide dedicated and consistent input to the service.

Variation in staffing has been highlighted previously (p. 341, Box 25.1). Table 25.1 shows staffing establishments identified in the London area in 2001 (Pereira *et al.* 2005) prior to the publication of the NMS and nationally subsequent to publication of the Standards (Pereira *et al.* 2006). Though the methods used were different (the 1997 survey identified units through pharmacists from the UK Psychiatric Pharmacists Group; the subsequent surveys, via The Mental Health Act Commission) and the distinction between PICUs and LSUs was not made in the 1997 survey, it is evident that multidisciplinary input into

PICUs and LSUs has remained poorly developed. Further research will no doubt allow more comparisons between different units and organisations.

Training and supervision

Standard 14.1: 'In a highly demanding and stressful work environment it is essential that staff be well trained. In the current climate of evidence-based practice, it is also important that clinicians keep up to date in the knowledge, skills and attitudes needed to provide high quality care'.

These sentiments cannot be argued with and the NMS further describe a structure within which this can be achieved, with an outline that training should cover:

- Management and administration
- Assessment
- Treatment and care management
- Interpersonal skills and collaborative working

These are further specified in an appendix to the Standards.

Within many organisations, general mandatory training is provided (e.g. fire prevention) and there is also often access to 'psychiatric-specific' training (e.g. cognitive-behavioural strategies, clinical risk management), but perhaps education regarding specific issues prevalent in PICU or other secure settings (e.g. impact, and importance of boundary setting), or how psychiatric skills acquired can be adopted within such an environment, is more limited or unavailable.

In the UK, the inception of an MSc in Psychiatric Intensive Care has gone some way to meeting the need for such training and NAPICU supports both this and the further development of more physically accessible courses (e.g. e-learning). However, the combination of individual personal development plans (through appropriate supervision) and in-house training remains an imperative for every unit and staff member.

Within some services, specific packages for staff working within psychiatric intensive care have been developed that utilise the NMS and other related guidance (e.g. NICE guidance on management of disturbed behaviour) as a basis. These include an appropriate induction programme for new staff and making use of training from the wider organisation and beyond.

No amount of training will have an impact upon care unless reflective practice occurs. It is up to individual units to implement procedures to ensure that this takes place effectively in a variety of ways; for example, through debriefing following incidents, robust audit mechanisms, useful team meetings, clinical discussion groups, etc. Through this, the care provided by all staff will be meaningful, effective and up to date.

Policies and protocols

A PICU treats the most acutely unwell patients, who often display challenging unpredictability. It needs to do so with consistent and transparent methods that each member of staff understands and adheres to. This will ensure confidence and caring amongst staff, which helps foster the patient's recovery. The use of policies and protocols that are agreed within the organisation (following appropriate consultation) should allow for such consistency and transparency. There are some organisation-wide policies and protocols that the PICU staff should lead upon (given their experience and knowledge), e.g. rapid tranquillisation, seclusion, high-dose medication, and control and restraint. There are others that PICU staff should be consulted heavily upon, e.g. observation and engagement as well as risk management.

Each PICU should have its own specific operational policy that reflects the local approach to psychiatric intensive care within the framework of the NMS in a realistic fashion. Not to do so could lead to inappropriate use of PICUs and difficulties that the NMS were introduced to avoid. Many PICUs have introduced their own working practice manual that includes not only the unit's operational policy, but also relevant policies and procedures. The NMS give a number of recommended areas for policy and procedure development: access and discharge, treatment and interventions, environment, legal and other issues, human resources and staff development, equality and anti-discriminatory practices. This is an excellent starting point for the development of such a manual (some units have posted their manuals within the members' section of the NAPICU website: www.napicu.org.uk).

Governance

Audit is integral to the monitoring and subsequent improvement of services in every organisation. The NMS give each unit a tool for benchmarking their own service and specifically highlight clinical audit and monitoring, with guidance given as to specific areas for audit. Higher levels of risk, loss of liberty, and greater rates of restraint and physical intervention suggest a greater need for clinical audit. For such audit to be successful the multidisciplinary team needs to give full cooperation and the process should be based upon reflective learning.

Following publication of the NMS, individuals and organisations (such as NAPICU) were asked to perform service reviews and continual monitoring of some units with respect to the Standards. However, this was a labour-intensive exercise and only benefited those individual units involved. Additional developments within secure services [e.g. publication of the Bennett report (Norfolk, Suffolk and Cambridgeshire Strategic Health Authority 2003), death of a nurse within a PICU (NHS London 2006) and publication of the NICE guidance on management of disturbed behaviour (National Institute for Clinical Excellence 2005)] continued to highlight the need for a more systematic approach to governance specifically within psychiatric intensive care.

Within the implementation section of the Standards, mention is made of the development of a PICU/Low Secure Practice Development Network as a useful way to monitor the implementation of the NMS. This recommendation was taken forward with the development of a Psychiatric Intensive Care/Low Secure Governance Network focusing upon four specific key areas (multidisciplinary working, diversity, service user/carer involvement and responding to emergencies) using the NMS

as a benchmark. Through project working this enables positive change in services for patients, with demonstrable benefits via a system of audit and review (Dye and Johnston 2005; Dye *et al.* 2005).

The collaborative nature of such a project allows PICUs/LSUs to share experiences and difficulties, and plan improvements drawing upon expertise from both within and outside the network. Through individual units demonstrating successful and sustainable improvements to patient care and being able to share these with other units in a similar position, the Governance Network helped in not only monitoring standards but also disseminating positive change occurring as a result of their development.

Despite the success of the Network, organisations continued to request assistance with many areas of governance, e.g. help in commissioning and performing service reviews, such as assistance in conducting reviews of untoward incidents. Some of these requests were unable to be fulfilled; others required greater timescales than the requesting organisation demands. This identified unmet need and subsequently a Psychiatric Intensive Care Advisory Service (PICAS) was developed, consisting of a team with expertise in working within psychiatric intensive care/low secure care, in commissioning units, in providing reviews and in working with organisations to implement positive changes. The function of such a service is shown in Box 25.6.

Summary and Conclusions

A clear and defined system of operating within any environment fosters good practice and confidence. The NMS provide a template that aids in the development of such a system: they demystify the role of the PICU/LSU, which leads to a transparency of practice and encourages self-critical and innovative methods of working rather than reinforcing traditional views of what constitutes PICU practice. The NMS are crucial for each unit to improve and monitor their own ways of working.

Box 25.6. Functions of PICAS

- Answer queries relating to psychiatric intensive care
- Facilitate and develop user involvement initiatives and engagement programmes
- Continue the psychiatric intensive care Governance Network on a rolling year-long programme for specific organisations
- Perform independent reviews of psychiatric intensive care services
- Project work aimed at meeting the NMS
- Support, inform and shape psychiatric intensive care service improvement within organisations
- Advise on commissioning of a new service
- Advise on improvements of physical environments of PICUs
- Provide workshops and practical guidance on development initiatives
- Give assistance with national policy advice
- Respond to any untoward incident that may occur within a particular service and give assistance with analysis of the incident from a clinical and systems-wide approach
- Suicide prevention and training/education
- Develop and implement risk assessment tools
- Troubleshoot various aspects of any psychiatric intensive care service and assistance in supporting units that are experiencing complex issues
- Provide specific training and education
- Assist with statutory inspections (e.g. Healthcare Commission visits) and the report compilation following these visits
- Assist in the development and delivery of learning material
- Aid the development of local policies relating to psychiatric intensive care
- Facilitate liaison with other services (e.g. criminal justice system)

It is true to say that at present the NMS are guidelines to 'inform' practice and not to 'instruct' it but they were developed with the best interests of both patients and staff in mind and should be commended for this. There is something for any stakeholder or staff member associated with PICUs/LSUs to take from the Standards (this is a testament to the wide ranging consultation and involvement of different groups of individuals in their formation); for instance, junior staff members may wish to concentrate on admission criteria and documentation, commissioners of services would find the physical environment of units and personnel service structure useful, and clinical governance departments can be guided by the section on clinical audit and monitoring. The Standards thus not only promote psychiatric intensive and low secure care but also provide a foundation from which to base good practice within any such unit.

Notwithstanding the NMS, the most recent study of PICU and Low Secure Services conducted (Pereira *et al.* 2006) demonstrates ongoing inconsistency in important areas of practice and standards of care. The underdevelopment of multidisciplinary team working in the psychiatric intensive care setting has already been highlighted in this chapter (LSUs were shown to have greater levels of input than PICUs from psychologists, occupational therapists and social workers). Despite the Standards, 57% of PICUs and 52% of LSUs are willing to admit informal patients and 82% of PICU managers report that they are also willing to accept patient admissions over 8 weeks in length. The survey also described the current use of policies and protocols in these settings. Whilst 90% of LSUs had protocols for referral, 99% had risk assessment protocols and 82% had policies regarding preadmission assessment, in PICU settings these figures were lower (76%, 92% and 61% respectively) and had not therefore been developed consistently and sufficiently. Research is not currently available to demonstrate the actual extent to which patients are admitted or receive care that contravenes or fails to meet the Standards.

As psychiatric services themselves mature and expand, the fluid nature of Standards must be appreciated and, with good practice remaining at the top of the agenda, 'our target now is to ensure that as this specialism [psychiatric intensive care] grows, it is not an ivory tower but bridges with other services and countries' (Pereira and Dalton 2006). The development of robust crisis, home treatment and outreach services will lead to robust intensive community services and the focus of psychiatric intensive care must shift accordingly away from the physical environment in which care is given to the specific type of care that is provided to the most unwell individuals treated within psychiatric services.

It is evident that publication of the NMS, in conjunction with other available guidance, has been immensely important in establishing and highlighting the standards to which all PICUs and LSUs should operate. It is essential that this valuable document be used appropriately and that, following its publication, standards of care improve. The Governance Network enabled some of the individual PICUs in the UK to implement and monitor the Standards, and PICAS will further aid service and practice development. However, evidence of current practice in the UK suggests that further work needs to follow. This should include a national strategy to ensure implementation (with essential auditing and monitoring) as well as ongoing revision of the Standards to ensure they reflect continued best practice as further developments are made in this subspecialty of psychiatry.

REFERENCES

Atakan Z. 1995 Violence on psychiatric inpatient units: what can be done? Psychiatr Bull 19: 119–122

Beck AT, Ward CH, Mendelson M, Mock J, Erbaugh J. 1961 An inventory for measuring depression. Arch Gen Psychiatry 4: 561–571

Beer MD, Paton C, Pereira S. 1997 Hot beds of general psychiatry; a national survey of psychiatric intensive care units. Psychiatr Bull 21: 142–144

Department of Health. 1983 Mental Health Act 1983. London: HMSO

Department of Health. 1999a Effective care co-ordination in mental health services: modernising the care programme approach – a policy booklet. London: HMSO

Department of Health. 1999b National Service Framework for Mental Health: Modern Standards and Service Models. London: HMSO

Department of Health. 1999c Safety, Privacy and Dignity in Mental Health Units. London: HMSO

Department of Health. 2002 National Minimum Standards for General Adult Services in Psychiatric Intensive Care Units (PICU) and Low Secure Environments. In: Pereira S, Clinton C (eds) Mental Health Policy Implementation Guide. London: Department of Health Publications

Dye S, Johnston A. 2005 After the standards . . . a gaping cavity filled by clinical governance? J Psychiatr Intensive Care 1(1): 3–5

Dye S, Johnston A, Pereira S. 2005 The national psychiatric intensive care governance network 2004–2005. J Psychiatr Intensive Care 1(2): 97–104

HL v. UK, European Court of Human Rights, C [2004] J 4269

Home Office. 2000 Race Relations (Amendment) Act 2000. London: HMSO

Krawiecka M, Goldberg D, Vaughan M. 1977 A standardised psychiatric assessment scale for rating chronic psychotic patients. Acta Psychiatr Scand 55: 209–308

Laidlaw J, Buckle D. 2006 Informal patients in secure wards; restriction of movement or deprivation of liberty? J Psychiatr Intensive Care 1(2): 61–63

National Institute for Clinical Excellence (NICE). 2005 Clinical Guideline 25: The Short-term Management of Disturbed/Violent Behaviour in In-patient Psychiatric Settings and Emergency Departments. London: NICE

NHS London. 2006 Report of the External Review of John Meyer Ward Following the Death of Eshan Chattun. Commissioned by South West London Strategic Health Authority. Review by Barnard M, Neill P.

Norfolk, Suffolk and Cambridgeshire Strategic Health Authority. 2003 Independent Inquiry into the death of David Bennett. Cambridge: Norfolk, Suffolk and Cambridgeshire Strategic Health Authority. Available online at www.irr.org.uk/pdf/bennett_inquiry.pdf

Overall JE, Gorham DR. 1962 The Brief Psychiatric Rating Scale. Psychol Rep 10: 799–812

Pereira S, Dalton D. 2006 Integration and specialism: complementary not contradictory. J Psychiatr Intensive Care 2(1): 1–5

Pereira SM, Sarsam M, Bhui K, Paton C. 2005 The London survey of psychiatric intensive care units. J Psychiatr Intensive Care 1(1): 17–24

Pereira S, Dawson P, Sarsam M. 2006 The national survey of PICU and low secure services: 2. unit characteristics. J Psychiatr Intensive Care 2(1): 13–19

Pierce DW. 1981 The predictive validation of a suicide intent scale: a five year follow-up. Br J Psychiatry 139: 391–396

Sugarman P, Moss J. 1994 The rights of voluntary patients in hospital. Psychiatr Bulletin 18: 269–271

UK Government. 2005 Disability Discrimination Act 2005. London: HMSO

Young RC, Biggs JT, Ziegler VE, Meyer DA. 1978 A rating scale for mania: reliability, validity and sensitivity. Br J Psychiatry 133: 429–435

Yudofsky SC, Silver JM, Jackson W, Endicott J, Williams D. 1986 The Overt Aggression Scale for the objective rating of verbal and physical aggression. Am J Psychiatry 143: 35–39

Wing JK, Beevor A, Curtis RH, Park SBG, Hadden S, Burns A. 1998 Health of the Nation Outcome Scales (HoNOS): research and development. Br J Psychiatry 172: 11–18

Index